THE
MEDICAL
BOOK

Books by Clifford A. Pickover

THE MEDICAL BOOK

FROM WITCH DOCTORS TO ROBOT SURGEONS,
250 MILESTONES IN THE HISTORY OF MEDICINE

Clifford A. Pickover

Author of *The Math Book* and *The Physics Book*

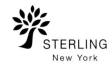

STERLING
New York

STERLING
New York

An Imprint of Sterling Publishing
387 Park Avenue South
New York, NY 10016

STERLING and the distinctive Sterling logo are registered trademarks of Sterling Publishing Co., Inc.

© 2012 by Clifford A. Pickover

ISBN 978-1-4027-8585-6 (hardcover)
ISBN 978-1-4027-9233-5 (ebook)

Library of Congress Cataloging-in-Publication Data

Pickover, Clifford A.
 The medical book : from witch doctors to robot surgeons : 250 milestones in the history of medicine / Clifford A. Pickover.
   p. ; cm.
 From witch doctors to robot surgeons : 250 milestones in the history of medicine
 ISBN 978-1-4027-8585-6 (hardcover) – ISBN 978-1-4027-9233-5 (ebook)
 I. Title. II. Title: From witch doctors to robot surgeons : 250 milestones in the history of medicine.
 [DNLM: 1. History of Medicine–Chronology. WZ 30]

 610.9–dc23
         2011050376

Distributed in Canada by Sterling Publishing
c/o Canadian Manda Group, 165 Dufferin Street
Toronto, Ontario, CanadaM6K 3H6
Distributed in the United Kingdom by GMC Distribution Services
Castle Place, 166 High Street, Lewes, East Sussex, England BN7 1XU
Distributed in Australia by Capricorn Link (Australia) Pty. Ltd.
P.O. Box 704, Windsor, NSW 2756, Australia

For information about custom editions, special sales, and premium and corporate purchases,
please contact Sterling Special Sales at 800-805-5489 or specialsales@sterlingpublishing.com.

Manufactured in China

2 4 6 8 10 9 7 5 3 1

www.sterlingpublishing.com

"Truly the gods have not from the beginning revealed all things to mortals, but by long seeking, mortals make progress in discovery."

—Xenophanes of Colophon, c. 500 B.C.

"Wherever the art of medicine is loved, there also is love of humanity."

—Hippocrates, c. 400 B.C.

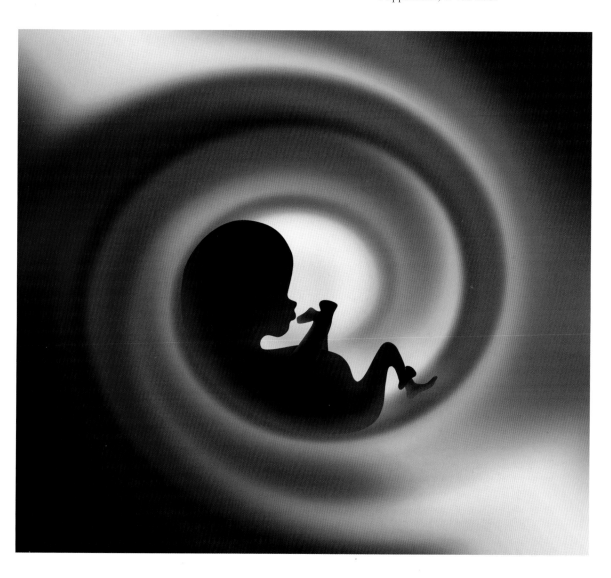

Contents

Introduction

The Scope of Medicine

Welcome to *The Medical Book*, a vast journey into the history of medicine that includes eminently practical topics along with the odd and perplexing. We'll encounter subjects that range from circumcision to near-death experiences and from witch doctors to robot surgeons. Educational content from The Great Courses provides a wonderful glimpse of the richness of medical history and the amazing progress humankind has made from the Stone Age until today:

> In today's era of modern Western medicine, organ transplants are routine, and daily headlines about the mysteries of DNA and the human genome promise that the secrets of life itself are tantalizingly within our reach. . . . Yet to reach this point took thousands of years. One step at a time . . . humanity's medical knowledge has moved forward from a time when even the slightest cut held the threat of infection and death, when the flow of blood within the body was a mystery, and "cells" were not even a concept, and when the appearance of a simple instrument allowing a physician to listen to the beat of a diseased heart was a profound advance.

Each entry in *The Medical Book* is short—at most only a few paragraphs. This format allows readers to jump in and ponder a subject without having to sort through a lot of verbiage. When was the first time physicians studied maggot therapy to clean wounds and save lives? Turn to the entry "Maggot Therapy" for a brief introduction. Do acupuncture and truth serum really work? When was the first eye surgery performed? Will humans ever be able to be frozen and resurrected a century later? What's the difference between yellow fever and sleeping sickness? We'll tackle these and other thought-provoking topics in the pages that follow. Health care is among the most significant issues of our time, and it will be more so in the future. This book should appeal to students and their parents, health-care practitioners, and even many of the exuberant fans of *Grey's Anatomy*, *House M.D.*, and the countless medical shows—past, present, and future—that capture our hearts and minds.

When colleagues ask me what I feel are the greatest milestones in medicine, I usually offer three events. The first involves the use of ligatures to stem the flow of blood during surgeries, for example, as performed by the French surgeon Ambroise Paré (1510–1590). He promoted the ligature (e.g., tying off with twine) of blood vessels to prevent hemorrhage during amputations, instead of the traditional method of burning the stump with a hot iron to stop bleeding. The second key milestone includes methods for decreasing pain through general anesthetics such as ether, attributed to several American physicians. The third breakthrough concerns antiseptic surgery, which was promoted by British surgeon Joseph Lister (1827–1912), whose use of carbolic acid (now called phenol) as a means of sterilizing wounds and surgical instruments dramatically reduced postoperative infections.

If pressed, I would add two additional key developments in the history of medicine. The use of X-rays was the first of several groundbreaking modern approaches for visualizing the interior of living humans. Also very important was the gradually increasing openness of physicians and authorities to the dissection of bodies in order to learn about human anatomy. In fact, several milestones in this book offer portrayals of the human body by such greats as Leonardo da Vinci (1452–1519), Bartolomeo Eustachi (1500–1574), Andreas Vesalius (1514–1564), Pietro da Cortona (1596–1669), William Cheselden (1688–1752), Bernhard Siegfried Albinus (1697–1770), William Hunter (1718–1783), and Henry Gray (1827–1861). In order to become seasoned dissectors and anatomists, surgeons of the past often were able to suppress normal emotional responses for their human brethren. For example, English physician William Harvey (1578–1657), famous for his elucidation of blood circulation, participated in dissections of both his sister and his father. In the early 1800s, the appetite for corpses was so great in England that anatomists frequently collaborated with grave robbers to secure needed specimens. As I mention later in this book, art historians Martin Kemp and Marina Wallace write, "The portrayal of the human body, however ostensibly neutral or technical the illustration, always involves a series of choices, and invariably brings into play strong sensations. Historical images of the dissected body range from the most flamboyant of the multicolored waxes, in which dissected figures assume the roles of expressive actors and actresses in their own timeless drama, to the remorselessly sober woodcuts in Henry Gray's famous *Anatomy*. All the images exhibit what an art historian would call 'style.'"

Historian Andrew Cunningham writes, "The problem underlying all illustrations of anatomical dissection is that they are all . . . idealizations. Indeed this is why engravings [and photographs] are attempts at solving the same problem: that of bringing into view . . . the things that the anatomist wishes to make visible. For anatomizing is not only a very messy business . . . but distinguishing all the structures that are visible to the eye of the trained anatomist is very difficult for those who are not yet anatomists."

On a personal note, I should mention that I've suffered from a strange case of anatophilia—that is, an extreme love of anatomy—since childhood. While I was growing up in New Jersey, my bedroom featured plastic anatomical models of the heart, brain, head, eye, and ear. My walls were covered with posters of organ systems rendered in exquisite precision. In college, I wore only anatomy T-shirts featuring circulatory systems, dissected frogs, and the like. It is this passion for understanding biology and the human body that led me to write this book.

Finally, we should note that before germ theory and the rise of modern science, a significant portion of medicine was based on superstition and the placebo effect. On this topic, medical experts Arthur and Elaine Shapiro write, "For example, the first three editions of the *London Pharmacopoeia* published in the seventeenth century included such useless drugs as usnea (moss from the skull of victims of violent death) and Vigo's plaster ([including] viper's flesh, live frogs, and worms)." Even the beloved doctor Ira Johnson in Robert Heinlein's novel *To Sail Beyond the Sunset* admits the limitations of medicine and the ubiquity of the placebo effect in rural America around 1900: "I don't do them much good. Iodine, calomel, and Aspirin—that's about all we have today that isn't a sugar pill. The only times I'm certain of results are when I deliver a baby or set a bone or cut off a leg." Even today, according to the Institute of Medicine, less than half the surgeries, drugs, and tests that doctors recommend have been proved effective.

Purpose and Chronology

My goal in writing *The Medical Book* is to provide a wide audience with a brief guide to important medical milestones, ideas, and thinkers, with entries short enough to digest in a few minutes. Many entries are ones that interest me personally. Alas, not all of the great medical milestones are included in this book, in order to prevent the book from growing too large. Thus, in celebrating the wonders of medicine in this short volume, I have been forced to omit many important medical marvels. Nevertheless, I believe that I have included a majority of those with historical significance and that have had a strong influence on medicine, society, or human thought. In 1921, British neurosurgeon Charles Ballance delivered a talk titled "A Glimpse into the History of Surgery of the Brain," in which he said that the history of brain surgery was so vast that he would not make an effort to touch upon all of it, but would merely, "like an alpine traveler, salute a few of the peaks and pass on." We will do the same for these medical milestones. Sometimes, snippets of information are repeated so that each entry can be read on its own. Occasional text in a bold font points the reader to related entries. For example, **sleeping sickness** may appear in bold because it has the index item *Sleeping sickness, cause*. Additionally, a small SEE ALSO section near the bottom of each entry helps weave entries together in a web of interconnectedness and may help the reader traverse the book in a playful quest for discovery.

The Medical Book reflects my own intellectual shortcomings, and while I try to study as many areas of medical history as I can, it is difficult to become fluent in all aspects; this book clearly reflects my own personal interests, strengths, and weaknesses. I am responsible for the choice of pivotal entries included in this book and, of course, for any errors and infelicities. This is not a comprehensive or scholarly dissertation, but rather is intended as recreational reading for students of science and interested laypersons. I welcome feedback and suggestions for improvement from readers, as I consider this an ongoing project and a labor of love.

This book is organized chronologically, according to the year associated with an entry. Many of the older dates in this book, including the B.C. dates, are only approximate. Rather than place the term *circa* in front of all of these older dates, which designates an approximate date, I inform the reader here that the ancient dates are only rough estimates.

For most entries, I used dates that are associated with a discovery or breakthrough. Of course, dating of entries can be a question of judgment when more than one individual made a contribution. Often, I have used the earliest date associated with a discovery or event, but sometimes, after having surveyed colleagues and other scientists, I decided to use the date when a concept gained particular prominence.

The famous Canadian physician William Osler once wrote, "In science, the credit goes to the man who convinces the world, not to the man to whom the idea first occurs." When we examine discoveries in medicine, in hindsight we often find that if one scientist did not make a particular discovery, some other individual would have done so within a few months or years. Most scientists, as Newton said, stood on the shoulders of giants to see just a bit farther along the horizon. Often, more than one individual creates essentially the same device or unravels the same medical mystery at about the same time, but for various reasons—including sheer luck—history remembers only the more famous discoverer and completely forgets the others. Perhaps the time was ripe for such discoveries, given humanity's accumulated knowledge at the time the discoveries were made. We may be reluctant to believe that great discoveries are part of a "discovery kaleidoscope" mirrored in numerous individuals at once. However, the history of science is replete with examples. Alexander Graham Bell and Elisha Gray, working independently, filed their own patents on telephone technologies on the same day. As sociologist of science Robert Merton remarked, "The genius is not a unique source of insight; he is merely an efficient source of insight.

Merton also suggested that "all scientific discoveries are in principle 'multiples'"— that is, the same discovery is often made by more than one person. Sometimes a discovery is named after the person who *develops* the discovery rather than the original discoverer. The great anatomist William Hunter frequently quarreled with his brother about who was first in making a discovery, but even Hunter admitted, "If a man has not such a degree of enthusiasm and love of the art, as will make him impatient of unreasonable opposition, and of encroachment upon his discoveries and his reputation, he will hardly become considerable in anatomy, or in any other branch of natural knowledge." When Mark Twain was asked to explain why so many inventions were invented independently, he said, "When it's steamboat time, you steam."

Readers may notice that a significant number of discoveries in basic physics also led to a range of medical tools and helped to reduce human suffering and save lives. Science writer John G. Simmons notes,

> Medicine owes most of its tools for imaging the human body to twentieth-century physics. Within weeks of their discovery in 1895, the mysterious X-rays of Wilhelm Conrad Röntgen were used in diagnoses. Decades later, laser technology was a practical result of quantum mechanics. Ultrasonography emerged from problem solving in submarine detection, and CT scans capitalized on computer technology. Medicine's most significant recent technology, used for visualizing the interior of the human body in three-dimensional detail, is magnetic resonance imaging (MRI).

Finally, I should note that war and violence often accelerated the pace of medical understanding. For example, when Galen of Pergamon (129–199) was a physician to the gladiators, he peered into horrific wounds to learn more about human anatomy. French surgeon Dominique Larrey (1766–1842) observed at the Battle of Eylau in Prussia that the pain of amputations was very much reduced when limbs were extremely cold, and he used snow and ice to dull the pain. Finally, today's International Red Cross and Red Crescent Movement owes its existence to the Swiss social activist Henri Dunant (1828–1910), who was appalled by the horrors he had witnessed at the 1859 Battle of Solferino in Italy. You can read about these and related topics throughout this book.

In some entries, science reporters and authors are quoted, but purely for brevity I don't list the source of the quote or the author's credentials in the entry. I apologize in advance for this occasional compact approach; references in the back of the book should help to make the author's identity clearer. Because this book has entries ordered chronologically, be sure to use the index when hunting for a favorite concept, which may be discussed in entries that you might not have expected.

In closing, let us note that the discoveries in this book are among humanity's greatest achievements. For me, medicine cultivates a perpetual state of wonder about the limits of biology and the workings of the tissues and cells—and provides hope that most of the horrific health ravages of humankind will one day be a thing of the past.

A Note on the Use of "Witch Doctor"

The first entry of this book is titled "Witch Doctor," a phrase that started to become popular when applied to African healers after its use by British author Robert Montgomery Martin, in his *History of Southern Africa Comprising the Cape of Good Hope, Mauritius, Seychelles, &c.*, published in 1836. Although the term can sometimes be considered pejorative today, I intend no disrespect and use the phrase to provide a sense of its history, and because numerous colleagues have asked about the etymology of this interesting phrase. While many authors use the term *shaman* in place of *witch doctor*, *shaman* can suggest a greater emphasis on knowledge of spirits, magic, divination, and myth rather than a focus on medical issues.

Disclaimer and Acknowledgments

The information provided in this book should not be used during any medical emergency or for the diagnosis or treatment of any medical condition. A licensed physician should be consulted for diagnosis and treatment of any and all medical conditions.

I thank Dennis Gordon, Teja Krašek, Jennifer O'Brennan, Melissa K. Carroll, Bryan Plaunt, Sue Ross, Rachel D'Annucci Henriquez, and Pete Barnes for their comments and suggestions. I would also like to especially acknowledge Melanie Madden, my editor for this book. While researching the milestones and pivotal moments in this book, I studied a wide array of wonderful reference works and websites, many of which are listed in the reference section at the end of this book.

Witch Doctor

"There are glaring hazards in venturing generalizations about the beliefs of myriad societies—from the Nuer [African tribes] to the Navajo," writes historian Roy Porter. "However . . . unlike modern Western medicine, traditional healing is disposed to see much sickness . . . as essentially personal." In old tribal settings, sickness was often viewed as targeted and caused by a supernatural agency.

Since ancient times, "medicine men" (also sometimes loosely referred to as witch doctors, shamans, or sangomas) have addressed the health needs of their people by performing ceremonies and minor surgical procedures and by providing charms and plant-based medicines.

Shamanic practices, involving healers who appear to be in contact with a spirit world, probably originated in Paleolithic (Old Stone Age) times. For example, evidence for Mesolithic (Middle Stone Age) shamanism was found in Israel in the form of an old woman from a burial dating to around 10,000 B.C. The importance of this woman, along with her possible close association with nature and animals, is suggested by the special arrangement of stones by her body, along with 50 complete tortoise shells, a human foot, and remains of birds, boars, leopards, cows, and eagles. Today, the vast majority of the traditional Nguni societies of southern Africa make use of *sangomas* who employ herbal medicine, divination, and counseling.

Several types of shamans may exist for a single people. For example, according to psychologist Stanley Krippner, who writes on the Cuna Indians of Panama, the "*abisua* shaman heals by singing, the *inaduledi* specializes in herbal cures, and the *nele* focuses on diagnosis."

Science journalist Robert Adler writes, "In many groups throughout the world, shamans or sorcerers are thought to possess the twin abilities to hurt or heal, kill or cure. Where they exist, shamans often possess detailed knowledge of the local psychedelic plants. They use [the plants] in healing rituals and to commune with the supernatural. . . . It is in the powerful figures of shamans and sorcerers that we find the predecessors of our white-coated physicians . . . whom we, like our ancestors, imbue with great powers."

SEE ALSO Trepanation (6500 B.C.), Dioscorides's *De Materia Medica* (70), and Placebo Effect (1955).

Two witch doctors from Lassa, Nigeria (courtesy of the U.S. Centers for Disease Control and Prevention).

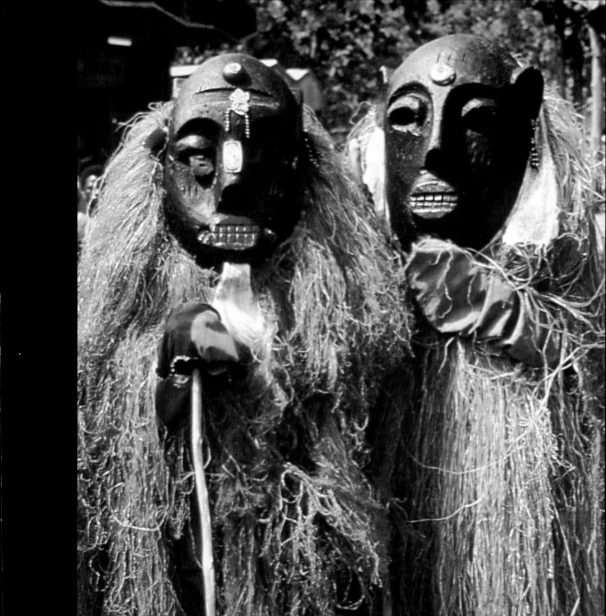

Trepanation

Albucasis (936–1013)

Neuroscientist and medical historian Stanley Finger writes, "The assertion that the brain may have been given a special role in higher functions prior to the advent of the great civilizations is based on the fact that skulls with holes deliberately cut or bored in them have been found in a number of Neolithic [New Stone Age] sites." Indeed, the act of creating a hole in the human skull through cutting, drilling, and/or scraping, called trepanation, was once quite common. In prehistoric times, the removed bone may have been worn as a charm to ward off evil spirits. Motivations for the procedure are unclear—perhaps ancient peoples attempted to relieve severe headaches and **epilepsy** or to let "evil spirits" escape from the head. Also unclear is whether recipients were anesthetized, for example, with coca leaves and alcohol. Interestingly, at one French burial site, dated to 6500 B.C., about a third of the 120 prehistoric skulls had trepanation holes. Many examples of trepanned skulls show healing of the surrounding bone, which suggests that individuals often survived this gruesome procedure. During the Middle Ages and beyond, people underwent trepanation in an attempt to relieve seizures and ameliorate head wounds such as skull fractures.

Trepanation has been practiced throughout the world, including Africa, pre-Columbian Mesoamerica, and in many parts of Europe. More than 10,000 trepanned skulls have been unearthed in Peru alone. The holes in European skulls range in size from a few centimeters in diameter to almost half of the skull.

Albucasis, one of Islam's greatest medieval surgeons, used a drill in such procedures. He wrote, "You cut through the bone in the confident knowledge that nothing inward can happen to the membrane even though the operator be the most ignorant and cowardly of men; yes, even if he be sleepy." However, if the dura (outer membrane of the brain) turned black, "you may know that he is doomed."

A number of quirky individuals in recent years have performed self-trepanation, believing that the procedure facilitates a path to enlightenment.

SEE ALSO Witch Doctor (10,000 B.C.), Treatment of Epilepsy (1857), and Modern Brain Surgery (1879).

Trepanated skull (c. 3500 B.C.) of a girl who survived the operation, as evidenced by smooth growth of bone around the hole (Muséum d'Histoire Naturelle de Lausanne).

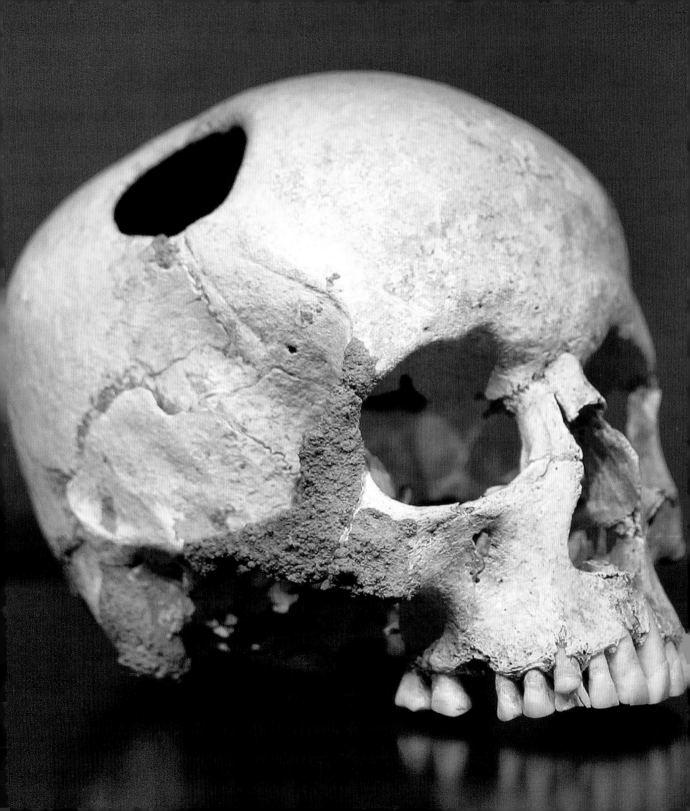

Urinalysis

The comedian Rodney Dangerfield once said, "I drink too much. The last time I gave a urine sample it had an olive in it." In fact, urinalysis, or the study of urine for medical diagnosis, has had both a zany and serious history.

Starting around 4000 B.C., Sumerian physicians recorded on clay tablets their analyses of urine. Sanskrit medical texts, roughly from 100 B.C., describe at least 20 different types of urine. In ancient India, physicians were aware that people affected by what we now refer to as diabetes produced urine that tasted sweet and to which ants were attracted.

Before modern medicine, visual inspection of the urine was referred to as uroscopy. Physicians of the Middle Ages elevated uroscopy to a near-magical art, with some physicians dressing in long robes, holding up and twirling the matula (a glass vessel shaped somewhat like a bladder) in front of the patient's eyes before making a prognosis. Some physicians began to diagnose without ever seeing the patient. During the Renaissance, uroscopy was even used to tell fortunes and predict the future.

Today, we know that white blood cells detected in a urine sample can be indicative of a urinary tract infection if present in large numbers. Hematuria, or the presence of red blood cells in the urine, may suggest the presence of a kidney stone, kidney trauma, or a tumor in the urinary tract (which includes the kidneys, ureters, urinary bladder, prostate, and urethra). Diabetes mellitus is the major cause of glucose (sugar) in the urine. Other urine tests can be used to help diagnose liver or thyroid disease.

Physiologist J. A. Armstrong writes, "From a liquid window through which physicians felt they could view the body's inner workings, urine led to the beginnings of laboratory medicine. As the role of physicians became elevated, the importance of urinary diagnosis became exaggerated [and by the seventeenth century] the uses of uroscopy had spiraled far beyond the edge of reason."

SEE ALSO Inborn Errors of Metabolism (1902) and "The Rabbit Died" (1928).

Physician peering into a flask of urine (1653), by Dutch painter Gerrit Dou (1613–1675). Oil on oak panel.

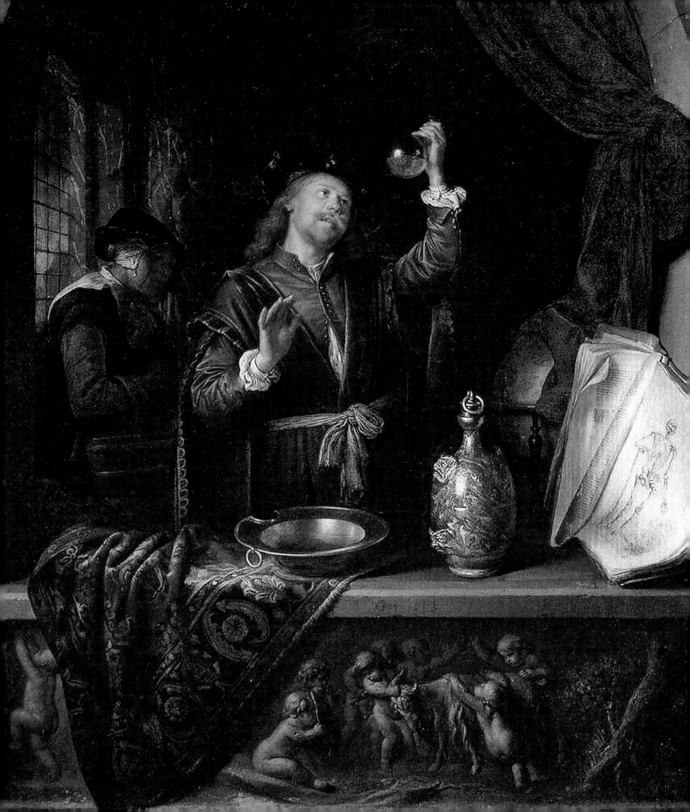

Sutures

Galen of Pergamon (129–199), **al-Zahrawi** (936–1013), **Joseph Lister** (1827–1912)

"In an era of escalating surgical technology," writes surgeon John Kirkup, "it is tempting to downgrade the minor craft of wound closure when compared to more sophisticated operating skills. Indeed, before **antiseptic** and aseptic procedures were established, closure was a source of many disasters. Even today, successful operations depend on prompt reliable healing of skin, bowel, bone, tendon and other tissues, and neither healing nor a cosmetically acceptable scar can be guaranteed."

Today, a surgical suture usually refers to a needle with an attached length of thread that is used to stitch together the edges of a wound or surgical cut. However, through history, the suture has taken many forms. Needles have been made of bone or metal. Sutures were made of materials such as silk or catgut (sheep intestines). Sometimes, large ants were used to pinch wounds together. After the ant's pincers had bitten into the flesh and closed an opening, the body of the ant was removed, leaving just the head and closed pincers behind. The ancient Egyptians used linen and animal sinew to close wounds, and the earliest reports of such suturing date back to 3000 B.C. Galen, the second-century Greco-Roman physician, used sutures made from animal materials, as did the Arab surgeon al-Zahrawi. British surgeon Joseph Lister investigated ways to sterilize catgut, a suture material the body gradually absorbed. In the 1930s, a major manufacturer of catgut sutures used 26,000 sheep intestines in a single day. Today, many sutures are made from absorbable or nonabsorbable synthetic polymer fibers, and eyeless needles may be premounted to the suture in order to lessen trauma to body tissues during the threading process. Adhesive liquids are also used to assist in wound closure.

Depending on use, sutures vary in width, with some smaller than the diameter of a human hair. In the nineteenth century, surgeons often preferred to cauterize (burn) wounds, an often gruesome process, rather than risk the patients dying from infected sutures.

SEE ALSO Edwin Smith Surgical Papyrus (1600 B.C.), Paré's "Rational Surgery" (1545), Tissue Grafting (1597), Antiseptics (1865), Vascular Suturing (1902), Halstedian Surgery (1904), Nanomedicine (1959), Laser (1960), and Laparoscopic Surgery (1981).

Surgeon's gloved hand holding a needle holder with an atraumatic curved cutting needle attached to a 4-0 monofilament nonabsorbable synthetic suture.

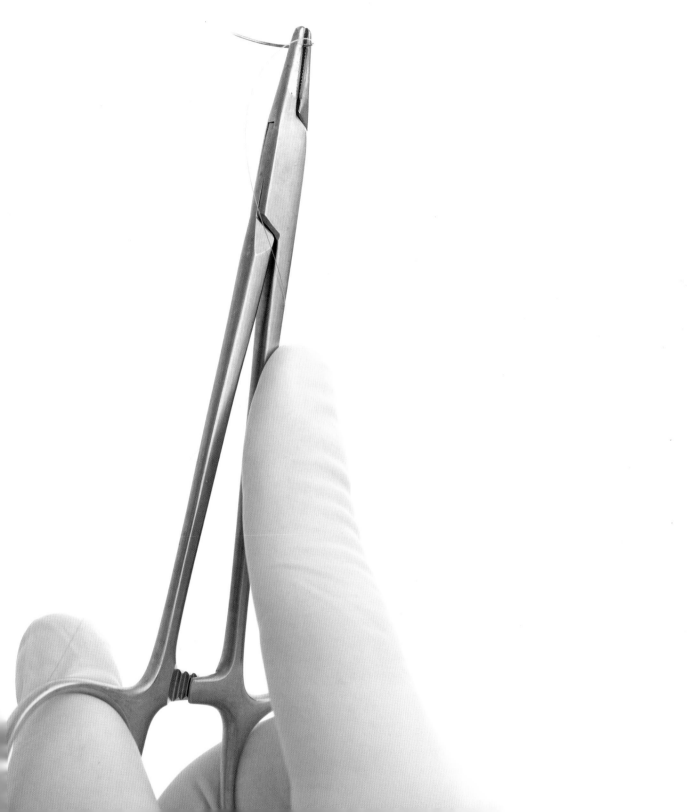

Glass Eye

"He had but one eye, and the popular prejudice runs in favor of two," wrote Charles Dickens of a nasty schoolmaster in *Nicholas Nickelby*. Indeed, the loss of an eye, whether due to disease, birth defect, or accident, is a deeply emotional experience for cosmetic, social, and functional reasons. Artificial eyes do not replace an individual's sight, but they can fill the eye socket and even be attached to muscles to provide natural eye movements. Today, more than 10,000 people each year lose an eye. Although often referred to as glass eyes, most artificial eyes are now made of plastic.

Interestingly, the oldest known artificial eye is nearly 5,000 years old, discovered in a six-foot-tall female skeleton in the remains of the Burnt City, an ancient city in southeastern Iran. The eye is hemispherical and seems to consist of a natural tar mixed with animal fat. Its surface is covered with a thin layer of gold, engraved with a circular iris and gold lines patterned like sun rays. The artificial eye was not intended to mimic a real eye, but had this tall woman been a prophetess, it might have glittered and given her the semblance of special powers. Holes on both sides of the eye probably held the eyeball in place, and microscopic studies of the eye socket indicated that the eyeball was worn during the woman's lifetime.

In 1579, the Venetians invented the first artificial eyes, made of thin shells of glass, to be worn behind the eyelids. In 1884, a glass sphere was sometimes implanted in the natural eyeball socket to restore lost volume and to allow the prosthesis to move. German craftsmen once toured the United States, custom-making eyes as needed, and ocularists began to keep hundreds of premade eyes in their stocks. In 1943, when Germany's superior kryolite glass could not be exported during World War II, U.S. Army technicians began fitting wounded soldiers with plastic eyes. Researchers are currently developing various implants affixed to the retina in order to provide eyesight through the use of advanced microelectronics that communicate with the optic nerve or the visual cortex of the brain.

SEE ALSO Greville Chester Great Toe (1000 B.C.), Eye Surgery (600 B.C.), and Cranial Nerves Classified (1664).

Orbital prosthesis made of glass and silicon used in a patient after enucleation (surgical removal) of the right eye due to carcinoma (a malignant tumor).

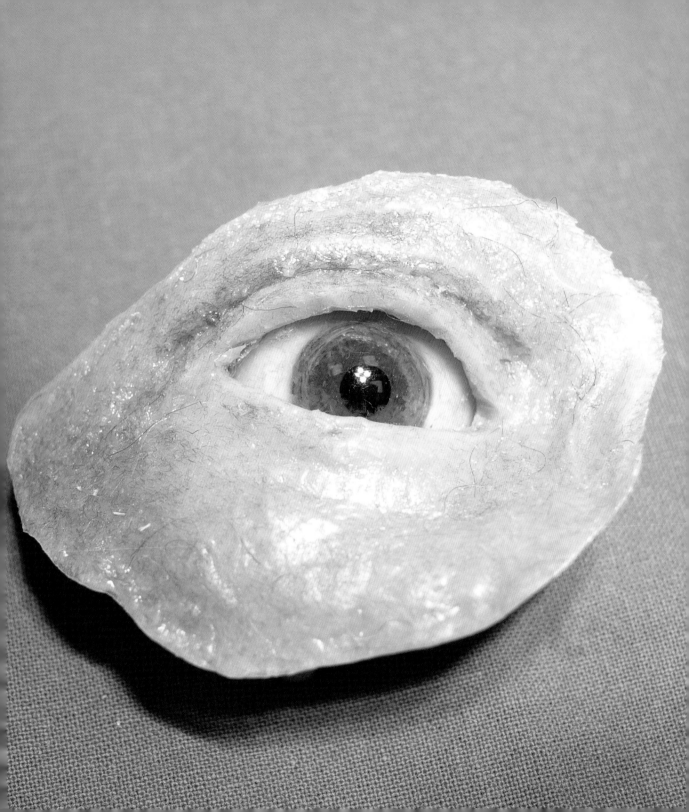

Circumcision

Felix Bryk (1882–1957), **David L. Gollaher** (b. 1949)

"Circumcision is the oldest enigma in the history of surgery," writes medical historian David Gollaher. "It is far easier to imagine the impulse behind Neolithic cave painting than to guess what inspired the ancients to cut their genitals or the genitals of their young. Yet millennia ago, long before medicine and religion branched into separate streams of wisdom . . . cutting the foreskin of the penis was invented as a symbolic wound; thus, circumcision became a ritual of extraordinary power."

The practice of male circumcision involves removal of a portion of the foreskin of the penis. Various theories have been suggested for its origination, such as its being used to aid in hygiene, to increase or decrease pleasure, or to differentiate groups of people. The earliest known depiction of circumcision is found on an Egyptian bas-relief (carved scene) from around 2400 B.C. The inscription reads, "Hold him and do not allow him to faint." According to the Book of Jeremiah in the Hebrew Bible, written in the sixth century B.C., Israelites and some of the nearby peoples practiced circumcision. In the Book of Genesis, God tells Abraham to undergo circumcision as a "sign of the covenant between me and you." Although not mentioned in the Koran, male circumcision is widely practiced in Islam. In 1442, the Catholic Church condemned circumcision as a mortal sin. Today, approximately 30 percent of the males in the world are circumcised. Although evidence suggests that male circumcision significantly reduces the risk of a man's acquisition of HIV (human immunodeficiency virus) during penile-vaginal intercourse, most major medical societies decline to recommend routine infant circumcision.

Swedish anthropologist Felix Bryk wrote in his *Circumcision in Man and Woman* (1934), "He who enters into the study of circumcision must cut a cross-section through all the spheres of culture; for here the very roots of the history of mankind are touched, since in this ancient custom . . . the origins of the formation of government, magic, religion, surgery, hygiene, and last but not least, sexual culture, intersect."

SEE ALSO Condom (1564), Discovery of Sperm (1678), and Reverse Transcriptase and AIDS (1970).

Circumcision being performed on a small boy in Turkestan, central Asia (c. 1870). (Illustration from Turkestanskiĭ al'bom, chast' ėtnograficheskaia.)

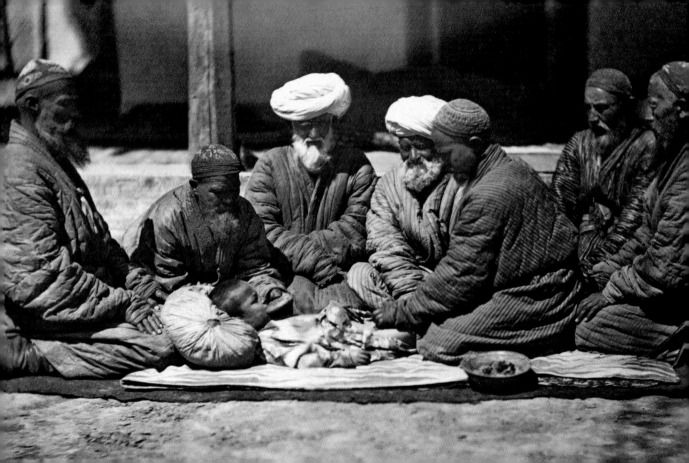

Ayurvedic Medicine

Ayurveda is a traditional system of medicine from the Indian subcontinent. Some of its earliest components may have originated as early as 3,000 years ago, during the Vedic Period of India. Though Ayurveda developed over time, the compendiums *Charaka Samhita* and *Sushruta Samhita*, and a later compendium of the physician Bhela, contain much of the early information related to diagnosis, therapy, and health recommendations. The Sanskrit word *Ayurveda* is roughly translated as "the science of life," and the system makes use of herbs (including spices), oils, massage, yoga, and meditation.

According to Ayurvedic medicine, three life forces called *doshas* control the health of the body, and an imbalance may lead to disease. The *vata dosha* is said to control cell division, the heart, and the mind; the *pitta dosha* controls hormones and digestion; and the *kapha dosha* concerns immunity and growth. Patients are classified by body types, which affect treatment plans that may include doing breathing exercises, rubbing the skin with herbal oil, and "cleansing" the body through bowel movements and even vomiting.

Today, numerous colleges in India offer degrees in traditional Ayurvedic medicine, and a large portion of the population uses this medicine alone or in combination with modern medicine. Certain Ayurvedic exercises, such as yoga and meditation, are helpful in reducing stress. Although some evidence exists for the beneficial use of certain herbs as antifungal agents, for wound healing, and for other purposes, the presence of toxic metals (e.g., lead, mercury, and arsenic) and toxic herbs in some Ayurvedic treatments has sometimes been a safety concern. More research is needed to determine the efficacy of many Ayurvedic practices.

Historian Lois N. Magner writes on Ayurvedic treatments, "Diseases caused by improper diet called for remedies that accomplished internal cleansing, but physicians often began treatment with a seven-day fast. Some patients recovered during this period and needed no other remedies; some died and also needed no further remedies."

SEE ALSO Acupuncture *Compendium* (1601) and Alternative Medicine (1796).

Ayurveda herbal and oil treatment equipment. Shirodhara is an Ayurvedic treatment involving liquids, such as sesame oil with oil of lavender, that are slowly poured over the patient's forehead.

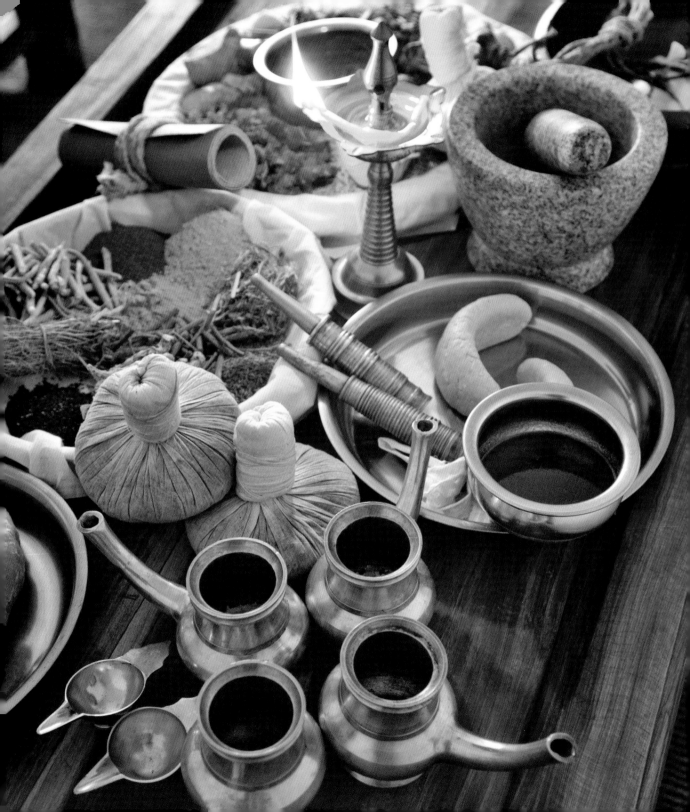

Edwin Smith Surgical Papyrus

Imhotep (2650 B.C.–2600 B.C.), **Edwin Smith** (1822–1906), **Georg Moritz Ebers** (1837–1898)

The Edwin Smith Surgical Papyrus is the world's oldest surgical document and part of an ancient Egyptian textbook. Written around 1600 B.C. in the Egyptian hieratic script, the papyrus incorporated content from more than 1,000 years earlier. The text discusses methods for closing wounds with **sutures** and the use of honey to prevent infections. The text also contains the first known descriptions of the cranial sutures (fibrous bands of tissue that connect the bones of the skull), the surface of the brain, and **cerebrospinal fluid**.

Imhotep, perhaps the first physician in history known by name, is often credited with the authorship of the content of the papyrus, but the papyrus was likely written and edited by more than one individual. Edwin Smith, an American collector of antiquities, purchased the manuscript from a dealer in 1862 while in Egypt. However, the papyrus was not fully translated until 1930. The Edwin Smith Surgical Papyrus stands in contrast with the more magic-laden Ebers Papyrus (c. 1550 B.C.)—another famous Egyptian document, purchased by German Egyptologist Georg Ebers in 1873—which is filled with superstitious elements, including incantations for repelling disease-causing demons.

As one example treatment from the Edwin Smith Surgical Papyrus, consider Case 25: "If you examine a man having a dislocation in his mandible [jawbone], should you find his mouth open, and his mouth cannot close, you should put your thumbs upon the ends of the two rami [vertical portions] of the mandible in the inside of his mouth and your fingers under his chin, and you should cause them to fall back so that they rest in their places." A similar treatment is still in use today for treating a dislocated jaw.

Of the 48 cases described in the Edwin Smith Surgical Papyrus, 27 concern head trauma (e.g., deep scalp wounds and fractures) and six deal with spine trauma. The papyrus often repeats the phrase "An ailment not to be treated," which indicated that the prognosis was hopeless for the afflicted individual.

SEE ALSO Sutures (3000 B.C.), *Huangdi Neijing* (300 B.C.), Dioscorides's *De Materia Medica* (70), Paré's "Rational Surgery" (1545), and Cerebrospinal Fluid (1764).

A fragment of the Edwin Smith Surgical Papyrus, written in hieratic script, a form of ancient Egyptian cursive writing. This particular section discusses facial trauma.

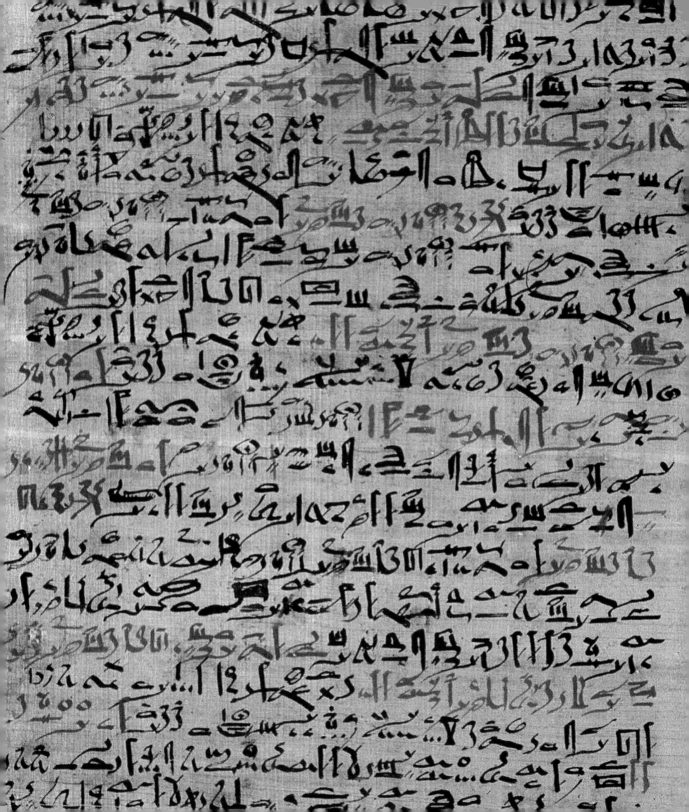

Bloodletting

Galen of Pergamon (129–199), **George Washington** (1732–1799), **William Osler** (1849–1919)

The practice of bloodletting—removal of blood from a patient to cure or prevent illness—has largely been ineffective or harmful. However, it has been one of the most common medical practices performed by physicians for more than 2,000 years. For example, an illustration from an ancient Egyptian tomb (c. 1500 B.C.) shows leeches being applied for bloodletting. Moreover, bloodletting has had extremely wide geographic distribution and has been practiced by the ancient Mesopotamians, Egyptians, Greeks, Mayans and Aztecs, and inhabitants of the Indian subcontinent (e.g., in ancient **Ayurvedic medicine**). Ancient Islamic medical authors recommended the practice, and the Talmud of the Jews suggested specific days of the week and month for bloodletting.

Bloodletting became increasingly popular after the time of Greek physician Galen, who subscribed to Hippocrates's ideas that illnesses resulted from an imbalance of four humors (liquids): blood, black bile, yellow bile, and phlegm. Galen made complex recommendations regarding the amount of blood to be removed based on patient age, the weather, symptoms, and so forth. The barber surgeons of Europe in the Middle Ages and Renaissance practiced bloodletting with great enthusiasm, and physicians continued to bleed patients for every ailment imaginable. A massive amount of blood was drained from President George Washington for his throat infection, accelerating his death. Bloodletting persisted into the twentieth century and was even recommended by Canadian physician William Osler in the 1923 edition of his textbook on the practice of medicine.

Bloodletting was accomplished through the use of lancets (fine knives), scarificators (spring-loaded devices with multiple blades), and leeches. Perhaps bloodletting remained popular due to a **placebo effect** during the centuries in which patients could receive few viable treatments. Today, bloodletting (therapeutic phlebotomy) has few clinical uses except, for example, in patients with hemochromatosis, in order to reduce the high levels of iron in the blood, or polycythemia, a disease characterized by an overabundance of red blood cells. In 2010, the California Department of Consumer Affairs forbade the common practice of Chinese bloodletting by licensed acupuncturists.

SEE ALSO Hippocratic Oath (400 B.C.), Galenic Writings (190), Barber Pole (1210), Leech Therapy (1825), and Placebo Effect (1955).

Medieval manuscript depicting bloodletting with a sharpened instrument. European barber-surgeons in the Middle Ages and Renaissance practiced bloodletting with great enthusiasm, bleeding patients for every aliment imaginable.

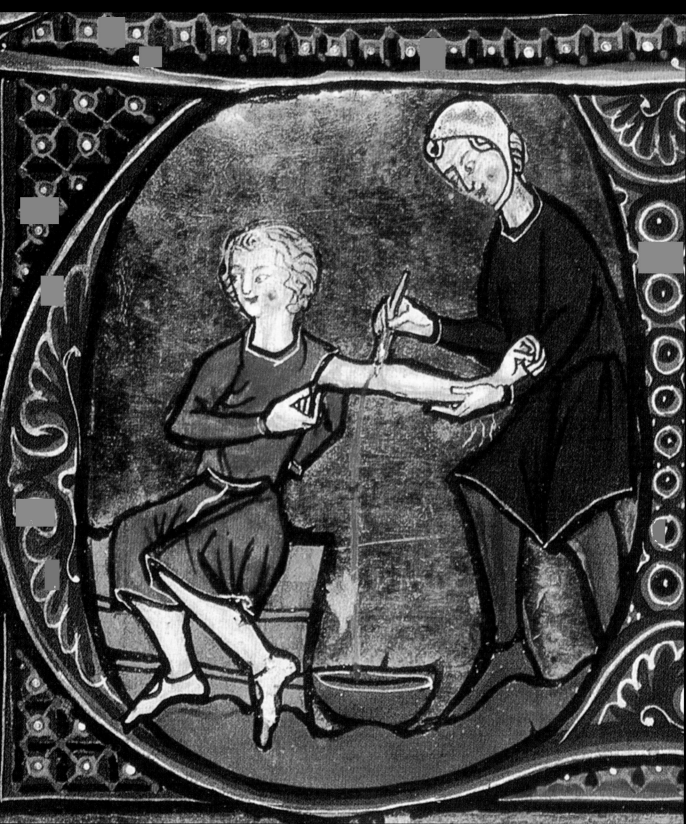

Greville Chester Great Toe

Ambroise Paré (1510–1590), **Greville John Chester** (1830–1892)

Journalist Haley Poland writes, "Whether they are helping a blind person see, a deaf person hear, or a double amputee walk, prostheses have come a long way since Captain Hook. What were once wooden limbs and glass eyes are now engineered electromechanical devices interfacing with human body systems and communicating, almost intelligently, with the human nerves and brain."

A prosthesis is a device that replaces or augments a missing or damaged part of the body. For example, the Greville Chester Great Toe, named after the Egyptologist and collector of antiquities who acquired the Egyptian artifact for the British Museum in 1881, is an artificial big toe made from linen, glue, and plaster dating from 1295 B.C. to 664 B.C. The Great Toe shows signs of wear, suggesting it was not something attached only after death during mummification. Another fake toe exhibiting signs of wear, the Cairo Toe, was discovered on an Egyptian mummy dated to 1069 B.C.–664 B.C. Jointed in three places, it was probably more functional than the Great Toe.

Medieval armor makers created artificial limbs out of iron for soldiers who had lost limbs. In the 1500s, the French surgeon Ambroise Paré developed an artificial leg with a movable knee joint and a spring-operated flexible foot. He also invented mechanical hands with springs.

In modern times, new plastics and materials, such as carbon fiber, have allowed prosthetics to be strong and light. Myoelectric limbs, controlled by converting muscle movements to electric signals, are also used today. Targeted muscle reinnervation is a method in which nerves that previously controlled muscles of an amputated limb are surgically rerouted so that they now control the function of a working muscle. Using this approach, when a person thinks about moving a particular finger, a small area of muscle on the chest, for example, may contract. Sensors placed atop the muscle can then control a robotic prosthesis. Neurocognitive prostheses that directly sense brain or nerve impulses for prosthetic control are being researched.

SEE ALSO Glass Eye (2800 B.C.) and Paré's "Rational Surgery" (1545).

Flexible leather-and-wood prosthetic big toe still attached to the foot of a 2,400-year-old female Egyptian mummy whose real toe was amputated. Toe and foot are displayed at the Cairo Museum.

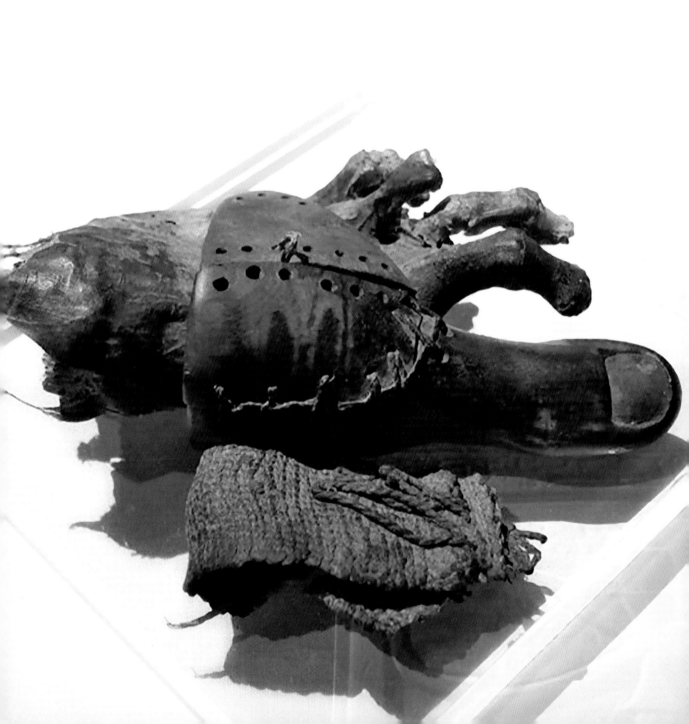

Eye Surgery

Ali ibn Isa (940–1010), **Ibn al-Haytham** (965–1039), **Ibn al-Nafis** (1213–1288), **Julius Hirschberg** (1843–1925)

"One of the most delicate parts of the body on which a surgeon can operate is the eye," write historian Peter James and archeologist Nick Thorpe. "Yet ophthalmic surgery was one of the most advanced areas of medicine in the ancient world." A common cause of near or total blindness is a cataract, a clouding that develops in the crystalline lens of the eye. Cataract surgery was known to the Indian physician Sushruta (very approximately 600 B.C.), who described an operation in *Sushruta Samhita* ("Treatise of Sushruta") in which a physician used a curved needle to actually push the lens into the eye and away from the line of vision. Although the eye can no longer properly focus, this surgery could be life-changing for those in which the very cloudy lens blocks nearly all light. After the procedure, the physician soaked the eye with warm butter and bandaged it. This basic approach to cataract surgery may have been used centuries earlier in Babylonia. Today, the procedure often involves removal of the lens and replacement with an artificial lens.

Ophthalmology—the branch of medicine concerning eye anatomy and function—was a very active area of interest in medieval Islamic medicine, with numerous experts, including Ammar ibn Ali of Mosul (c. 1000 A.D.), who used a syringe and suction for extraction of cataracts (see his *Choices in the Treatment of Eye Diseases*); Ibn al-Haytham (Alhazen), whose *Book of Optics* (1021) discussed eye anatomy and optics; Ibn al-Nafis, who wrote a large textbook on ophthalmology titled *The Polished Book on Experimental Ophthalmology*; and Ali ibn Isa, author of the famous ophthalmology textbook *Notebook of the Oculists*. During the period of medieval Islam, ophthalmologists were often required to have licenses in order to practice.

German ophthalmologist Julius Hirschberg writes, "From 800–1300 C.E., the World of Islam produced not less than 60 renowned eye specialists or oculists, authors of textbooks and producers of monographs in ophthalmology. Meanwhile, in Europe prior to the twelfth century, an oculist was unheard of."

SEE ALSO Sutures (3000 B.C.), Glass Eye (2800 B.C.), Ayurvedic Medicine (2000 B.C.), Ophthalmoscope (1850), Corneal Transplant (1905), and Laser (1960).

An illustration from Anatomy of the Eye, *an Arabic manuscript (c. 1200 A.D.), by al-Mutadibih.*

اخرى ولقد بقيت لها ولابد ما لابد ... به ... لها ... ملتم من بها
فنا يلتم حول الطبقة القرنية ورد بعضها ... بعضى بساير الطبقة لبعضها
بعضها بعضا لانه لوغشاه كله لمنع البصر من ان يتفتد ه
وهو على هذا المثال

والمبتدى بالاخبار عن منافع كل واحد من الرطوبات والطبقات التي وصف معى
انشانها وكونها ومنتها ومواضعها وركنت تقدمت في اخبارك
الرطوبة الجليدية في وسط الجزء وان خلفها رطوبة واحده وتلث طبقا
فاخبارط واحده ... ... طبقان ... ... الله بالاخبار

Sewage Systems

Given the very large variety of diseases that can be caused by sewage or sewage-contaminated water, the development of effective sewage systems deserves an entry in this book. As an example, the following sewage-related diseases are possible dangers in the United States today, and many can cause severe diarrhea: campylobacteriosis (the most common diarrheal illness in the United States, caused by the bacterium *Campylobacter*, which can spread to the bloodstream and cause a life-threatening infection in people with weakened immune systems), cryptosporidiosis (caused by the microscopic parasite *Cryptosporidium parvum*), diarrheagenic *E. coli* (different varieties of the *Escherichia coli* bacteria), encephalitis (a viral disease transmitted by mosquitoes that often lay eggs in water contaminated by sewage), viral gastroenteritis (caused by many viruses, including rotavirus), giardiasis (caused by the one-celled microscopic parasite *Giardia intestinalis*), hepatitis A (a liver disease caused by a virus), leptospirosis (caused by bacteria), and methaemoglobinaemia (also known as blue-baby syndrome, triggered when infants drink well-water high in nitrates from septic systems).

Other sewage-related diseases include poliomyelitis (caused by a virus) and the following diseases caused by bacteria: salmonellosis, shigellosis, paratyphoid fever, typhoid fever, yersiniosis, and cholera.

This entry is dated to around 600 B.C., which is traditionally thought to be the date of the initial construction of the Cloaca Maxima, one of the world's most famous early and large sewage systems, constructed in ancient Rome in order to drain local marshes and channel wastes to the River Tiber. However, older sewage disposal systems were built in ancient India, prehistoric Middle East, Crete, and Scotland. Today, sewage treatment often involves various filters and the biological degradation of wastes by microorganisms in a managed habitat, followed by disinfection to reduce the number of microorganisms before the water is discharged into the environment. Disinfectants may include chlorine, ultraviolet light, and ozone. Chemicals are sometimes used to reduce the levels of nitrogen and phosphorus. Prior to sewage systems, city dwellers often threw waste into the streets.

SEE ALSO Zoo Within Us (1683), *The Sanitary Condition of the Labouring Population of Great Britain* (1842), Broad Street Pump Handle (1854), and Chlorination of Water (1910).

The latrines of Housesteads Roman Fort along Hadrian's Wall in the ancient Roman province of Britannia. The flow of water from adjacent tanks flushed away waste matter.

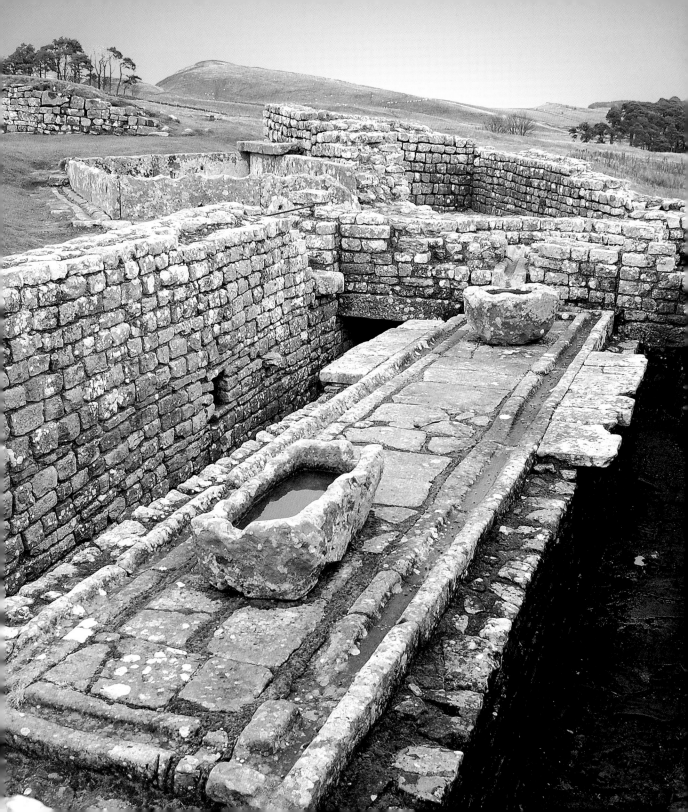

Hippocratic Oath

Hippocrates of Cos (460 B.C.–377 B.C.), **Sun Simiao** (581–682)

Hippocrates of Cos, sometimes referred to as the father of Western medicine, was a Greek physician famous for his dismissal of ancient beliefs involving the supernatural origin of disease. The code of medical ethics bearing his name is still of relevance even today.

We know very little of Hippocrates himself. His body of writings, the Hippocratic Corpus, was actually written by several authors mostly between 420 B.C. and 370 B.C., providing advice on **epilepsy**, head wounds, and gynecology, among other topics. The Hippocratic School suggested that illness was the result of an imbalance of four humors (liquids): blood, black bile, yellow bile, and phlegm. Doctors relied on therapy and dietary recommendations in an attempt to restore the balance. As one example, citrus fruit was considered to be useful when phlegm was in abundance. Recording of patient medical histories was also considered to be important during treatment.

The Hippocratic Oath, written by Hippocrates and/or other ancient Greeks, was taken by physicians who swore to practice medicine ethically. Modernized versions have been used through the centuries. In the original oath, the physician swears to a number of gods to revere his medical teachers, respect patient privacy, and keep patients from harm—and to never give a lethal drug, cause an **abortion** using a pessary (vaginal suppository), perform certain kinds of surgery, or have sex with patients.

"Within a few centuries of his death," writes science journalist Robert Adler, "his writings and teachings became indiscriminately mixed with those of his followers and other Greek physicians. . . . The thread that bound the Hippocratic Corpus together was the conviction that health and disease are strictly natural phenomena—no gods need apply. As civilizations rose and fell over the next fifteen hundred years, the kernel of medical knowledge passed from the Greeks to the Romans, from the Romans to the Muslims, and from the Muslims to medieval Europe."

Ancient Chinese physician Sun Simiao is known for the text "On the Absolute Sincerity of Great Physicians," often referred to as the Chinese equivalent of the Hippocratic Oath.

SEE ALSO Abortion (70), Galenic Writings (190), Paracelsus Burns Medical Books (1527), and Aspirin (1899).

Portion of the Paneth codex, completed in Bologna in 1326 A.D. Shown here is a demon blowing a horn, perhaps a metaphor for disease, perched near text relating to Hippocrates's aphorisms.

...fier.

...ate ati

...eunte

...farinā

...botoma

...cōueit.

...peruc

...hec in

...chdau.

...eum oð

...et fell...

eus. ꝗ claudicā...

Particula se[q]...

...g aer...

...ortatō...

...not...

...g ietm...

T...n u...

...ingultus et cū...

...Et fiat ergo...

N minia diffen...

aut excessus bon...

Huangdi Neijing

The *Huangdi Neijing* (*The Yellow Emperor's Inner Canon*) is the oldest and most famous medical classic of China, compiled by various unknown authors around 300 B.C.– 200 B.C. The work consists of two main texts, the *Su Wen* (*Basic Questions*) and *Ling Shu* (*Spiritual Pivot*), each consisting of 81 chapters. According to scholar Paul Unschuld, the *Huangdi Neijing* "plays a role in Chinese medical history comparable to that of the Hippocratic writings in ancient Europe. Progress and significant paradigm changes have reduced Hippocrates to the honored originator of a tradition that has become obsolete. In contrast, many practitioners of Chinese medicine still consider the *Su Wen* a valuable source of theoretical inspiration and practical knowledge in modern clinical settings."

The text contains questions posed by the legendary Yellow Emperor, which are then answered. The first text, the *Su Wen*, discusses medical theories and diagnostic methods. The second text, the *Ling Shu*, discusses **acupuncture** therapy.

Unlike older works that stressed demonic influences upon health, the *Neijing* addresses more natural causes, including diet, age, lifestyle, and emotions. In addition to considering other forces and concepts, such as yin and yang, as well as qi (a life process or "flow" of energy), the *Neijing* also addresses many aspects of normal and abnormal functioning of the human body, along with diagnoses and therapies.

According to the *Neijing*, humans have five "viscera" (heart, spleen, lungs, liver, and kidneys) and six "bowels" (gallbladder, stomach, small intestine, large intestine, bladder, and Triple Burner). The Triple Burner does not appear to have a strict anatomical form, but nevertheless some acupuncturists believe it plays a role in the circulation of various fluids. The various organs are connected by channels that are not visible structures, but rather are functional connections into which needles may be inserted during acupuncture.

Several passages in the *Neijing* use the metaphor of a bureaucratic division of labor in which parts of the body are assigned specific tasks. Sometimes, the organs are cast as rivals for supremacy. If the organs are victorious over the mind, this may lead to poor health and even death.

SEE ALSO Edwin Smith Surgical Papyrus (1600 B.C.) and Acupuncture *Compendium* (1601).

Acupuncture (inserting and manipulating needles at various points on the body) is discussed in Huangdi Neijing. *Shown here is an acupuncture chart from Chinese physician Hua Shou (1304–1386), which appeared in his* Shi si jing fa hui (Expression of the Fourteen Meridians).

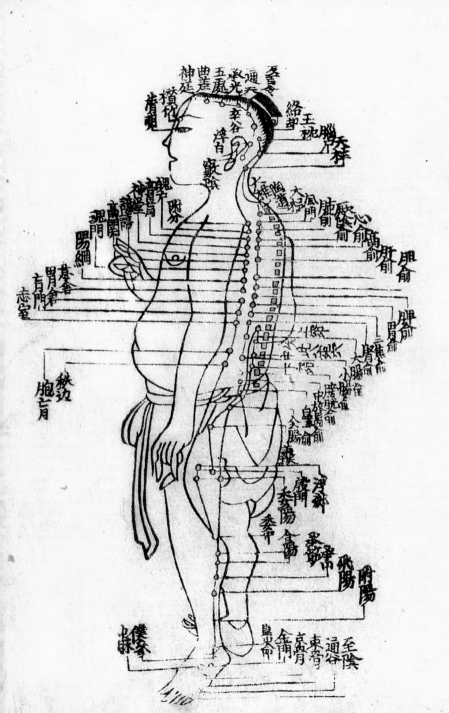

Mithridatium and Theriac

Mithridates VI (132 B.C.–63 B.C.), **Nero Claudius Caesar Augustus Germanicus** (37–68)

Since antiquity, people have been fascinated by poisons and fearful of their consequences. For example, in ancient Greece and Rome, poisons were used for assassinations and state-sanctioned executions, which stimulated quests to find a universal antidote. Two well-known supposed antidotes, which for centuries were widely regarded to be protective against a range of poisons, were Mithridatium (second century B.C.) and Theriac (first century A.D.). The number and diversity of ingredients in these compounds boggles the mind. Mithridatium is said to have been developed by Mithridates VI, King of Pantus (now in Turkey), who was of Persian and Greek Macedonian ancestry. Fearful of being assassinated by poisoning, he perfected his Mithridatium by testing it on criminals and slaves. He believed that its 45 or more ingredients protected him against animal venom and other poisons.

In the first century A.D., Andromachus the Elder, physician to Roman Emperor Nero, "improved" upon Mithridatium by adding viper flesh and increasing the amount of opium. The resultant Theriac, also known as Venice Treacle in the twelfth century, contained at least 64 ingredients, including minerals, poisons, animal flesh, herbs, flowers, squills ("sea onions"), and honey. Through time, Theriac was claimed not only to protect against poisoning but also to treat various diseases, including **bubonic plague**. By the Middle Ages, Theriac sometimes contained more than 100 ingredients that were required to "mature" for several years, and in the early twentieth century it was still available for use in Europe.

Researcher John Griffin writes, "The two ancient products, Mithridatium and Theriac Andromachus, held central places in therapeutics for nearly two millennia. Concern for the quality of these products was the stimulus for requiring the public compounding of these preparations, later replaced by inspection of manufacture and examination of finished product. . . . Perhaps in the final analysis, the contribution of Mithridatium and Theriac to modern medicine was that concerns about their quality stimulated the earliest concepts of medicine's regulation."

SEE ALSO Dioscorides's *De Materia Medica* (70), Paracelsus Burns Medical Books (1527), Antitoxins (1890), Cause of Bubonic Plague (1894), Patent Medicines (1906), and Placebo Effect (1955).

Illustration of an apothecary mixing Theriac, from Hortus sanitatis (Garden of Health), *1491, compiled by printer Jacob Meydenbach. Note the use of snakes.*

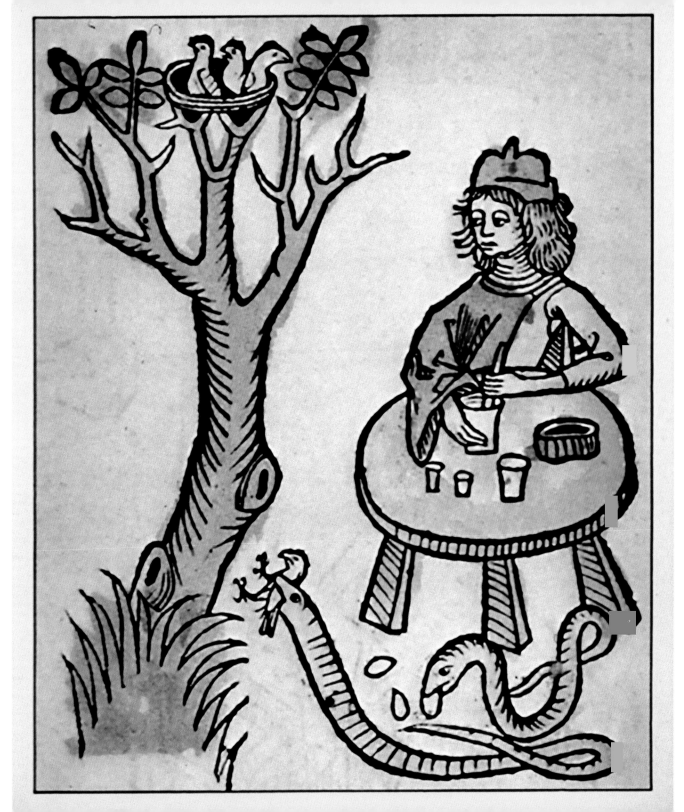

Abortion

Pedanius Dioscorides (c. 40–90)

The practice of abortion started thousands of years ago with a large variety of effective and ineffective means, ranging from herbs and firm abdominal massage to the insertion of sharpened instruments. For example, the Greek pharmacologist Dioscorides recommended "abortion wine" made from hellebore, squirting cucumber, and scammony—which are all plants—around 70 A.D. Soranus, a second-century Greek physician, prescribed riding animals, or leaping energetically so that the woman's heels touched her buttocks, to induce abortion. Today, the removal or expulsion of an embryo or fetus from the uterus is accomplished by various procedures. For example, medical abortions are nonsurgical and make use of certain drugs. Vacuum aspiration employs a manual syringe or electric pump. Dilation and curettage makes use of a scraping tool.

Abortion is a source of considerable debate, with some suggesting that the destruction of a fertilized egg is murder of a human being. However, as discussed by ethicist Louis Guenin, "zygotic personhood" (the idea that a fertilized egg is a person) is a recent concept. For example, before 1869, the Catholic Church accepted the notion that the embryo was not a person until it was 40 days old, at which time the soul entered. Aristotle also presumed this 40-day threshold. If the early embryo was soulless, perhaps early abortion was not murder. Pope Innocent III in 1211 determined that the time of ensoulment was anywhere from three to four months. In Jewish law, the fetus becomes a full-fledged human being when its head exits the womb. Before the embryo is 40 days old, it is *maya b'alma* or "mere water" (Talmud, Yevamoth 69b).

In the 1973 case *Roe v. Wade*, the U.S. Supreme Court invalidated state laws banning abortion, ruling that such laws violated a woman's right to privacy. In particular, a state cannot restrict a woman's right to an abortion in any way during the first trimester (first three months of pregnancy).

SEE ALSO Hippocratic Oath (400 B.C.), Condom (1564), Discovery of Sperm (1678), Separation of Conjoined Twins (1689), Cesarean Section (1882), Sterilization of Carrie Buck (1927), "The Rabbit Died" (1928), IUD (1929), Amniocentesis (1952), Birth-Control Pill (1955), Thalidomide Disaster (1962), and First Test-Tube Baby (1978).

Soviet poster from 1925 warning midwives not to perform abortions and showing that abortions often lead to death of the mother. The poster also warns that midwives who perform abortions are committing crimes.

ВЫКИДЫШ, ПРОИЗВЕДЕННЫЙ БАБКОЙ ИЛИ АКУШЕРКОЙ, НЕ ТОЛЬКО КАЛЕЧИТ ЖЕНЩИНУ, НО ЧАСТО ВЕДЕТ К СМЕРТИ.

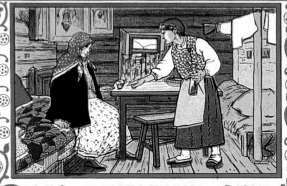

• У ПОВИТУХИ •

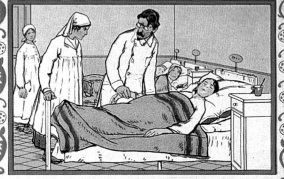

• ПОСЛЕДСТВИЯ ВЫКИДЫША •

ВСЯКИЙ ВЫКИДЫШ ВРЕДЕН.

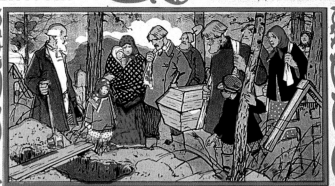

• СМЕРТЬ ОТ ВЫКИДЫША •

БАБКА И АКУШЕРКА, ПРОИЗВОДЯЩАЯ ВЫКИДЫШ, СОВЕРШАЕТ ПРЕСТУПЛЕНИЕ.

Издание Отдела Охраны Материнства и Младенчества Н.К.З.

Dioscorides's *De Materia Medica*

Pedanius Dioscorides (c. 40–90)

For millennia, the history of pharmacy—the art of preparing and dispensing medical drugs—was identical with the history of pharmacognosy, which involves the study of medicines derived from natural sources. In the first century A.D., army surgeon Pedanius Dioscorides began his remarkable quest to consolidate all the known medical information on plants and other natural substances into a work that would be read and translated for 1,500 years. The Arabs initially preserved and copied the work, which was a foundation for Islamic pharmacology and which was eventually recopied in Latin.

Dioscorides—a Greek physician born in what is now Turkey who practiced in Rome at the time of Nero—traveled extensively and described around 600 plants in his five-volume work *De Materia Medica* ("Regarding Medical Matters," c. 70 A.D.), in which he included precise drawings. His explanations were practical and included dosages and recipes for preparation, as well as instructions for administration to patients. In addition to describing uses of opium for pain, he also discussed such plants as cannabis (marijuana), peppermint, and wild blackberries. His treatments concerned ulcers, roundworms, antidotes to poisons, and much more.

Chemist John Mann writes, "The major triumph and novelty of Dioscorides's herbal [book] was his ordering of plants according to their pharmacological properties, rather than their botanical family. Many of his plant extracts were undoubtedly effective, for example those of henbane and mandrake containing tropane alkaloids [naturally occurring nitrogen-containing organic molecules], which were used for pain relief; but his use of hemlock is less convincing: 'it prevents the breasts of a virgin growing larger.'" Other superstitions included applying bedbugs to treat **malaria**.

Note that in modern times, physicians have often prescribed medicines that were originally related to compounds found in plants. For example, **aspirin** has an active ingredient found in willow bark and treats fever, pain, and inflammation. **Digitalis** from a common garden flower can control the heart rate.

SEE ALSO Witch Doctor (10,000 B.C.), *Huangdi Neijing* (300 B.C.), Mithridatium and Theriac (100 B.C.), Digitalis (1785), Cause of Malaria (1897), and Aspirin (1899).

Page from an Arabic translation of the De Materia Medica *of Dioscorides (1224).*

فاذا ازداد العصير نصفه فهذا الشراب موافق لوجع الحلق والجنب والرئتين

والاسر والراقف والمزنه بلغم غليظ في حلقه يصفي اللون وكثر النوم

وليس له غايلة موافق للمثانه والكلا م ع م ع

صنعه شراب للزكام والسعال

ووزم البطر واسترخاه المعدن خذ مر ربع اوقيه واصول سوس ثرااوقيه

وفلفل ابيض ربع ثمن اوقيه دقه جميعا واربطه بخرقه واجعله في قسطا اشراب

طيب واتركه ثلثه ايام ثم نصفه وارفعه في آناء نظيف اشرب منه بعد العشا

Galenic Writings

Galen of Pergamon (129–199)

Aside from Hippocrates six centuries earlier (see entry "**Hippocratic Oath**"), probably no other Greek physician has influenced the path of Western medicine for a longer period of time than Galen. Born in the second century A.D.—at the height of the Roman Empire—Galen's medical knowledge, anatomical studies, and tremendous collection of writings dominated his successors for more than a millennium. According to reports, he sometimes employed 20 scribes to keep pace with his dictations! Additionally, his animal dissections led to new understandings of organ systems.

Born in what is today the western coast of Turkey, he traveled extensively before settling in Rome. Because human dissection was illegal, his vast anatomical research was based on pigs, dogs, and monkeys ("Barbary apes"). Through vivisections (live dissections), he was able to cut various nerves to demonstrate that the brain controlled muscle motions in the body. Loss of vocalizations became apparent after cutting of a laryngeal nerve. To demonstrate that kidneys produced urine, he tied the ureters and observed kidney swelling. As a physician to the gladiators, he peered into horrific wounds to learn more about human anatomy. Eventually, he became physician of the Roman Emperor Marcus Aurelius, among others.

Not all of Galen's medical findings and theories were sound. After considering Hippocrates's ideas that illness was the result of an imbalance of four humors (liquids)—blood, black bile, yellow bile, and phlegm—he extrapolated the concepts to suggest that an imbalance of each humor corresponded to a human temperament (for example, an abundance of black bile corresponded to a melancholic personality). He also incorrectly suggested that venous blood was created and pumped by the liver and that arterial blood originated in the heart, and he believed that blood passed from the left and right sides of the heart through invisible pores.

For Galen, philosophy was an essential component in the training of each physician. After the Roman Empire fell, his influence continued, with his writings and ideas moving through the Arabic world and later into the European Middle Ages and beyond.

SEE ALSO Hippocratic Oath (400 B.C.), Al-Razi's *Comprehensive Book* (900), Al-Nafis's Pulmonary Circulation (1242), Paracelsus Burns Medical Books (1527), *De Humani Corporis Fabrica* (1543), and Circulatory System (1628).

Gladiators' wounds gave Galen crucial glimpses of the anatomy of muscles and internal organs. Pollice Verso *(1872), by French painter Jean-Léon Gérôme (1824–1904).*

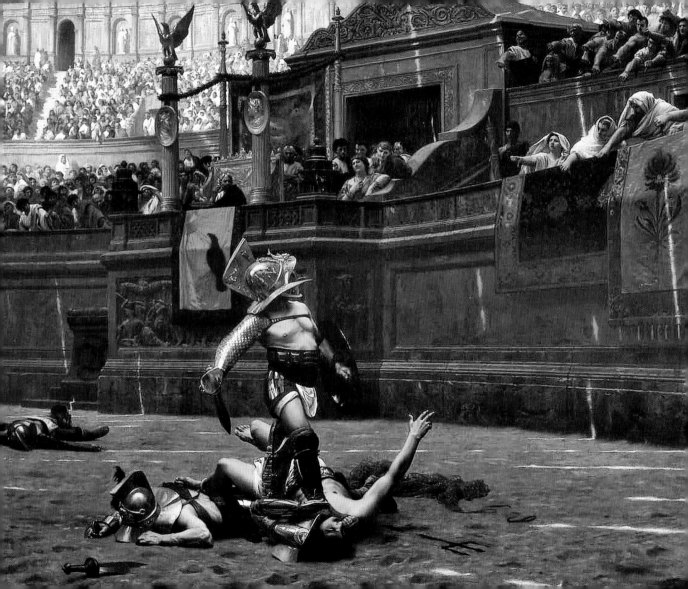

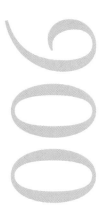

Al-Razi's *Comprehensive Book*

Abu Bakr Muhammad ibn Zakariya al-Razi (865–925), Abu 'Ali al-Husayn ibn 'Abd-Allah Ibn Sina (Avicenna) (980–1037)

One of the greatest physicians in medieval medicine and of the Islamic world was al-Razi, who was born in Persia (modern-day Iran) and known in the West as Rhazes. During his life, he wrote nearly 200 books on topics ranging from philosophy and alchemy to medicine. He was the author of the first book on pediatrics and is famous for extensive observations that differentiated smallpox and measles. He was among the first to study lesions of the nervous system and to correlate them with clinical symptoms. In addition to his scholarly works, he also wrote for ordinary people seeking help. When discussing medical ethics, he wrote, "The doctor's aim is to do good, even to our enemies. . . . My profession forbids us to do harm to our kindred, as it is instituted for the benefit and welfare of the human race."

Rhazes frequently contradicted previous famous physicians, such as Galen, when he found them to be wrong, and he also offered harsh criticism of religious prophets and religions, including Islam. According to legend, he turned away a physician offering to remove his cataracts, saying, "I have seen enough of the world." He died embittered and blind.

Among his landmark works is *Kitab al-hawi fi al-tibb* (*Comprehensive Book of Medicine*, c. 900), a vast compilation of medicine and observations that his students accumulated after his death. This work inspired subsequent physicians of the Islamic world, including the famous Avicenna, author of the five-volume *Canon of Medicine*. Jewish physician Faraj ben Salim translated *Kitab al-hawi* into Latin in 1279, and after it was printed in 1486 under the title *Liber continens*, its influence spread. *Kitab al-hawi* is notable not only for its size but for its discussions of Greek, Arabian, and Indian physicians, whose work would otherwise have been lost. Also influential in Europe was al-Razi's book *Al-tibb al-Mansuri* (*Medicine Dedicated to Mansur*), a medical textbook that eventually became one of the most widely read medieval manuals in Europe.

SEE ALSO Hippocratic Oath (400 B.C.) and Avicenna's *Canon of Medicine* (1025).

European depiction of al-Razi, in Collection of Medical Treatises *by Gerard of Cremona (1114–1187). Gerard was an Italian translator who journeyed to Toledo, Spain, to learn Arabic and translate numerous Arabic scientific works found there.*

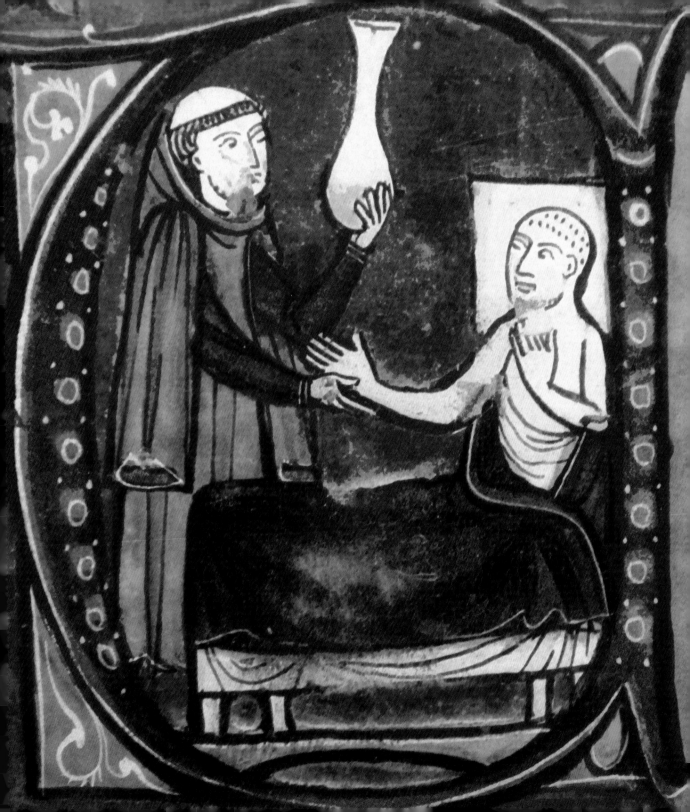

Avicenna's *Canon of Medicine*

Hippocrates of Cos (460 B.C.–377 B.C.), **Aristotle** (384 B.C.–322 B.C.),
Galen of Pergamon (129–199), **Abu Bakr Muhammad ibn Zakariya al-Razi**
(865–925), **Abu 'Ali al-Husayn ibn 'Abd-Allah Ibn Sina (Avicenna)** (980–
1037)

Islamic physicians of the Middle Ages helped preserve and expand the medical
traditions of Greece and Rome, and the most influential of the great Islamic physician-
philosophers was Ibn Sina, known to the West as Avicenna. His most famous work was
the five-book encyclopedia *Al-Qanun fi al-Tibb* (*The Canon of Medicine*), completed
in 1025, which provided a basis for medical teaching for more than 700 years and was
used in European medical schools. His work, written in Arabic and later translated into
Latin, was influenced by Hippocrates, Galen, and Aristotle. Like his famous Islamic
predecessor al-Razi, Avicenna stressed the importance of observation, experimentation,
and evidence-based medicine for making clinical decisions.

In the *Canon*, Avicenna discusses **cancer** surgery and also helps elucidate the nature of
infectious diseases (including tuberculosis) and the usefulness of quarantine. Remarkably,
he was able to make the distinction between mediastinitis (inflammation of the tissues in
the mid-chest) and pleurisy (inflammation of the lining of the pleural cavity surrounding
the lungs). He wrote that during drug testing, the drug must be pure and tested on multiple
diseases to understand its intended and "accidental" effects, and that its action must be
timed. Additionally, he advised that clinical trials be repeated on multiple patients to judge
medical efficacy and that drug tests on animals are not sufficient to determine effects in
humans. Avicenna was very interested in psychiatric conditions, ranging from hallucinations
and depression to the behaviors of stroke victims. Of course, the *Canon* has flaws. For
example, Avicenna wrote that the heart had three ventricles instead of two.

Historian Lawrence Conrad writes that the *Canon* "covered the various fields of
medicine with a precision and thoroughness that gave it authoritative sway over the
discipline for hundreds of years, and it ranks as one of the most impressive and enduring
achievements of Islamic science." Canadian physician William Osler described
Avicenna as the "author of the most famous medical textbook ever written" and noted
that the *Canon* persisted as "a medical bible for a longer time than any other work."

SEE ALSO Hippocratic Oath (400 B.C.), Galenic Writings (190), Al-Razi's *Comprehensive Book* (900),
Al-Nafis's Pulmonary Circulation (1242), Panum's "Measles on the Faroe Islands"(1846), and Randomized
Controlled Trials (1948).

Internal organs according to Avicenna's Canon of Medicine, *published in Ishfahan, Persia.*

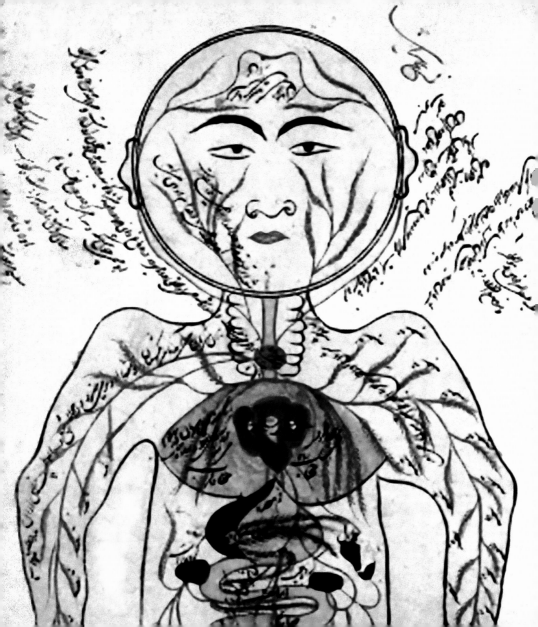

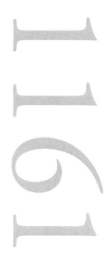

Persecution of Jewish Physicians

Martin Luther (1483–1546)

The persecution of Jewish physicians and their colleagues is a pervasive theme in the history of medicine. For example, in 1161, 86 Jews were burned alive as punishment for an alleged plot by Jewish physicians to poison the citizens of Bohemia in central Europe. Around 1348, many Jews were exterminated for supposedly causing the Black Death in Europe, despite the fact that many Jews perished from the plague. According to the medical faculty of the University of Vienna in 1610, Jewish law forced Jewish physicians to murder every tenth Christian through poisoning. Martin Luther, the German theologian, wrote, "If they [the Jews] could kill us all, they would gladly do so. . . . They do it often, especially those who pose as physicians." Luther also urged people to "burn down their synagogues."

Several popes in the European Middle Ages forbade Christians from seeking help from Jewish physicians, and later, in the seventeenth century, the clergy of Hall in Württemberg declared that "it were better to die with Christ than to be cured by a Jew doctor aided by the devil." In 1938, Germany revoked the licenses of Jewish physicians. The ensuing physician shortage compelled Germany to reduce the period of medical education by two years.

In the years before World War II, quotas limited the number of Jewish medical students and physicians at U.S. medical schools. In order to assess an applicant's Jewishness, administrators examined student names and asked about religious affiliation on medical school applications. In 1940, the dean of Cornell University's medical college limited the number of Jews allowed to enter each class, and applications of Jewish candidates at Yale Medical School were marked with an *H* for *Hebrew*. The head of Columbia University's Neurological Institute was told, in 1945, to fire all the Jews in his department or resign. He resigned.

Even today, Jewish health-care professionals are sometimes the subject of strange allegations. In 1988, a Chicago mayoral assistant charged that Jews injected the AIDS virus into African Americans, and in 1997, a prominent Palestinian representative suggested that the Israelis injected Palestinian children with HIV (human immunodeficiency virus).

SEE ALSO Cause of Bubonic Plague (1894), Informed Consent (1947), and Reverse Transcriptase and AIDS (1970).

Illustration showing Jews being burned alive during the Black Death, by German physician, historian, and cartographer Hartmann Schedel (1440–1514).

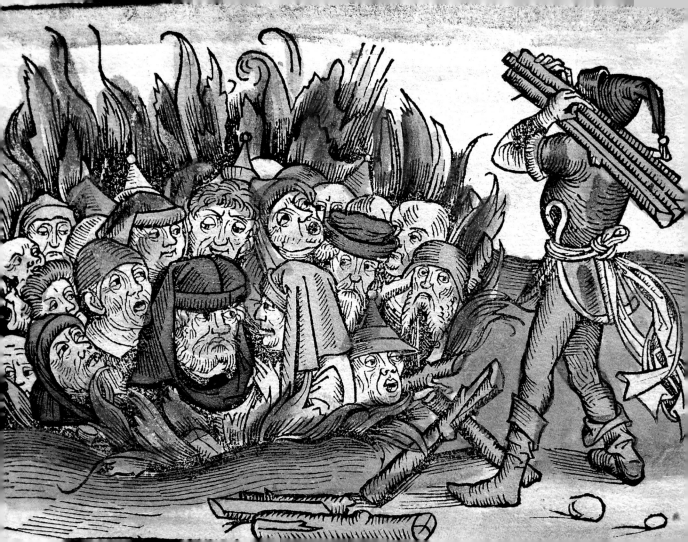

Barber Pole

Ambroise Paré (1510–1590)

The barber pole with its red and white helical stripes has been used for centuries as a symbol of the barber's trade. This emblem dates to an era in which a barber, in addition to cutting hair, also pulled teeth and performed various surgical procedures, including **bloodletting**, a practice in which blood was drained from the body in a questionable effort to improve health. The red bloody bandages, perhaps only partially cleaned, were placed outside the barber shop to dry. As they blew in the wind around a pole, they created a pattern that was eventually transformed into an advertising symbol in the form of a striped helical pole.

In 1096, the barber-surgeons formed their first official organization in France. Around 1210, in order to distinguish between academic surgeons and barber-surgeons, the Collège de Saint Côme et Saint Damien of Paris required that the former wear long robes and the latter wear short robes. Note that barber-surgeons should not all be considered crude practitioners—the French surgeon Ambroise Paré started as a barber-surgeon and became the most celebrated surgeon of the European Renaissance.

In 1540, the barber-surgeons and academic surgeons in England united to form a single guild—the United Barber-Surgeons Company—but the two classes of surgeons had different jobs. The barbers displayed blue and white poles and were prohibited from carrying out advanced surgery, although they still could pull teeth and perform bloodletting. Academic surgeons displayed poles with red and white stripes and were not allowed to cut hair or shave clients.

During bloodletting, clients would tightly clutch a staff to make their veins visible and encourage blood flow, and barbers would cut clients' arms and bleed them. Blood-drawing leeches were also used. The early barber pole was topped with a brass basin representing a container of leeches.

In the United States, the most famous manufacturer of motorized spinning barber poles was the William Marvy Company of St. Paul, Minnesota, founded in 1950. By 1967, the company had sold 50,000 poles.

SEE ALSO Bloodletting (1500 B.C.), Paré's "Rational Surgery" (1545), Leech Therapy (1825), Caduceus (1902), and Band-Aid Bandage (1920).

The stripes on the barber pole date to an era in which a barber performed surgical procedures and bloodletting. The red stripes represent the bloody bandages. (Blue may partly be an homage to the colors of the U.S. flag.)

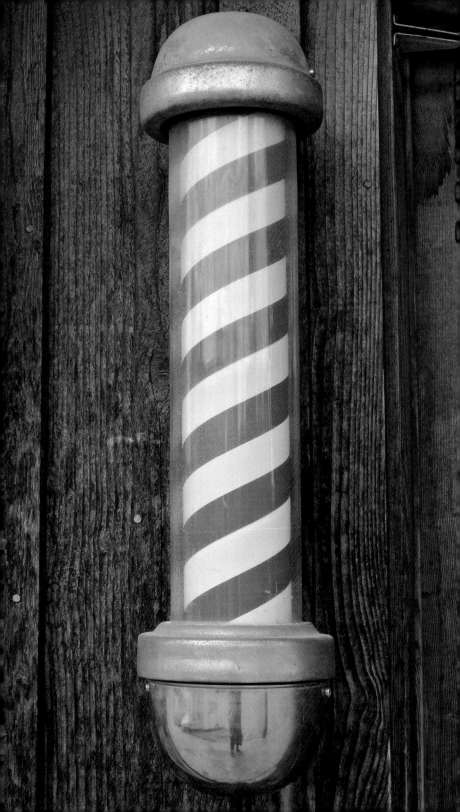

Al-Nafis's Pulmonary Circulation

Abu 'Ali al-Husayn ibn 'Abd-Allah Ibn Sina (Avicenna) (980–1037), Ala al-Din Abu al-Hassan Ali ibn Abi-Hazm al-Qurashi al-Dimashqi (known as Ibn al-Nafis;1213–1288), William Harvey (1578–1657)

The first person known to have correctly described pulmonary circulation is Muslim physician Ibn al-Nafis, who was born near Damascus, Syria, and worked in Cairo, Egypt. Pulmonary circulation refers to the path of blood between the heart and lungs. In particular, oxygen-depleted blood leaves the heart, traveling from the right ventricle (lower chamber) into the pulmonary arteries leading to the lungs. After the blood is oxygenated by the lungs, it travels through the pulmonary veins and returns to the heart's left atrium (upper chamber), then moves to the left ventricle before being pumped to the aorta and into the rest of the body.

Al-Nafis was adamant about not relying on the entrenched ideas of past physicians, writing in his 1242 treatise *Commentary on Anatomy in Avicenna's Canon*: "In determining the use of each organ we shall rely necessarily on verified examinations and straightforward research, disregarding whether our opinions will agree or disagree with those of our predecessors." For example, he denied the prevailing wisdom of the Greek physician Galen and the Persian physician Avicenna, both of whom believed that blood passed from one side of the heart to the other through invisible pores in the heart wall. Al-Nafis knew there were no pores. Instead, al-Nafis wrote, "The blood from the right chamber must flow through the vena arteriosa [pulmonary artery] to the lungs, spread through its substances, be mingled there with air, pass through the arteria venosa [pulmonary vein] to reach the left chamber of the heart and there form the vital spirit." His radical observation was developed around age 29 and was not dramatically surpassed until about 1628, when English physician William Harvey published his complete theory of the continuous cycle of blood throughout the entire body.

Al-Nafis also wrote notes for 300 volumes of the medical encyclopedia *The Comprehensive Book on Medicine*, of which 80 volumes, discussing surgical and other medical techniques, were published.

SEE ALSO Eye Surgery (600 B.C.), Galenic Writings (190), Avicenna's *Canon of Medicine* (1025), *De Humani Corporis Fabrica* (1543), Circulatory System (1628), Lavoisier's Respiration (1784), and Blalock-Taussig Shunt (1944).

Ibn al-Nafis described the pulmonary circulation of blood between the heart and lungs. In the depiction, the pulmonary arteries and veins, seen at the upper part of the heart, branch horizontally to the left and right, making their way to the lungs.

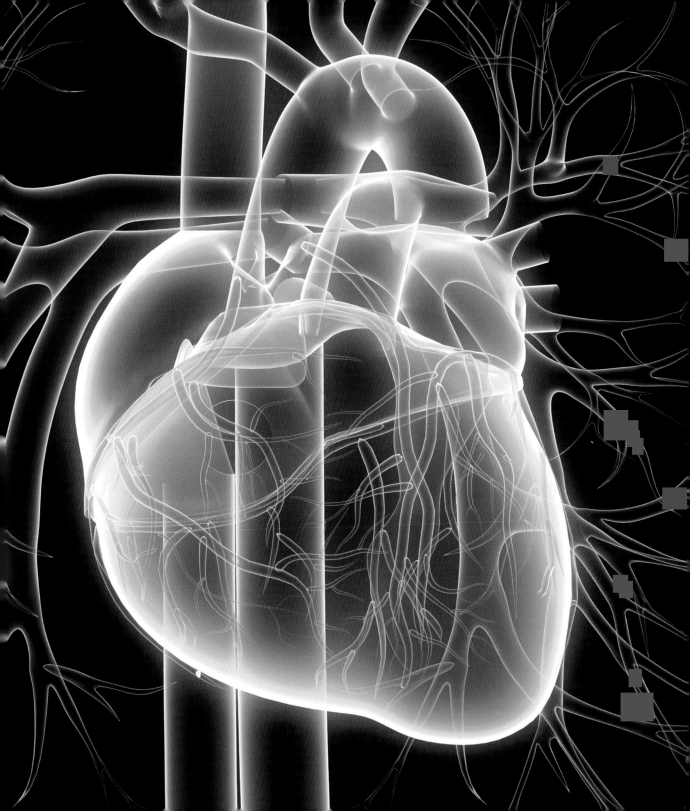

Eyeglasses

Salvino D'Armate of Florence (1258–1312), Giambattista della Porta (1535–1615), Edward Scarlett (1677–1743)

Historian Lois N. Magner writes, "The use of spectacles must have occasioned a profound effect on attitudes towards human limitations and liabilities. Spectacles not only made it possible for scholars and copyists to continue their work, they accustomed people to the idea that certain physical limitations could be transcended by the use of human inventions."

Today, the terms *eyeglasses* and *spectacles* usually refer to lenses attached to a frame to correct vision problems. Various forms have existed through history, including the pince-nez (supported only by pinching the bridge of the nose, with no earpieces), monocle (a circular lens over one eye), and lorgnette (spectacles with a handle).

By 1000 A.D., "reading stones"—crystals or segments of a glass sphere placed on reading material to magnify the text—were common. Eyeglasses were in use in China by the time of Marco Polo's journey, around 1270, and they may have been used in Arabia even earlier. In 1284, the Italian Salvino D'Armate became perhaps the most famous inventor of eyeglasses in Europe. The earliest eyeglasses made use of convex glasses for the correction of hyperopia (farsightedness) and presbyopia (age-related farsightedness). One early reference to concave lenses for nearsightedness (also called myopia, in which distant objects appear blurred and near objects are clear) occurred in *Natural Magick* (1558), by Italian scholar Giambattista della Porta. Convex lenses were used to see text that was close to the eye.

Spectacles were once so expensive that they were listed in wills as valuable property. Around 1727, British optician Edward Scarlett developed the modern style of glasses, held by rigid arms that hook over the ears. The American scientist Benjamin Franklin invented bifocals in 1784 to address his combination of myopia and presbyopia.

Today, many eyeglasses are made of the plastic CR-39 due to its favorable optical properties and durability. Lenses are generally used to change the focus location of light rays so that they properly intersect the retina, the light-sensitive tissue at the back of the eye.

SEE ALSO *Micrographia* (1665), Ophthalmoscope (1850), Hearing Aids (1899), Laser (1960), and Cochlear Implants (1977).

A lorgnette is a pair of spectacles with a handle. It was invented in the 1700s by English optical designer George Adams. Some owners did not need glasses to see better, but carried ornate lorgnettes to be fashionable.

dubitavisset, miseric... ...otus ...
...fensissimum propter ...
Octavius in Italiam ...
ingressus est. Tùm ...
Jani gemini portas ...
dò bis anteà clau...fuerant,
iterùm post pri...um Punicum
præteritorum malorum oblivi...
Romanus præsentis otii lætitiâ ...
...tavio maxi... honores à senatu de...
Augustus co...nominatus est et in ejus honorem mensis
Sextilis eo...m nomine est appellatus, quòd illo
mense belli...civilibus finis esset impositus. Equi-
tes Romani ...alem ejus bidu... semper celebrârunt ;
senatus popul...que Romanus universus cognomen
Patris patriæ ma...consensu ei tribuerunt. Augustus præ gaudio...cymans respondit his verbis :
"Compos factus...votorum meorum ; neque
aliud mihi optan...est, quàm ut hunc consensum
vestrum ad ultim...vitæ finem videre possim."

Dictaturam, ...am populus magnâ vi offerebat,
Augustus, genu...xâ dejectâque ab humeris togâ,
deprecatus est. ...omini appellationem semper ex-
horruit, ea...tribui edicto vetuit, imò de re-
stituend...republicâ n...semel cogitavit ; sed repu-
tans ...se privatum n...sine periculo fore, et rem-
publi...m plurium arbit...o commissum iri, summam
reti...it potestatem, id ...erò studuit, ne quem novi
stat...s pœniteret. Ben...de iis etiam, quos adver-
sari...s expertus fuerat et sentiebat et loquebatur.
Legentem aliquandò ...num è nepotibus invenit :
quum...que puer terri...s volumen Ciceronis, quod
manu...tenebat, veste...tegeret, Augustus librum ce-

pit, eoque statìm reddito : "Hic vir, inquit, fili mi,
doctus fuit et patriæ amans."

Pedibus sæpè per urbem incedebat, summâque
comitate adeuntes excipiebat : undè quum quidam
libellum supplicem porrigens, præ metu et reve-
rentiâ nunc manum proferret, tunc retraheret ;
Putasne, inquit jocans Augustus, assem te ele-
...ta dare?" Eum aliquandò convenit veteranus
...catus in jus periclitabatur, rogavitque
ut ...... Statim Augustus unum è comitatu
suo ele... qui litigatorem commendaret.
Tùm veteran...vit : "At non ego, te peri-
clitante bello Actiaco, ...ium quæsivi, sed ipse
pro te pugnavi ;" simulque ...trices Eru-
buit Augustus, atque ipse veni...em.

Quum post Actiacam victoriam ...mam
ingrederetur, occurrit ei inter g...te
quidam corvum tenens, quem instituer...
Ave, Cæsar victor, imperator. Augustus ave...o...
ciosam miratus, eam viginti millibus nummorum
emit. Socius opificis, ad quem nihil ex illâ liberal-
itate pervenerat, affirmavit Augusto illum habere
et alium corvum, quem afferri postulavit. Allatus
corvus verba quæ didicerat expressit : Ave, Antoni
victor, imperator. Nihil eâ re exasperatus Augustus jussit tantummodò corvorum doctorem dividere
acceptam mercedem cum contubernali. Salutatus
similiter à psittaco emi eum jussit.

Exemplo incitatus sutor quidam, corvum instituit
ad parem salutationem ; sed, quum parùm profice-
ret, sæpè ad avem non respondentem dicebat : Ope-
ra et impensa periit. Tandem corvus cœpit pro-
ferre dictatam salutationem : quâ audità dùm transi-
ret, Augustus respondit : "Satis domi talium salu-

M

Biological Weapons

Hannibal (248 B.C.–183 B.C.)

Physicians play central roles in responding to the menace of biological weapons. They maintain an awareness of risks, quickly recognize an event, and institute appropriate responses such as antibiotics and vaccines. In the twenty-first century, bioweapons pose a growing threat of causing devastating epidemics as expertise in biotechnology grows and methods for the genetic manipulation of pathogens become simpler.

Biological warfare includes the use of bacteria, viruses, fungi, and other biological agents to kill humans, livestock, and plants. For example, *Bacillus anthracis*, the bacterium that causes anthrax, is an effective biological weapon because it forms resilient spores that are easily dispersed. Additionally, pulmonary anthrax infection can kill 90 percent of untreated individuals within a week. Terrorist sympathizers can be protected with antibiotics and thus avoid being killed themselves.

Other potential bioweapons include *Yersinia pestis* (a bacterium that can cause **bubonic plague**), viruses (such as Rift Valley fever and Ebola), and toxins (such as ricin, extracted from the castor bean, and botulinum toxin, a protein produced by the bacterium *Clostridium botulinum*).

Biological warfare has been conducted for millennia. In 184 B.C., the soldiers of Hannibal of Carthage threw clay pots filled with venomous snakes onto enemy ships. In 1346, Tartar forces threw warriors who died of plague over the walls of Kaffa, a Crimean city, and an outbreak of plague followed. In 1763, representatives of the Delaware Indians were given blankets exposed to smallpox. In 1940, Japanese warplanes flew over China and dropped ceramic bombs filled with fleas carrying bubonic plague.

Today, various field equipment is being developed that employs antibodies aimed at a number of specific pathogens to detect a possible bioterrorist attack. The World Medical Association writes, "The consequences of a successful biological attack, especially if the infection were readily communicable, could far exceed those of a chemical or even a nuclear event. Given the ease of travel and increasing globalization, an outbreak anywhere in the world could be a threat to all nations."

SEE ALSO Antitoxins (1890), Cause of Bubonic Plague (1894), and Common Cold (1914).

A gas mask and protective clothing. Physicians play central roles in responding to the menace of both chemical and biological weapons.

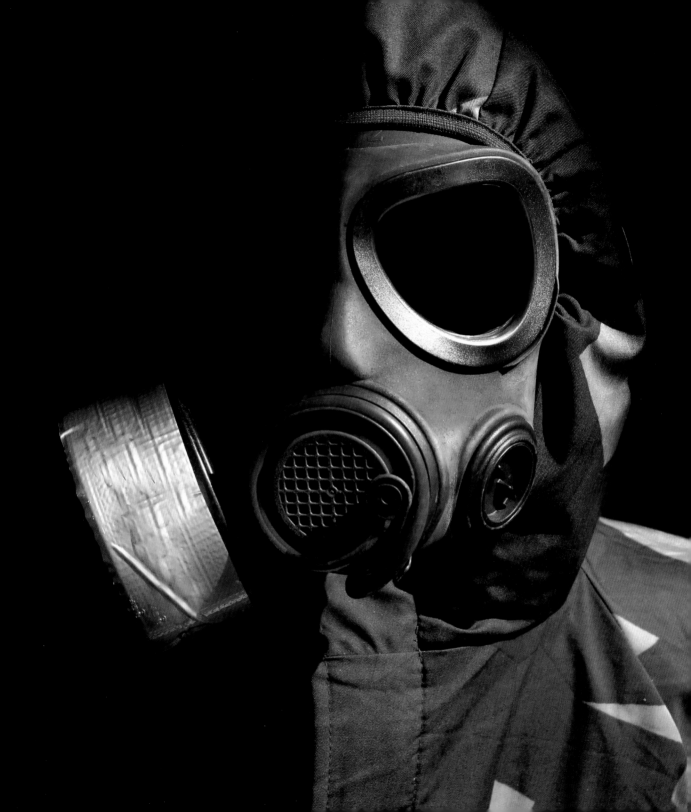

Leonardo's Anatomical Drawings

Leonardo da Vinci (1452–1519), **Louis d'Aragon** (1475–1519)

Many readers may be familiar with Leonardo da Vinci, the Italian genius who was both a scientist and an artist, famous for his paintings of the *Mona Lisa* and *The Last Supper*. As early as 1489, while he was in Milan, Leonardo established his grand plan for a *Treatise on Anatomy*, a comprehensive set of drawings and explanations concerning the human body. Although Leonardo outlined his plan, he never completed his work.

During his anatomical studies for the *Treatise*, Leonardo made one of the first scientific drawings of a fetus within the womb. Also fascinating were his groundbreaking methods of injecting wax into the ventricles of the brain in order to better understand their shapes. According to curators at the Museum of Science in Boston, "One cannot exaggerate the unpleasantness of Leonardo's anatomy studies. . . . Leonardo, in his fervor for knowledge, held countless creepy vigils with the local corpses, and their annoying tendency to decay forced him to work as quickly as possible. He described it as 'living through the night hours in the company of quartered and flayed corpses fearful to behold,' but as usual his curiosity pushed him ever onward."

Journalist Katie Lambert writes, "His notebooks are both gorgeous and grotesque [with] flayed body parts, [and] fetuses, and couples in the midst of sexual encounters. Notes crowd the drawings, allowing you to peek inside the brain of da Vinci himself as he questioned how a fetus breathes and what testicles do."

In 1517, near the end of his life and partially paralyzed, Leonardo was visited by Cardinal Louis d'Aragon and his secretary Antonio de Beatis. After Leonardo showed his various anatomical sketches to his visitors, Beatis recorded in his journal: "Leonardo has compiled a special treatise of anatomy with pictorial demonstrations of the limbs as well as of the muscles, nerves, veins, joints, intestines, and whatever can be imagined in the bodies of men as well as women, such as never have been made before by any person."

SEE ALSO *De Humani Corporis Fabrica* (1543), Eustachi's Rescued Masterpieces (1552), Drawings of Pietro da Cortona (1618), Cheselden's *Osteographia* (1733), Albinus's *Tables of the Human Body* (1747), Hunter's *Gravid Uterus* (1774), Anatomy Act of 1832 (1832), and *Gray's Anatomy* (1858).

Leonardo da Vinci's illustration of a fetus in the womb, with the umbilical cord visible (c. 1510).

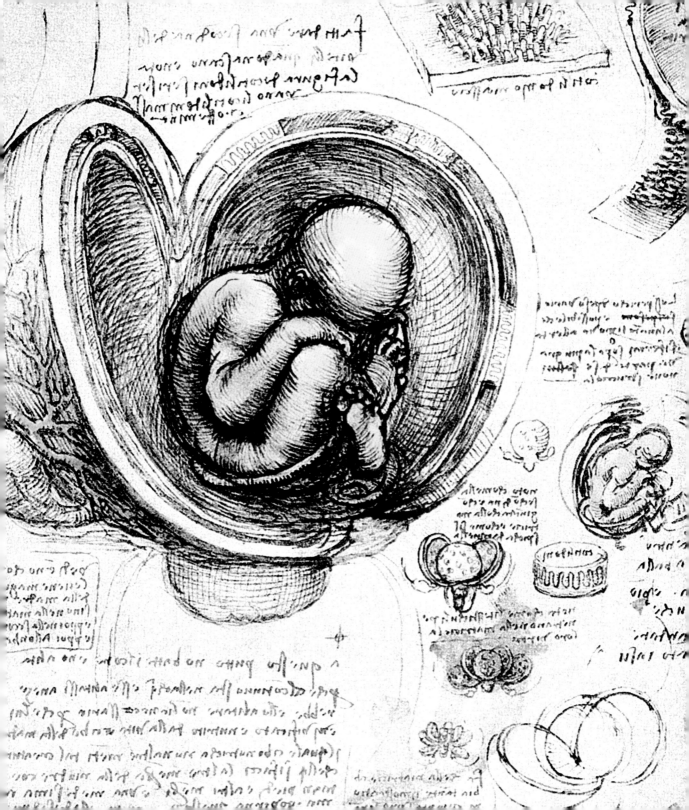

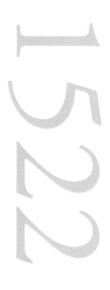

Burning of Dr. Wertt

Percival Willoughby (1632–1669), **John Hunter** (1728–1793), **George III** (**George William Frederick**; 1738–1820), **George IV** (**George Augustus Frederick**; 1762–1830)

Although male midwives started to become common in the West in the eighteenth century as men began to control the profession, the earlier taboos that kept men away from births played an important role in the history of medicine. No story exemplifies the early gender taboo concerning midwives greater than the punishment of Dr. Wertt of Hamburg. In 1522, the physician Wertt disguised himself as a woman so that he could observe the birthing process and learn firsthand about delivering babies. Alas, intrusion of men into the birthing room was unthinkable at that time. A midwife recognized Wertt dressed in woman's clothes and raised cries of protests. Wertt was burned at the stake while other physicians watched.

Several other stories are illustrative of the gender taboo. In 1646, Francis Rayus of Wells, Massachusetts, was arrested for a similar crime as Wertt. Luckily for Rayus, his punishment was a fine of only 50 shillings. In 1658, English physician Percival Willoughby asked to consult with a midwife on a difficult delivery, and was required to crawl into the patient's darkened room, examine her while she remained covered, and crawl out again to discuss the situation with the midwife. Also, consider that in 1762, John Hunter, a Scottish surgeon who was regarded as one of the most distinguished surgeons of his day, had to sit in an adjacent room while a Mrs. Stevens attended the wife of George III, King of England, to deliver George IV.

The disengagement of husbands from the birth process has been common in many cultures at different times in history. For example, when wives went into labor on Lukunor, an island in the South Pacific, men left for a month and stayed with other men. On the other hand, men have sometimes been more engaged. Among the Huichol tribe of Mexico, supposedly a string would be tied around the husband's testicles. During delivery, the wife pulled the string with each contraction so that he could participate in her pain.

SEE ALSO Obstetrical Forceps (1580), Mary Toft's Rabbits (1726), Hunter's *Gravid Uterus* (1774), and Modern Midwifery (1925).

A woman giving birth on a birth chair, by German physician Eucharius Rösslin (1470–1526). His book on childbirth, Der Rosengarten (The Rose Garden), *published in 1513, became a standard medical text for midwives.*

Rosegarten

Das vierd Capitel sagt wie

sich ein yede fraw/in/voz/vnd nach der geburt halte soll
vnd wie man ir in harter geburt zů hilff kommen soll.

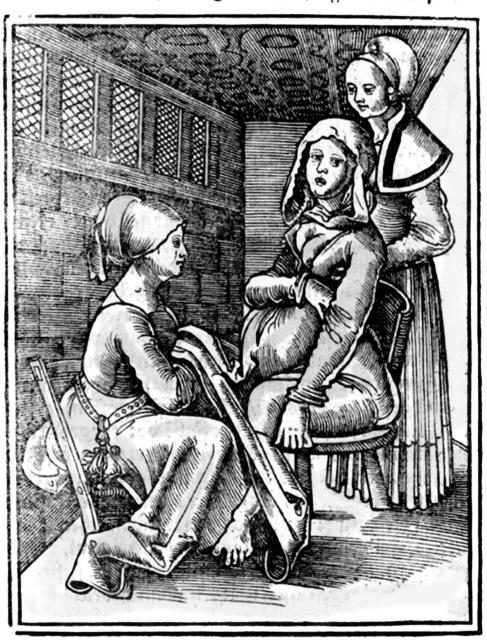

Paracelsus Burns Medical Books

Hippocrates of Cos (460 B.C.–377 B.C.), **Galen of Pergamon** (129–199), **Abu 'Ali al-Husayn ibn 'Abd-Allah Ibn Sina (Avicenna)** (980–1037), **Paracelsus (born Phillippus Aureolus Theophrastus Bombastus von Hohenheim; 1493–1541)**

Swiss physician, wandering mystic, and alchemist Paracelsus pioneered the use of chemicals and minerals in medicines. Science journalist Philip Ball writes, "Paracelsus lived from 1493 to 1541: a fulcrum of Western history, the dawn of the modern age. This was a world where magic was real, where demons lurked in every dark corner, where God presided over all creation, and yet it was also a time when humankind was beginning to crack nature's codes and map the geography of heaven and earth."

Paracelsus is famous for his railing against the ancient ideas of Hippocrates and Galen, both of whom suggested that illness was the result of an imbalance of four humors (liquids): blood, black bile, yellow bile, and phlegm. Paracelsus believed that illness resulted from the body being attacked by agents outside the body or by other abnormalities that could be treated with chemicals. In 1527, he publicly burned the standard medical texts of the day, which included the works of Galen and Avicenna. This burning, on a bonfire lit by students, could "justifiably be viewed as a turning point in the history of medicine," according to author Hugh Crone. Physicians had to destroy the foundations of Galenic medicine, be free to question authority, and use fresh observations and experiments while seeking *new* medicines.

One of Paracelsus's major works documented occupational hazards of metalworking and mining, and he is sometimes called the father of toxicology. He wrote, "All things are poison, and nothing is without poison—only the *dose* permits something not to be poisonous." In other words, he emphasized that toxicity depended upon dosage.

Paracelsus proposed the notion of "like cures like," and that if a poison caused a disease, then the same poison might be used as a cure if given in the correct dosage and form. In some ways, this was the forerunner of homeopathy, an alternative medicine still popular today in which practitioners use extremely diluted preparations. However, most highly controlled studies have concluded that homeopathy is no more effective than a **placebo**.

SEE ALSO Hippocratic Oath (400 B.C.), Mithridatium and Theriac (100 B.C.), Galenic Writings (190), Alternative Medicine (1796), and Placebo Effect (1955).

Paracelsus, by Flemish painter Quentin Massys (1466–1530).

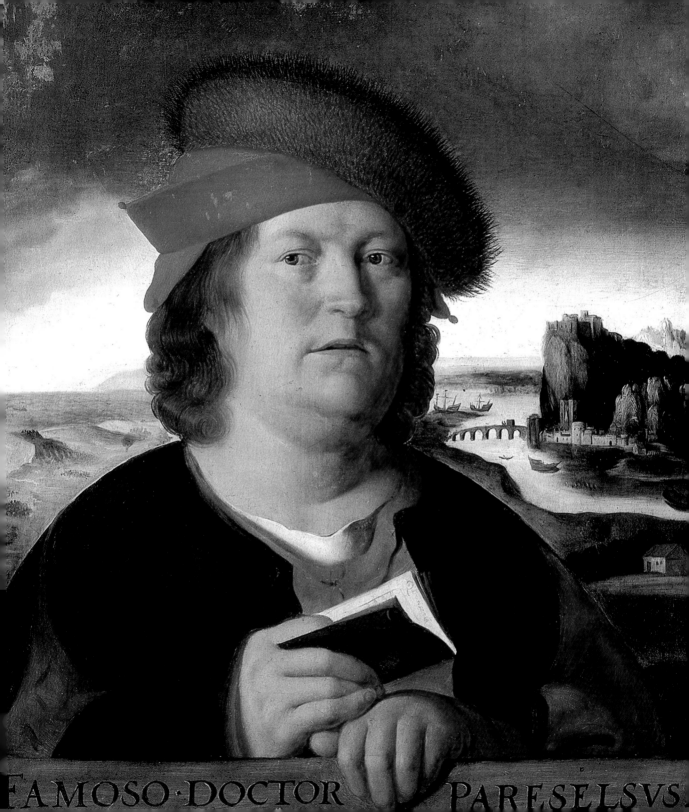

FAMOSO·DOCTOR   PARESELSVS

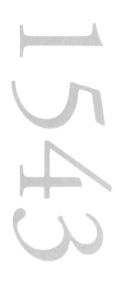

De Humani Corporis Fabrica

Jan Stephan van Calcar (1499–1546), **Andreas Vesalius** (1514–1564)

"The publication of *De Humani Corporis Fabrica* [*On the Fabric of the Human Body*] of Andreas Vesalius in 1543 marks the beginning of modern science," write medical historians J. B. de C. M. Saunders and Charles O'Malley. "It is without doubt the greatest single contribution to medical sciences, but it is a great deal more, an exquisite piece of creative art with its perfect blend of format, typography, and illustration."

Physician and anatomist Andreas Vesalius of Brussels performed dissections as a primary teaching tool and showed that many previous ideas about the human body, from such great thinkers as Galen and Aristotle, were demonstrably incorrect. For example, in contradiction to Galen, Vesalius showed that blood did not pass from one side of the heart to the other through invisible pores. He also showed that the liver had two main lobes. His challenges to Galen made him the enemy of many, and a detractor even claimed that the human body must have *changed* since Galen's studies to explain Vesalius's observations! In actuality, Galen had based nearly all of his observations on animal dissections, which led to significant errors about humans.

As a medical student, Vesalius braved feral dogs and horrible stenches in his feverish attempts to obtain rotting corpses from cemeteries or the remains of executed criminals hanging from beams until they disintegrated. He even kept specimens in his bedroom for weeks while dissecting them.

Fabrica, Vesalius's groundbreaking anatomy book, was probably illustrated by Jan Stephan van Calcar or other pupils of the famous Italian painter Titian. The book revealed the inner structures of the brain as never before. Science journalist Robert Adler writes, "With the *Fabrica*, Vesalius effectively ended the slavish scholastic worship of the knowledge of the ancient world and demonstrated that a new generation of scientists could forge ahead and make discoveries the ancients never dreamed of. Along with a few other Renaissance giants such as Copernicus and Galileo, Vesalius created the progressive, science-driven world in which we live."

SEE ALSO Galenic Writings (190), Leonardo's Anatomical Drawings (1510), Eustachi's Rescued Masterpieces (1552), Drawings of Pietro da Cortona (1618), Cheselden's *Osteographia* (1733), Albinus's *Tables of the Human Body* (1747), Hunter's *Gravid Uterus* (1774), Anatomy Act of 1832 (1832), and *Gray's Anatomy* (1858).

Delineation of spinal nerves from Vesalius's De Humani Corporis Fabrica.

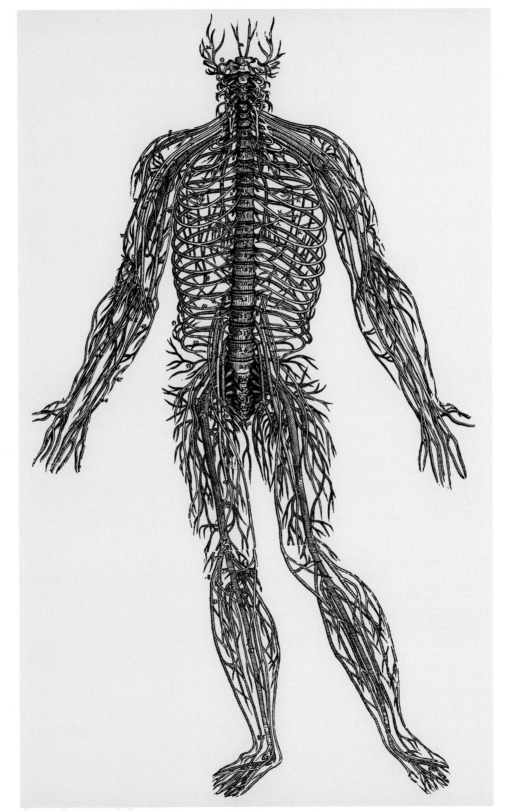

Paré's "Rational Surgery"

Ambroise Paré (1510–1590)

The French surgeon Ambroise Paré is one of the most celebrated surgeons of the European Renaissance. Surgeon and biographer Geoffrey Keynes writes, "Ambroise Paré was, by virtue of his personality and his independent mind, the emancipator of surgery from the dead hand of dogma. There was no comparable practitioner, during his time, in any other country, and his influence was felt in every part of Europe. He left in his collected 'Works' a monument to his own skill and humanity which is unsurpassed in the history of surgery." Paré's humble credo of patient care was "I dressed him, God cured him."

Paré lived during a time when physicians generally considered surgery beneath their dignity, and cutting of the body was left to the less prestigious "barber-surgeons." However, Paré elevated the status of surgeons and spread his surgical knowledge by writing in French rather than the traditional Latin.

Paré made his first significant medical discovery while treating gunshot wounds, which were considered to be poisonous and were usually dealt with by pouring boiling oil into the wound to burn it closed. One day, Paré ran out of oil and was forced to improvise with an ointment that contained turpentine. The next day, he discovered that the soldiers treated with boiling oil were in agony, with swollen wounds. However, the patients who had been treated with the more soothing ointment rested relatively comfortably with little signs of infection. From that day on, Paré vowed never again to use the cruel hot oil to treat wounds.

In 1545, Paré popularized his wound treatments in his *Method of Treating Wounds*, thus leading the development of the humane "rational" practice of surgery. Another important contribution to medicine was his promotion of the ligature of blood vessels (e.g., tying off with twine) to prevent hemorrhage during amputations, instead of the traditional method of burning the stump with a hot iron. Paré also facilitated progress in obstetrics, using practices that ensured safer delivery of infants.

SEE ALSO Sutures (3000 B.C.), Edwin Smith Surgical Papyrus (1600 B.C.), Greville Chester Great Toe (1000 B.C.), Tissue Grafting (1597), Ligation of the Abdominal Aorta (1817), Vascular Suturing (1902), and Halstedian Surgery (1904).

Artificial hand, from Ambroise Paré's Instrumenta chyrurgiae et icones anathomicae (Surgical Instruments and Anatomical Illustrations), *1564, Paris.*

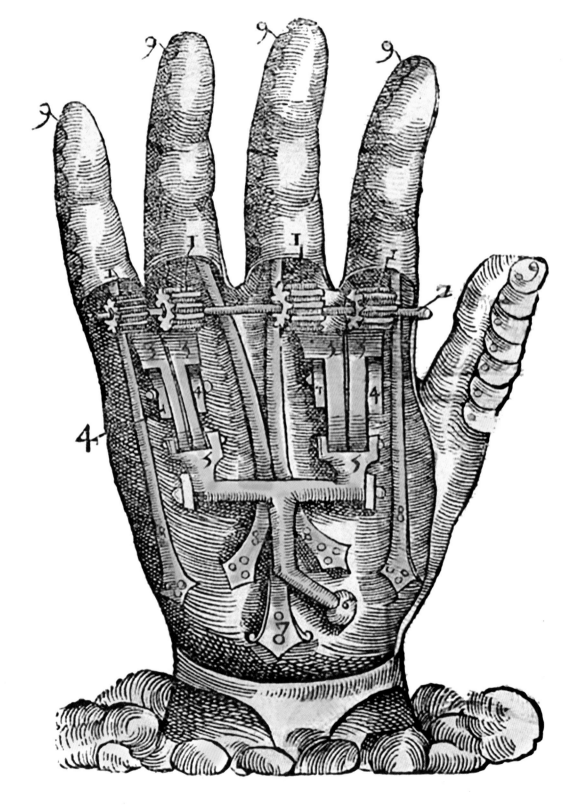

Eustachi's Rescued Masterpieces

Bartolomeo Eustachi (1500–1574)

Historian Andrew Cunningham writes, "The problem underlying all illustrations of anatomical dissection is that they are all . . . idealizations. Indeed this is why engravings [and photographs] are attempts at solving the same problem: that of bringing into view . . . the things that the anatomist wishes to make visible. For anatomizing is not only a very messy business . . . but distinguishing all the structures that are visible to the eye of the trained anatomist is very difficult for those who are not yet anatomists."

Italian anatomist Bartolomeo Eustachi was one of the founders of the study of human anatomy. Because he was affiliated with two hospitals in Rome, he was able to obtain and dissect cadavers of fetuses, infants, and adults. In 1552, with the help of artist Pier Matteo Pini, Eustachi created a great work of anatomical depictions. Alas, most of the illustrations were lost until the early eighteenth century. Ultimately, the missing masterpieces were discovered after 162 years in the possession of one of Pini's descendants, and in 1714, the entire series of 47 engravings was published under the title *Tabulae anatomicae Bartholomaei Eustachi quas a tenebris tandem vindicatas (Anatomical Illustrations of Bartholomeo Eustachi Rescued from Obscurity)*. The engravings depict the kidneys, brain, spinal cord, muscles, and various other organs.

Medical historian Ole Daniel Enersen writes, "Although from an artistic point of view they are not as well done as the anatomical plates of Vesalius, from the point of view of anatomy they are sometimes more accurate than Vesalius's. Had the plates been published at the time they were executed, Eustachi would undoubtedly have ranked with Vesalius as founder of modern anatomy, and anatomical studies would have reached maturity in the seventeenth rather than in the eighteenth century."

Eustachi is also famous for his discussion of the Eustachian tube, named in his honor, which links the nasopharynx (upper throat) to the middle ear. This tube allows air to pass and equalizes pressure between the middle ear and the atmosphere.

SEE ALSO Leonardo's Anatomical Drawings (1510), *De Humani Corporis Fabrica* (1543), Drawings of Pietro da Cortona (1618), Cheselden's *Osteographia* (1733), Albinus's *Tables of the Human Body* (1747), Exploring the Labyrinth (1772), Hunter's *Gravid Uterus* (1774), Anatomy Act of 1832 (1832), and *Gray's Anatomy* (1858).

Drawing from Bartholomeo Eustachi's Tabulae anatomicae *(1714) .*

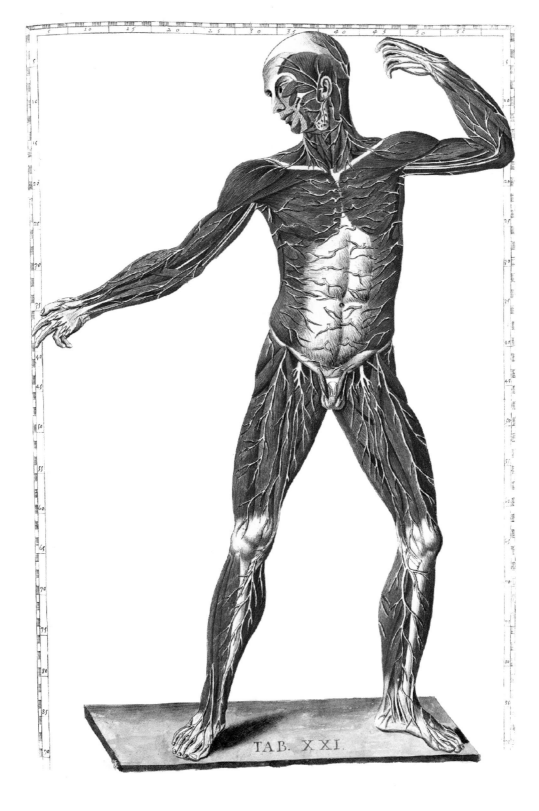

TAB. XXI.

De Praestigiis Daemonum

Johann Weyer (c. 1515–1588)

"Madness comes in many forms," writes psychologist Richard Adler. "We are all familiar with the kinds of mental disorders that strike individuals—depression, post-traumatic distress, phobias, obsessions, paranoia and psychoses. Sometimes, however, whole societies go mad. . . . As the medieval world order slowly crumbled . . . witches were everywhere, and right-minded people hurried to watch them burn."

One of the most fascinating physicians who studied the behavior of women accused of witchcraft was Dutch physician Johann Weyer, who lived during the time when suspected witches were tortured. Many science historians have probably gone too far in calling Weyer the "father of psychiatry," but some sections of his 1563 *De Praestigiis Daemonum et Incantationibus ac Venificiis* (*On the Illusions of the Demons and On Spells and Poisons*) did discuss witchcraft mania from a psychological perspective, and he also rejected some of the outlandish beliefs in the supernatural powers and activities of so-called witches. In particular, Weyer criticized the cruel witch-hunting and persecution by Christian authorities, and he may have been the first to use the term *mentally ill* when referring to some of the quirkier women accused of practicing witchcraft.

Weyer never denied the existence of the devil. In fact, in some sections of *De Praestigiis*, he suggests that some reckless or melancholic women were psychologically predisposed to become prey of the devil, who could make them imagine being involved in wild rituals that they did not actually take part in. Weyer believed that it was necessary to consult physicians when women were accused of witchcraft. According to medical historian George Mora, "By including a brief history, a report of his findings, and his rationale regarding treatment, he 'anticipated' the modern psychiatric examination. [His treatments] included medications, physical procedures, support, suggestions, and, in cases of mass hysteria in convents, removal of the most disturbed nuns." As might be expected, Weyer was criticized for his psychotherapeutic approach, and his book was placed on the Catholic Church's *Index* of banned books.

SEE ALSO Unchaining the Lunatics (1793), Psychoanalysis (1899), Jung's Analytical Psychology (1933), and Cognitive Behavioral Therapy (1963).

Witches (*woodcut, 1508*), by German Renaissance artist Hans Baldung Grien (1484–1545).

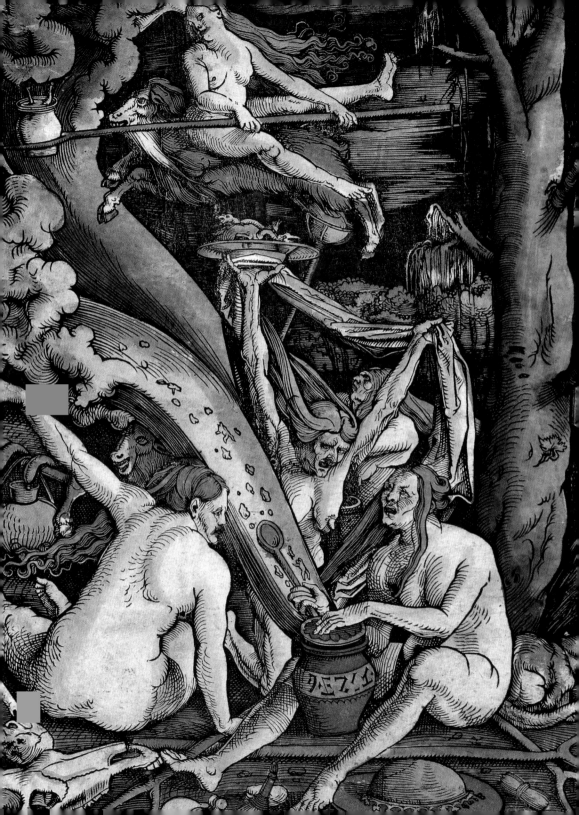

Condom

Gabriele Falloppio (1523–1562), Giacomo Girolamo Casanova de Seingalt (1725–1798)

Methods for preventing fertilization and pregnancy have had a long history. The ancient Egyptians placed crocodile dung mixed with honey in the vagina in an attempt to prevent conception. Condoms and other barrier devices have been popular throughout history to reduce the incidence of pregnancy and the spread of sexually transmitted diseases such as syphilis and gonorrhea (both caused by bacteria) as well as acquired immunodeficiency syndrome (AIDS) caused by the human immunodeficiency virus (HIV). Today, condoms made from latex, polyurethane, lamb intestine (called lambskin), or other materials are generally placed over the penis.

One of the first officially published descriptions of the condom occurred in 1564, when Italian physician Gabriele Falloppio described a linen sheath that served as a protection against syphilis. In *De Morbo Gallico* (*The French Disease*), he writes of his trials, "I tried the experiment on eleven hundred men, and I call immortal God to witness that not one of them was infected." The famous Venetian adventurer, author, and womanizer Giacomo Casanova used natural skin condoms, referring to them as "English riding coats, which puts one's mind at rest." The first rubber condom was produced in 1855, and the *New York Times* published its first condom advertisement in 1861. Latex condoms, developed in the 1920s, were thinner than rubber ones and required less labor to produce. In the 1930s, automated condom-production lines using machinery were in operation.

Condom use has been restricted or illegal throughout history. As brief examples, in 1873, the U.S. Comstock Law allowed the post office to confiscate condoms sold through the mail. In 1890, Julius Schmidt, who ran a famous New York business that initially manufactured skin condoms, was arrested for having nearly 700 condoms in his house. Germany outlawed civilian use of condoms in 1941. Condoms could not legally be sold in Ireland until 1978.

SEE ALSO Circumcision (2400 B.C.), Discovery of Sperm (1678), Pap Smear Test (1928), IUD (1929), Birth-Control Pill (1955), and Reverse Transcriptase and AIDS (1970).

Giacomo Casanova (left) and a colleague test their condoms for holes by inflating them. Engraving in Mémoires, écrits par lui-même *(1872).*

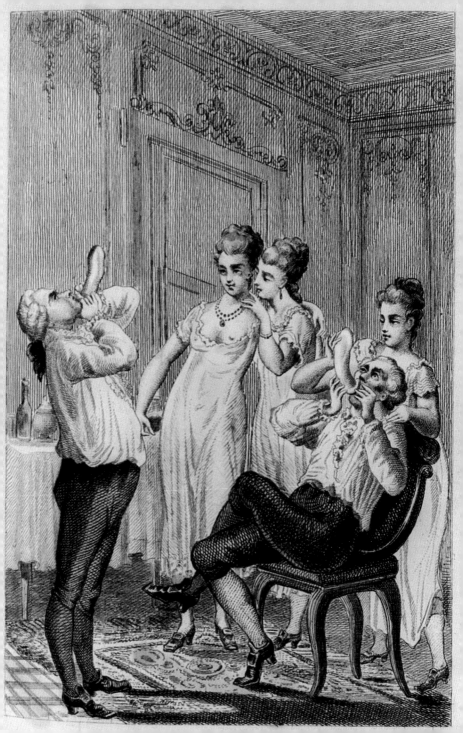

Large

— smal

Large

Large

Obstetrical Forceps

Peter Chamberlen (1560–1631)

Obstetrical forceps consist of two curved "blades"—vaguely reminiscent of two large spoons—that cradle the baby's head. The blades are then locked together so that they cannot crush the baby's head and so that the physician can pull the baby through the birth canal during difficult deliveries and when the fetus or mother is in distress. Today, **medical ultrasound** can be helpful in confirming the precise position of the fetal head.

British surgeon and obstetrician Peter Chamberlen is credited with the invention of particularly effective obstetrical forceps. The Chamberlen family members were careful to keep their method of successful delivery a secret, so the precise date of the invention is unknown. For example, when one of the Chamberlens arrived at the home of a woman trying to give birth, two people carried a massive box with gilded carvings that contained the secret forceps, and the pregnant patient was blindfolded so that even she would never see the forceps. Eventually these forceps, each loop-shaped blade of which could be inserted separately to ensure an optimal fitting, had a profound influence on successful deliveries.

Medical journalist Randi Epstein writes, "What the Chamberlens gave the world, as opposed to the devices made earlier, was a gentler sort of instrument, one trumpeted to get the baby out in one piece—and alive. One Chamberlen commented that forceps dispelled the old adage that 'when a man comes, one or both must necessarily die.' He meant that before forceps, men entered the birthing room only if the parturient woman, the baby, or both were near death."

Historian Rebecca Vickers, however, stresses the potentially lifesaving importance of sharing new technologies with the world: "The Chamberlens' development of forceps was a great success with an innovative design that has stood the test of time. It was also a huge failure. By keeping such an important breakthrough to themselves and a small number of patients in one country, the Chamberlen family slowed medical progress and probably allowed many thousands of women and children to die. Money and desire for fame won out over human life."

SEE ALSO Mary Toft's Rabbits (1726), Hunter's *Gravid Uterus* (1774), Cesarean Section (1882), Modern Midwifery (1925), and Medical Ultrasound (1957).

Drawing of childbirth with forceps, by British obstetrician William Smellie (1697–1763) in A Set of Anatomical Tables with Explanations and an Abridgement of the Practice of Midwifery *(1754).*

82

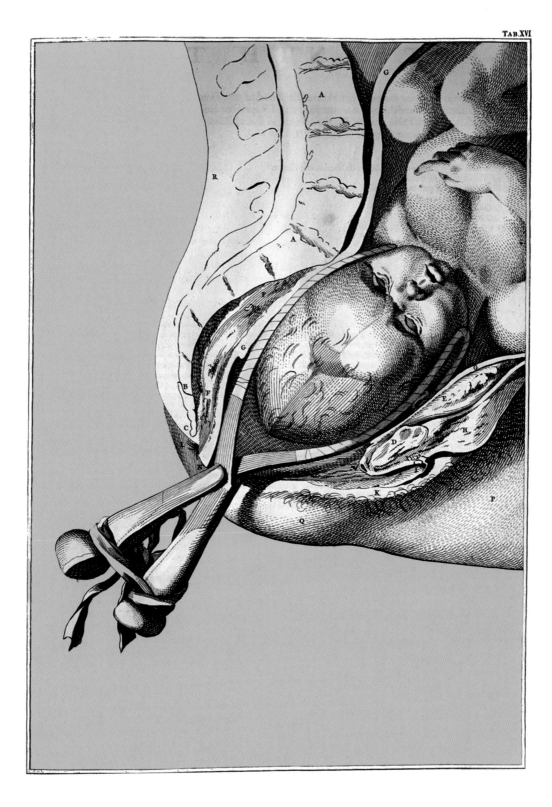

TAB.XVI

Tissue Grafting

Gaspare Tagliacozzi (1546–1599), Karl (or Carl) Thiersch (1822–1895), Jacques-Louis Reverdin (1842–1929), Sir Peter Brian Medawar (1915–1987)

In 1597, Italian surgeon Gaspare Tagliacozzi wrote, "We assemble and reconstruct and create whole parts of the face which nature has given and which fate has taken away, not only for the joy of the eye but also to build up the spirit and help the soul of the affected person." In addition to several ancient Indian surgeons before him, Tagliacozzi worked on creating an artificial nose, marking an intriguing milestone in the history of skin grafts, which are surgical procedures to transplant tissues to replace tissue lost as a result of burns and wounds. Tagliacozzi had partially cut a flap of skin on a patient's arm and sutured the flap to the area of the missing nose. For more than a week, the patient's arm was also secured to the face with a strap. After healing had occurred, the flap was removed from the arm, and the new nose was trimmed to the desired shape.

In 1869, Swiss surgeon Jacques-Louis Reverdin used completely detached small pieces of skin from one area of the body as "seeds" at a site that was missing skin. From these tiny grafts, the skin gradually grew and spread. In 1874, German surgeon Carl Thiersch published a paper describing a method of skin grafting that used a very thin donor slice of epidermis (outer layer of the skin) and underlying dermis (layer of skin between the epidermis and subcutaneous tissues).

British surgeon Peter Medawar performed pioneering research showing that skin grafts are more successful when the donor is in the recipient's immediate family. For example, skin from a sibling is more likely to be useful than that of a more distant relative. But in the early 1950s, he injected mouse embryos with tissue cells from unrelated adult mice and found that when the mice were born, they could accept skin grafts from the donor mice. Thus, he discovered how to change the immune systems of the embryos so that the donor tissue would not be rejected as foreign tissue.

SEE ALSO Sutures (3000 B.C.), Corneal Transplant (1905), Maggot Therapy (1929), Kidney Transplant (1954), Hand Transplant (1964), Face Transplant (2005), and Growing New Organs (2006).

Drawing from Gaspare Tagliacozzi's De curtorum chirurgia per insitionem *(1597). The blue strap secures the arm to the patient's face, giving skin tissue time to grow around the nose.*

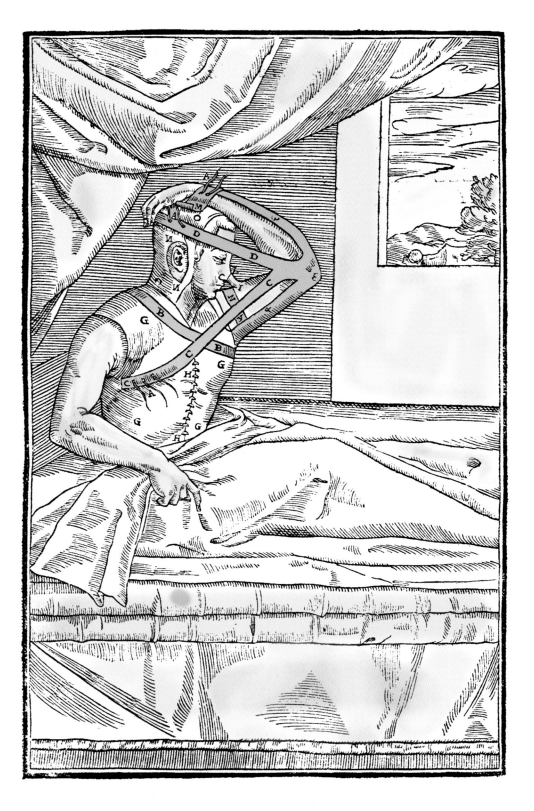

Acupuncture *Compendium*

Acupuncture usually involves the shallow insertion of needles into various points on the body referred to as acupoints. Although the practice appears in ancient Chinese writings (see entry "*Huangdi Neijing*") and may even date back to the Stone Age, physician Yang Jizhou's 1601 publication of *The Great Compendium of Acupuncture and Moxibustion* during the Ming Dynasty (1368–1644) is the basis for modern acupuncture and modern Chinese texts that describe a large set of acupoints. (Moxibustion involves the burning of the mugwort herb to generate heat.)

Although acupuncture has been used with some success for controlling certain maladies, such as nausea and pain, a number of scientific papers have concluded that this may be achieved mostly through a **placebo effect** and that further research is needed. For example, studies using sham treatments, with needles placed at "improper" locations or with needles that did not penetrate the skin, can sometimes produce the same effects as placing the needles at proper acupoints. Nevertheless, placebos can provide real relief, perhaps partly through the triggering of endorphins (natural painkillers) in the brain.

According to classical acupuncture theory, health is controlled by a balance between two complementary forces or principles—the yin and yang—along with qi, a kind of flowing "vital energy." Traditional Chinese Medicine uses pressure, heat, and acupuncture applied to acupoints to manipulate the qi. Classical texts describe most of the acupoints as being on 12 main meridians and two additional meridians through which qi flows. It is interesting to note that Chinese medicine forbade dissection and that meridians do not appear to have a precise counterpart in modern biological concepts.

The Great Compendium synthesized past texts and unwritten traditions. According to Yang Jizhou, "The more swiftly the qi comes, the more swiftly the effect is brought. If qi fails to come in the end, the case is beyond cure." Acupuncture was outlawed in China in 1929 in favor of Western medicine, but in 1949, the Chinese government reinstated the practice. In the United States, a significant number of employer health-insurance plans cover acupuncture treatments.

SEE ALSO Ayurvedic Medicine (2000 B.C.), *Huangdi Neijing* (300 B.C.), Health Insurance (1883), and Placebo Effect (1955).

Model of human head, showing several acupuncture points.

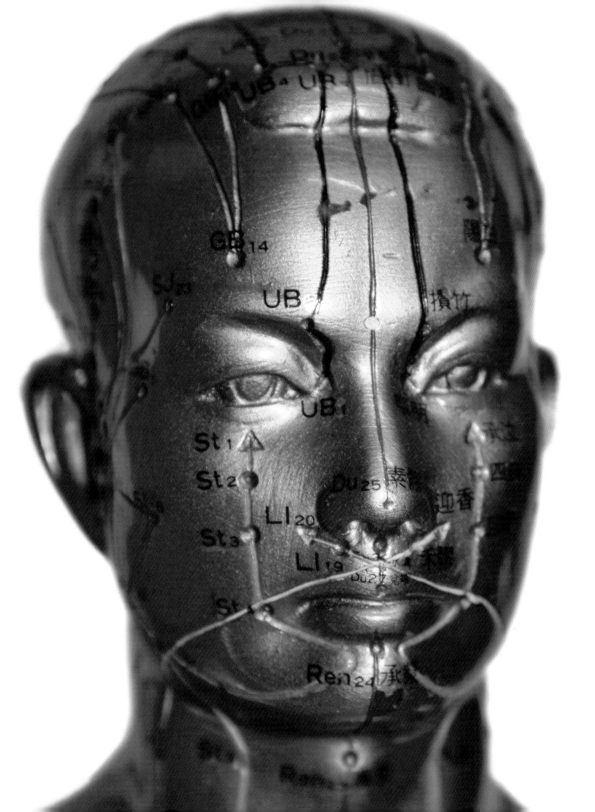

Drawings of Pietro da Cortona

Pietro da Cortona (born Pietro Berrettini; 1596–1669)

Pietro da Cortona was an Italian architect and painter who exemplified the Baroque style of art that often involved complex ornamentation and dramatic emotions. The Catholic Church often encouraged this artistic movement because it emphasized tradition and spirituality. Pietro studied in Rome, and from the mid-1620s until his death received commissions for major architectural and pictorial pieces, which he worked on simultaneously.

According to medical historian Jeremy Norman, Pietro's anatomical plates are "among the most exotic and dramatic anatomical studies ever created," yet they are also a profound mystery. For example, we do not know how his *Tabulae anatomicae* fit into his famous career of architecture and painting. Norman writes, "Why were they published 72 years after the artist's death and perhaps 100 years after their execution? For whom did Pietro make these studies?" Because many of the plates illustrate nerves, one might hypothesize that they were originally intended to illustrate a neurology book.

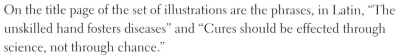

On the title page of the set of illustrations are the phrases, in Latin, "The unskilled hand fosters diseases" and "Cures should be effected through science, not through chance."

Occasionally, Pietro inserts classical buildings in the background along with various landscapes. Everywhere are flayed cadavers in various states of dissection, posed as if the bodies are still alive. Many of his subjects hold framed images of themselves to reveal additional details. Plate 27 of Pietro's collection is particularly haunting. A woman stands facing the viewer with her hands holding open her own womb in order to exhibit her uterus and urogenital system. In the wall to her right is a magnification of her open womb that protrudes from the wall, revealing a tiny baby squatting in her uterus, with its hands over its eyes. Is the baby crying or simply shielding its eyes from the viewer? Is the artist deliberately covering the baby's eyes so that it cannot see the dissection of its mother?

SEE ALSO Leonardo's Anatomical Drawings (1510), *De Humani Corporis Fabrica* (1543), Eustachi's Rescued Masterpieces (1552), Cheselden's *Osteographia* (1733), Albinus's *Tables of the Human Body* (1747), Hunter's *Gravid Uterus* (1774), Anatomy Act of 1832 (1832), and *Gray's Anatomy* (1858).

LEFT: *Two views of the female urogenital system (one with a fetus), by Pietro da Cortona.* RIGHT: *Nerves of the limbs and thorax.*

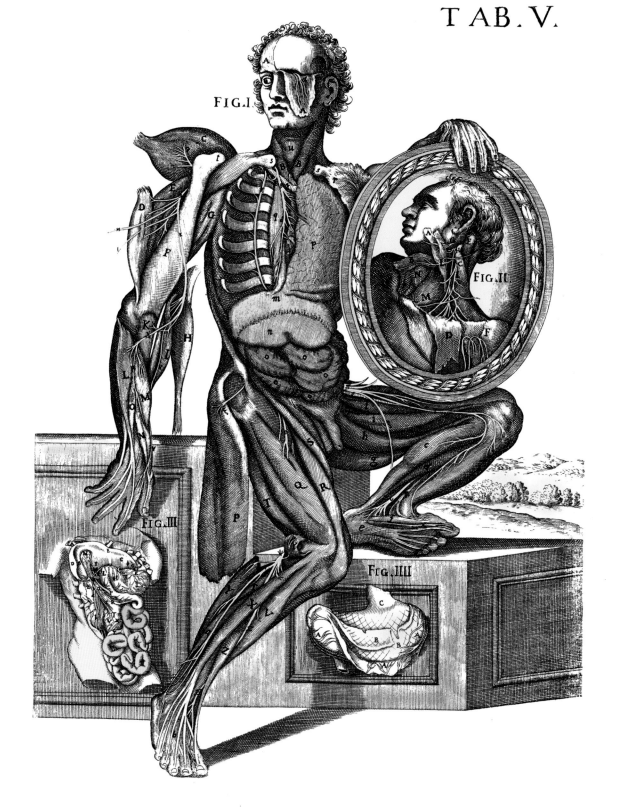

TAB. V.

FIG. I.

FIG. II.

FIG. III.

FIG. IIII.

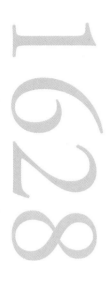

Circulatory System

Praxagoras (340 B.C.–280 B.C.), **Ibn al-Nafis** (1213–1288), **Hieronymus Fabricius** (1537–1619), **William Harvey** (1578–1657), **Marcello Malpighi** (1628–1694)

Science journalist Robert Adler writes, "Today, the basics of how blood circulates through the body seem trivial. . . . Grade-school children learn that the heart pumps oxygen-rich blood through the body via the arteries, that the veins return oxygen-depleted blood to the heart, and that tiny capillaries link the finest arteries and veins. Yet . . . the functioning of the heart and blood vessels remained a profound mystery from ancient times until the first quarter of the seventeenth century."

English physician William Harvey was the first to correctly describe, in detail, the circulation of blood through the body. In his 1628 work, *De motu cordis* (fuller title in English: *On the Motion of the Heart and Blood in Animals*), Harvey traced the correct route of blood through his study of living animals, in which he could pinch various blood vessels near the heart (or could cut vessels) and note directions of flow. He also applied pressure to veins near the skin of human subjects and noted blood-flow direction by observing swelling, along with the parts of the arms that grew congested or pale. In contrast to physicians of the past, who conjectured that the liver produced blood that was continually absorbed by the body, Harvey showed that blood must be recycled. He also realized that the valves that exist in veins, discovered by his teacher Hieronymus Fabricius, facilitated one-way blood flow to the heart.

Harvey traced the blood through smaller and smaller arteries and veins but did not have a microscope and, thus, could only conjecture that connections must exist between arteries and veins. Just a few years after Harvey died, Italian physician Marcello Malpighi used a microscope to observe the tiny capillaries that provided the elusive connections.

Various related work in blood circulation predates Harvey. For example, the Greek physician Praxagoras discussed arteries and veins, but he suggested that arteries carried air. In 1242, the Arab Muslim physician Ibn al-Nafis elucidated the flow of blood between the heart and lungs.

SEE ALSO Galenic Writings (190), Al-Nafis's Pulmonary Circulation (1242), Blalock-Taussig Shunt (1944), and Angioplasty (1964).

William Harvey correctly described, in detail, the circulation of blood through the body, including the path of oxygenated blood away from the heart and the return of deoxygenated blood back to the heart.

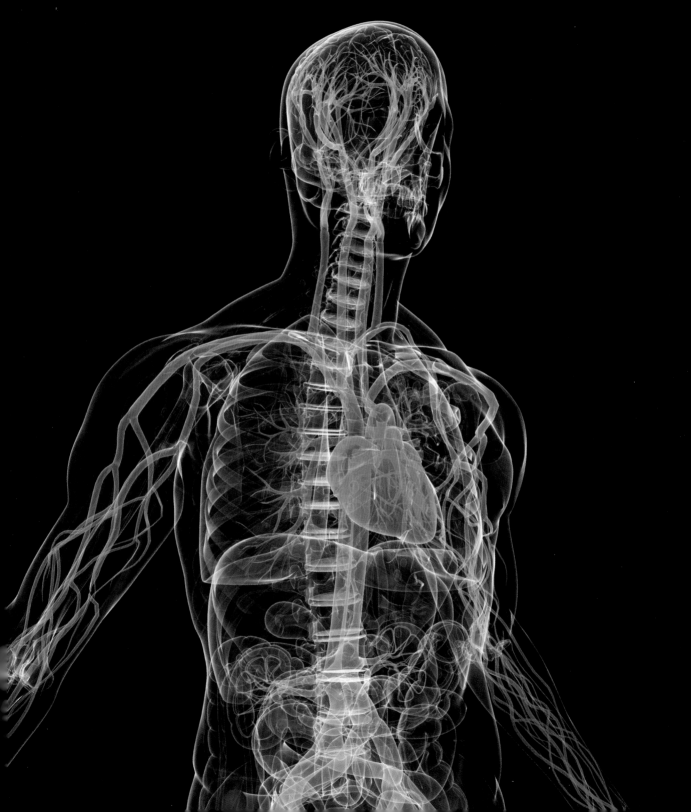

Murder and Wirsung's Duct

Johann Georg Wirsung (1589–1643), **Johann Wesling** (1598–1649), **Moritz Hoffmann** (1622–1698)

Pancreatic surgeons John Howard and Walter Hess write, "The discovery of the pancreatic duct in Padua by the German [Johann Georg] Wirsung was to prove one of the great milestones in the history of our knowledge of the pancreas; indeed, it proved a milestone in the history of medicine." Discovered in 1642 by anatomist Johann Wirsung while he was dissecting the body of a murderer, the pancreatic duct joins the pancreas to the common bile duct, and together these two ducts dump their contents into the duodenum, the beginning part of the small intestine. The duct, also called the duct of Wirsung in his honor, is the tube through which pancreatic enzymes flow to aid in the digestion of food.

The pancreas had always been somewhat of a mystery to physicians. Although Wirsung himself was unsure of the purpose of his duct, his finding was important because it established the role of the pancreas as a gland that secreted a fluid. Instead of publishing his finding, Wirsung sent illustrations to European anatomists for their comments. A year later, Wirsung was shot and killed while chatting with his neighbors near his home. Wirsung's mentor, the anatomist Johann Wesling, was accused of the crime because he was said to be jealous of Wirsung's discovery. However, Wesling was acquitted, and many conflicting stories about the identity of the assassin still exist in history books today.

Some accounts suggest that medical student Moritz Hoffmann, who was present at Wirsung's famous dissection, was his killer. Five years after Wirsung's murder, Hoffmann claimed to have discovered the duct of Wirsung in a turkey a year before Wirsung's human dissection; he also claimed to have informed Wirsung of this finding. The most likely suspect, however, is Giacomo Cambier. Just a week before the assassination, Cambier had been forced to resign his position as Procurator of the German Nation of Artists due to "doubts about his character," and Wirsung was involved with the decision process.

SEE ALSO Brunner's Glands (1679) and Pancreas Transplant (1966).

The pancreatic duct (central brown-orange tube in the yellowish pancreas) joins the pancreas to the common bile duct (green tube), and together these two ducts discharge their contents into the duodenum (brown tube at left).

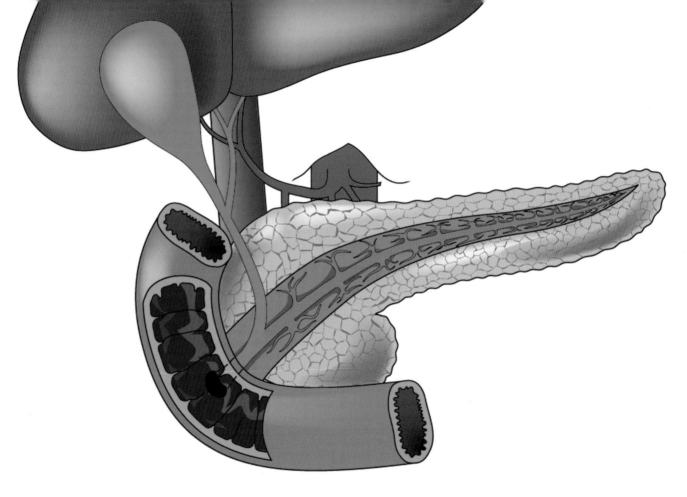

Lymphatic System

Thomas Bartholin (1616–1680), Olaus Rudbeck (1630–1702)

Physician David Weissmann praises the defensive power of the body's lymphatic system (LS) when he writes, "Lymph nodes are a combination of burglar alarm and West Point [Military Academy]. Like a burglar alarm, they are on guard against intrusive antigens. Like West Point, the nodes are in the business of training a militant elite: lymphoid cells that respond to the intruder by making antibodies and forming a corps of B and T cells that will remember the intruder's imprint for years."

The LS includes a network of vessels, nodes, and organs that: (1) serves as part of the immune system (to protect the body from invaders such as bacteria); (2) absorbs excess fluid from body tissues and returns it to the bloodstream; and (3) facilitates the absorption of dietary fat in the tiny villi (fingerlike projections) of the small intestine. The lymphatic vessels, in which the clear lymph fluid travels, contain a one-way system of valves that help channel fluids from body tissues to the left and right subclavian veins (blood vessels near the collarbones). Before the lymph fluid enters the bloodstream, the fluid passes through small bean-shaped lymph nodes that contain T-lymphocytes and B-lymphocytes (white blood cells) to help destroy and filter out bacteria. Because the LS is intimately associated with virtually all body tissues, the LS sometimes spreads **cancer** cells. The lymph nodes can also trap cancer cells, but if they are not able to destroy the cells, the nodes can become sites of tumors.

The spleen, located in the abdomen, is part of the LS and is one site of lymphocytes that engulf pathogens. The **thymus** gland, located in the chest, controls the development and maintenance of T-lymphocytes. The LS also includes bone marrow, in which B cells mature, and the tonsils.

In 1652, Danish physician Thomas Bartholin published a comprehensive description of the human LS and coined the term *lymphatic vessels*. At about the same time, the Swedish scientist Olaus Rudbeck made similar discoveries.

SEE ALSO Causes of Cancer (1761), Structure of Antibodies (1959), and Thymus (1961).

A portion of the lymphatic system (green), with the spleen at lower right.

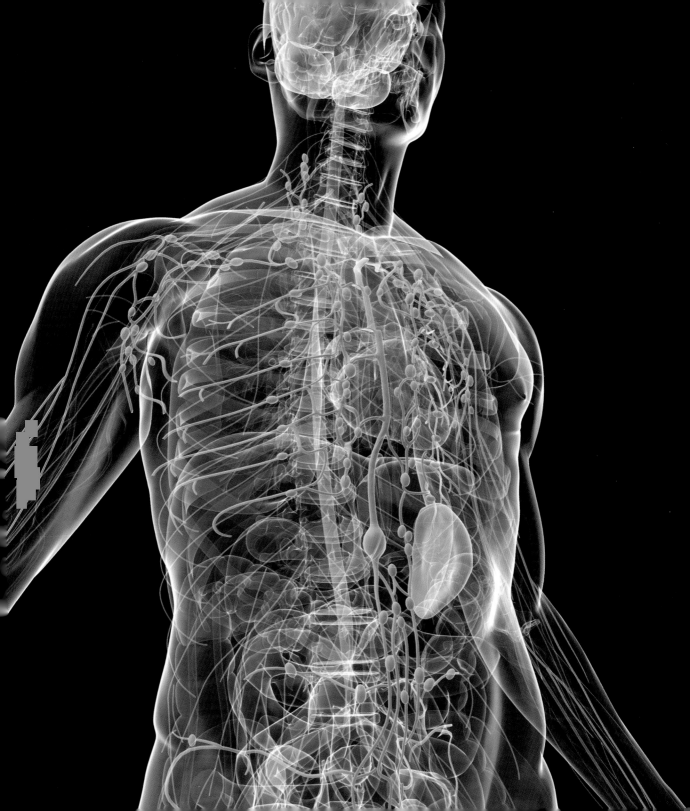

Cranial Nerves Classified

Thomas Willis (1621–1675)

In contrast to the spinal nerves that emerge from the spinal cord, cranial nerves are special in that they connect directly to the brain. Humans have 12 pairs of cranial nerves that enter and exit the cranium (the part of the skull that encloses the brain). Students often remember the first letter in each nerve name with a mnemonic such as "On Occasion, Our Trusty Truck Acts Funny—Amazingly Good Vehicle Any How."

The 12 pairs of cranial nerves, along with some of the functions of each, are the (I) *olfactory* (sensations of smell from the nose), (II) *optic* (sensations of vision from the eye), (III) *oculomotor* (eye-movement control), (IV) *trochlear* (eye-movement control), (V) *trigeminal* (sensations from face; chewing-muscle control), (VI) *abducens* (eye-movement control), (VII) *facial* (sensations of taste from the front of the tongue; facial and neck muscle control), (VIII) *auditory* (sensations of hearing and balance), (IX) *glossopharyngeal* (sensations of taste from the back of the tongue; neck muscle control), (X) *vagus* (interface with the heart, lungs, intestines, larynx, and other organs), (XI) *accessory* (neck muscle control), and (XII) *hypoglossal* (tongue muscle control).

In 1664, English physician Thomas Willis published *Cerebri Anatome*, a monumental work on the brain. His classification of the cranial nerves was used for more than 100 years, and he numbered the first six nerves precisely as we do today. Willis cut the nerves and vessels at the base of the brain so that it could be turned upside down, in order to carefully study the cranial nerves. His obsession with the brain was partly a result of his attempt to understand the soul based on brain investigations. The remarkable differences between the cerebral cortex of humans and other animals led Willis to suggest that the cerebrum (upper part of the brain) was the primary seat of the "rational soul" in man. He also hypothesized that the higher functions of the human brain arise from the convolutions of the cerebral cortex.

SEE ALSO Cerebrospinal Fluid (1764), Cerebellum Function (1809), Bell-Magendie Law (1811), Cerebral Localization (1861), Neuron Doctrine (1891), Searches for the Soul (1907), Cochlear Implants (1977), and Face Transplant (2005).

Depiction of some of the cranial nerves at the bottom of the brain, from Andreas Vesalius's De Humani Corporis Fabrica *(1543). The olfactory nerves are highlighted in bright yellow at top, and the optic nerves are represented in green.*

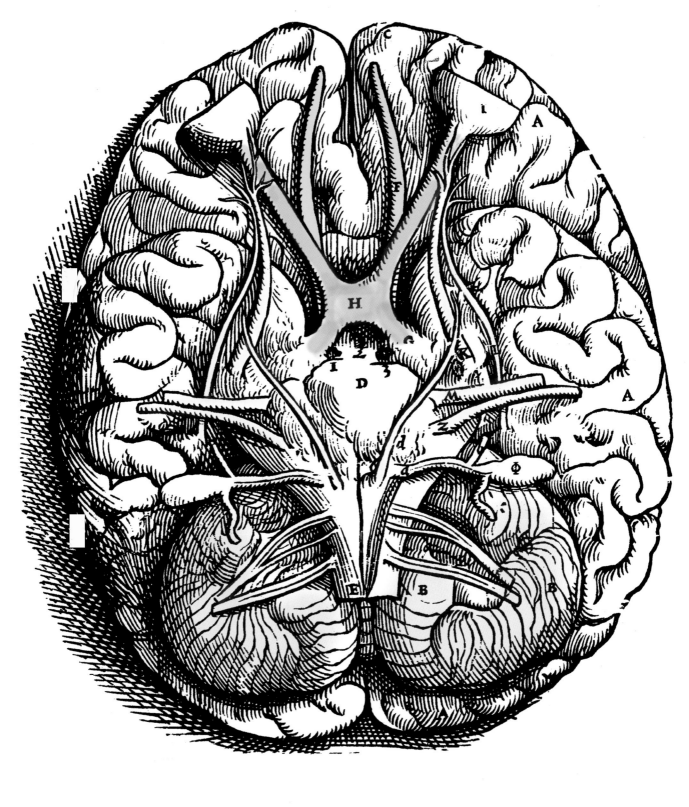

Micrographia

Marcello Malpighi (1628–1694), **Anton Philips van Leeuwenhoek** (1632–1723), **Robert Hooke** (1635–1703), **Georgios Nicholas Papanikolaou** (1883–1962)

Although microscopes had been available since about the late 1500s, the use of the compound microscope (a microscope with more than one lens) by English scientist Robert Hooke represents a particularly notable milestone, and his instrument can be considered an important optical and mechanical forerunner of the modern microscope. For an optical microscope with two lenses, the overall magnification is the product of the powers of the ocular (eyepiece lens) and the objective lens, which is positioned closer to the specimen.

Hooke's 1665 book *Micrographia* featured breathtaking microscopic observations and biological speculation on specimens that ranged from plants to fleas. The book also discussed planets, the wave theory of light, and the origin of fossils, while stimulating both public and scientific interest in the power of the microscope.

Hooke was first to discover biological cells and coined the word *cell* to describe the basic units of all living things. The word *cell* was motivated by his observations of plant cells that reminded him of cellulae, which were the quarters in which monks lived. About this magnificent work, the historian of science Richard Westfall writes, "Robert Hooke's *Micrographia* remains one of the masterpieces of seventeenth century science, [presenting] a bouquet of observations with courses from the mineral, animal and vegetable kingdoms."

In 1673, Dutch biologist Anton van Leeuwenhoek discovered living organisms in a drop of pond water, opening up the possibility of using the microscope in medical research. He later published pictures of red blood cells, bacteria, spermatozoa, muscle tissue, and capillaries, the last of which were also observed by Italian physician Marcello Malpighi. Through the years, the microscope has become essential in research into the causes of diseases, such as **bubonic plague**, **malaria**, and **sleeping sickness**. The device also plays a crucial role in the study of cells, such as when used in the **Pap smear test** (invented by Greek physician Georgios Papanikolaou) to detect premalignant and malignant (cancerous) cervical cells. Before this test became widely used around 1943, cervical cancer was the leading cause of death in American women.

SEE ALSO Eyeglasses (1284), Discovery of Sperm (1678), Zoo Within Us (1683), Cell Division (1855), Germ Theory of Disease (1862), Cause of Bubonic Plague (1894), Cause of Malaria (1897), Cause of Sleeping Sickness (1902), and Pap Smear Test (1928).

Flea, from Robert Hooke's Micrographia *(1665).*

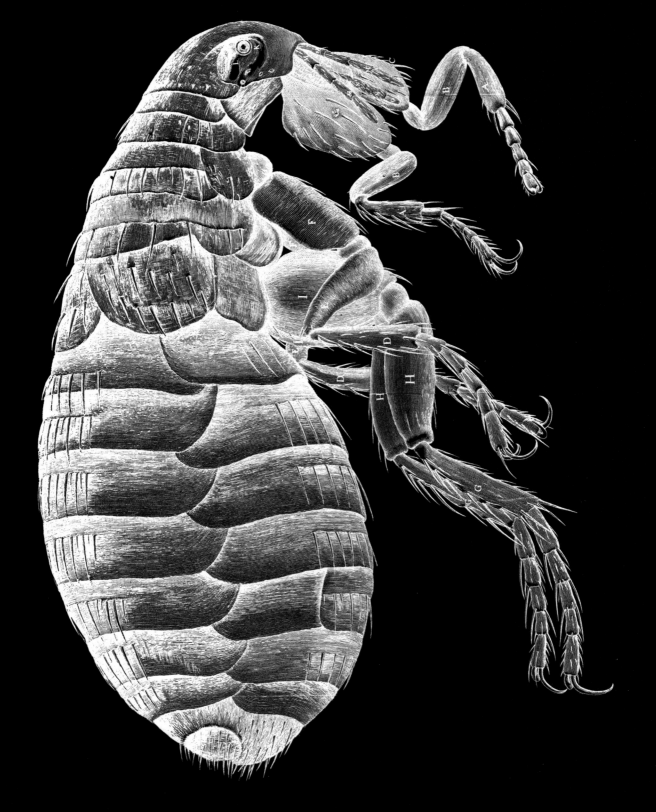

Discovery of Sperm

Anton Philips van Leeuwenhoek (1632–1723), Nicolaas Hartsoeker (1656–1725)

In 1678, Dutch scientist Anton van Leeuwenhoek reported to the Royal Society on the discovery of human spermatozoa, which resembled innumerable wormlike animals. He wrote, "What I investigate is only what, without sinfully defiling myself, remains as a residue after conjugal coitus. And if your Lordship should consider that these observations may disgust or scandalize the learned, I earnestly beg your Lordship to regard them as private and to publish or destroy them as your Lordship thinks fit." Van Leeuwenhoek eventually suggested that the minute microscopic creatures swimming in semen played a role in fertilization. Other scientists believed that the sperm were simply parasites and had nothing to do with the reproductive process.

Around 1677, van Leeuwenhoek and his student Johan Ham had used a microscope that magnified 300 times to examine spermatozoa, which he described as animalcules (little animals)—suggestive of his belief in preformation, a version of which posited that the head of each sperm cell contained a tiny, fully formed human. Dutch microscopist Nicolaas Hartsoeker claimed to have seen spermatozoa in 1674, but he was uncertain about his observations and, at first, thought the wriggling cells were parasites.

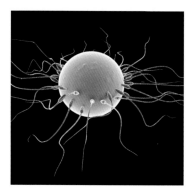

His famous drawing of a homunculus, or little human, crammed within the head of a sperm suggested preformation as well. Hartsoeker did not claim to have seen actual homunculi, but other researchers did! Some suggested that the homunculi in sperm might have smaller sperm of their own, in an infinite regress of homunculi within homunculi. Of course, when researchers began to show how organs in creatures such as chicks gradually appear in the process of development, it became clear that animals are not in a near-final form from the start.

The word *sperm* generally refers to the male reproductive cell, and *spermatozoan* refers specifically to a mobile sperm cell with an attached, whiplike tail. Today we know that in humans, the sperm cell has 23 chromosomes (threadlike carriers of genetic information) that join with the 23 chromosomes in the female egg when fertilization occurs.

SEE ALSO Condom (1564), *Micrographia* (1665), and Chromosomal Theory of Inheritance (1902).

LEFT: *Sperm surrounding an egg just prior to fertilization.* RIGHT: *Illustration of a sperm, emphasizing the head, whiplike tail, and joining midpiece, which contains a filamentous core with many energy-producing mitochondria for tail movement and propulsion.*

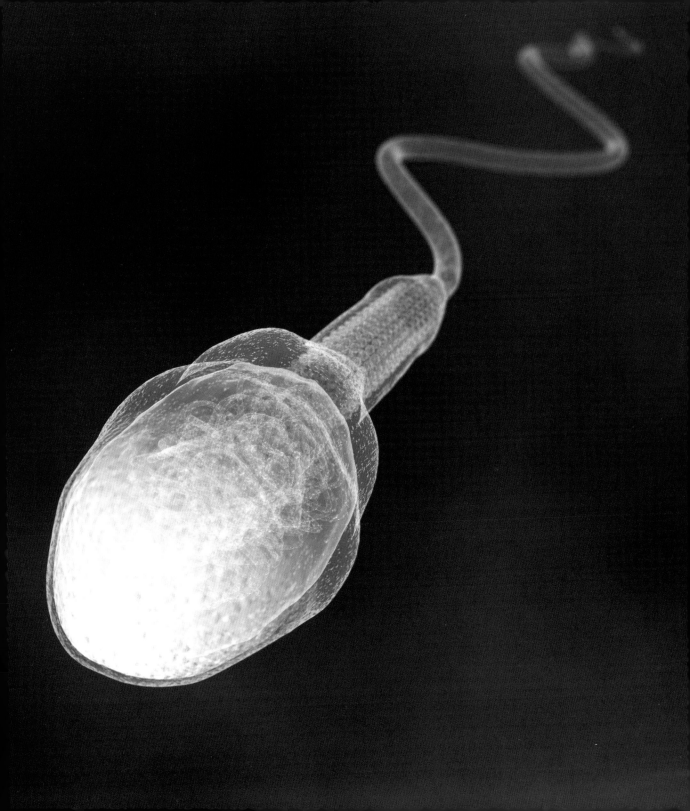

Brunner's Glands

Andrés Laguna de Segovia (1499–1559), **Johann Jakob Wepfer** (1620–1695), **Johann Conrad Brunner** (1653–1727), **Abraham Vater** (1684–1751), **Václav Treitz** (1819–1872), **Ruggero Oddi** (1864–1913)

The small intestines have fascinated humans since they saw intestines spilled on ancient battlefields, like a nest of twisting snakes. In the old Mediterranean cultures that practiced divination by animal-entrail reading, the intestines sometimes represented the complex movements of planets. Diviners would count the number of major twists. An even number of twists was good; an odd number, bad. Spanish physician Andrés Laguna poetically wrote in 1535, "Indeed the intestines are rightly called ships since they carry the chyle and all the excrement through the entire region of the stomach as if through the Ocean Sea."

The duodenum, the first section of the small intestine, is particularly fascinating, thanks to its range of functions, structures, and place in the history of anatomy. In 1679, Swiss pathologist Johann Wepfer first discovered the duodenal glands, but alas, they are now called Brunner's glands after the 1687 descriptions of his son-in-law Johann Brunner.

Brunner's glands secrete a mucus-rich alkaline fluid, containing bicarbonate, which protects the duodenum from the stomach's acidic contents. These glands also lubricate the intestinal walls and provide a more alkaline environment in which intestinal enzymes can be active. When the duodenum contains the partially digested food expelled by the stomach, it also produces secretin and cholecystokinin hormones, which trigger the liver and gallbladder to release bile and the pancreas to release its enzymes.

The duodenum wall also contains three important features. The Ampulla of Vater is formed by the union of the pancreatic duct and the common bile duct (from the liver) and is named after German anatomist Abraham Vater. The Sphincter of Oddi is a muscular valve that controls the flow of digestive juices (bile and pancreatic juice) through the Ampulla of Vater. This valve is named after Italian anatomist Ruggero Oddi, whose use of narcotics caused him to become mentally unstable. The Ligament of Treitz connects the duodenum to the diaphragm and is named after Czech pathologist Václav Treitz, who committed suicide by ingesting potassium cyanide.

SEE ALSO Murder and Wirsung's Duct (1642), Observations of St. Martin's Stomach (1833), Peptic Ulcers and Bacteria (1984), and Small Bowel Transplant (1987).

Visualization of the stomach (center), with attachment to the duodenum, the yellow-orange tube starting at the bottom of the stomach (at left in the visualization). The duodenum has a range of functions and structures and contains Brunner's glands.

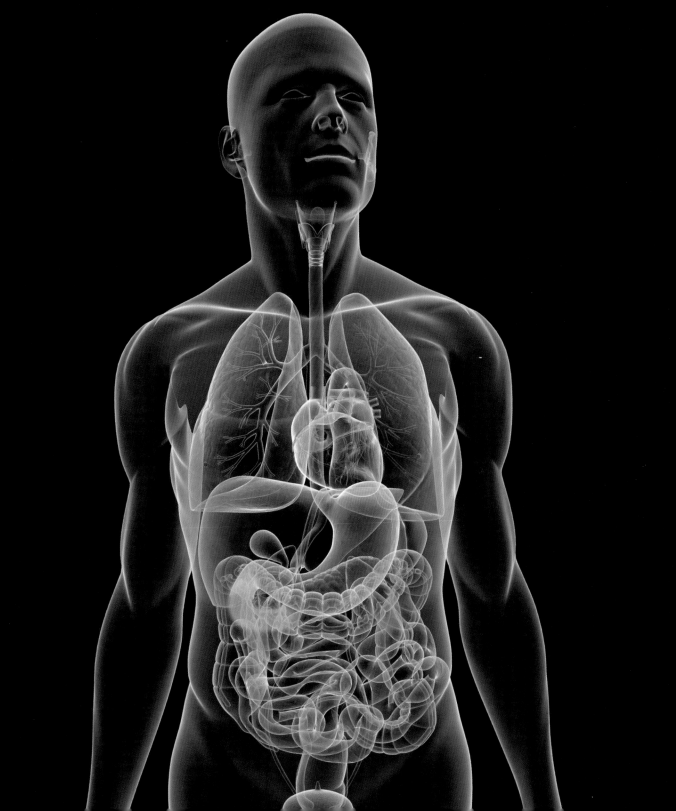

Zoo Within Us

Anton Philips van Leeuwenhoek (1632–1723)

Even healthy bodies contain a vast zoo of microbes affecting our health. The proper balance and functioning of this diverse ecosystem of bacteria, fungi, and viruses may hold cures to maladies ranging from inflammatory bowel diseases to various skin disorders. Interestingly, our bodies contain at least ten times as many of these tiny microbes (mostly in our intestines) than human cells, making our individual bodies behave like "superorganisms" of interacting species that, together, affect our well-being. One of the earliest discoveries of this microbiome zoo occurred in 1683, when Dutch microbiologist Anton van Leeuwenhoek used his home-built microscope to study scrapings of his own dental plaque and, to his surprise, found "little living animalcules, very prettily a-moving" in the specimen.

Beneficial and harmful microbes typically reside on and in the skin, mouth, gastrointestinal tract, vagina, nose, and other various orifices. More than 500 species of bacteria live in the human intestines, motivating researchers to think of this population as comprising a "virtual organ." The creatures in our gut can ferment food to aid in digestion, produce vitamins for our bodies, and prevent the growth of harmful species. Such bacteria rapidly colonize a baby's intestines starting from birth. Researchers are studying the possible role of different bacterial populations in diseases of the intestine (e.g., ulcerative colitis), tumor formation, and obesity. Researchers have also shown the importance of microbial diversity in the progression of cystic fibrosis (a genetic disease that can cause lung scarring) and continue to study possible roles of the microbial zoo in affecting the severity of eczema, psoriasis, Parkinson's, diabetes, and a variety of autoimmune diseases.

Using helminthic therapy, physicians and their patients experiment with the deliberate infestation of the intestines with helminths (parasitic worms such as hookworms and whipworms), which, in some cases, may have a beneficial role in ameliorating inflammatory bowel diseases, multiple sclerosis, asthma, and certain skin diseases by helping to modulate the functioning of the body's immune system.

SEE ALSO Sewage Systems (600 B.C.), *Micrographia* (1665), Appendectomy (1848), Allergies (1906), Imprisonment of Typhoid Mary (1907), Maggot Therapy (1929), Medical Self-Experimentation (1929), and Small Bowel Transplant (1987).

Electron micrograph of a cluster of salami-shaped E. coli *bacteria.* E. coli *normally colonize an infant's gastrointestinal tract within a day or two after birth.*

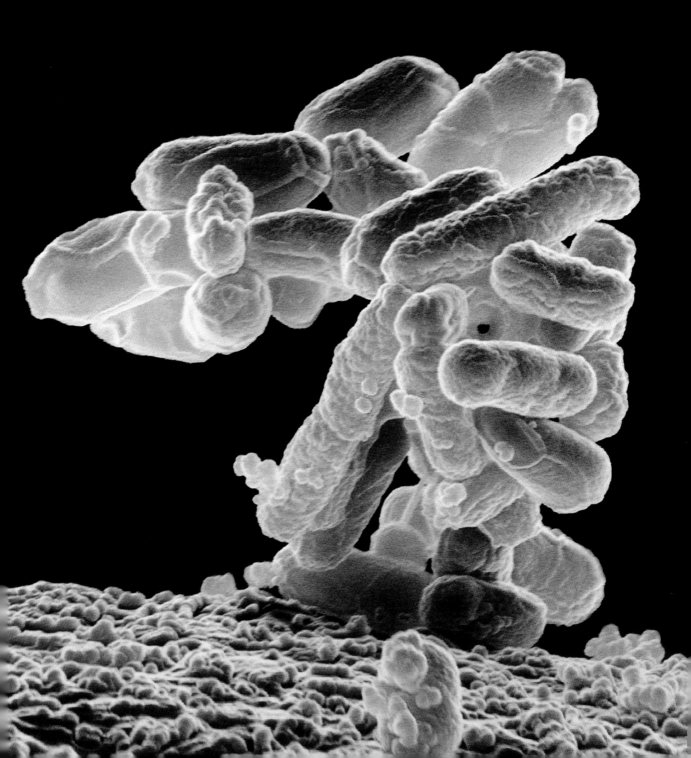

Discovery of *Sarcoptes Scabiei*

Francesco Redi (1626–1697), **Diacinto (or Giacinto) Cestoni** (1637–1718),
Giovanni Maria Lancisi (1654–1720), **Giovanni Cosimo Bonomo**
(1663–1696)

Italian researcher Giovanni Cosimo Bonomo, in collaboration with pharmacist
Diacinto Cestoni, discovered the cause of the scabies skin infection, suggesting that it
spread through the union of male and female mites, and observed a mite laying an egg,
which led him to infer that the disease was transmitted to and between humans through
contaminated clothing. He also speculated on treatments for scabies, such as sulfur.
Professor of dermatology Marcia Ramos-e-Silva writes, "Their study, even though not
immediately recognized, marked the first notice of the parasitic theory of infectious
diseases, demonstrating for the first time that a microscopic organism could be the cause
of a disease. It may even be said without doubt that Bonomo's and Cestoni's discovery
initiated a new era in medicine."

Although the microscopic mite *Sarcoptes scabiei* (just barely visible to the naked
eye) was observed before Bonomo's detailed descriptions in a 1687 letter to the
physician and naturalist Francesco Redi, the mite was not considered to be the *cause* of
scabies; rather, the disease was often thought to be related to the bodily humors of Galen
(see entry "**Galenic Writings**"). Bonomo wrote, "[From the skin] I took out a very small
white globule scarcely discernible; observing this with a microscope, I found [the larva]
to be a very minute living creature, in shape resembling a tortoise of whitish color, a
little dark upon the back, with some thin and long hairs, of nimble motion, with six feet,
a sharp head, with two little horns at the end of the snout."

Immediately after the publication of Bonomo's letter, Giovanni Lancisi, the Pope's
chief physician, rejected the parasite as the single cause of scabies. Bonomo decided to
avoid debate when Lancisi suggested a humoral origin and referenced the Scriptures.

Scabies is manifested as a very itchy skin rash. Severe forms are sometimes found
on individuals with compromised immune systems. Subsequent researchers discovered
that parasitic mites are also the source of other skin diseases, such as mange in domestic
animals, and that mites may infest plants and honeybees.

SEE ALSO Galenic Writings (190) and Cause of Rocky Mountain Spotted Fever (1906).

*In 1687, mites were difficult to study because of their small size. However, today, scientists at the U.S.
Agricultural Research Service freeze mites and use scanning electron microscopy for observation. Shown here is a
yellow mite,* Lorryia formosa, *among fungi.*

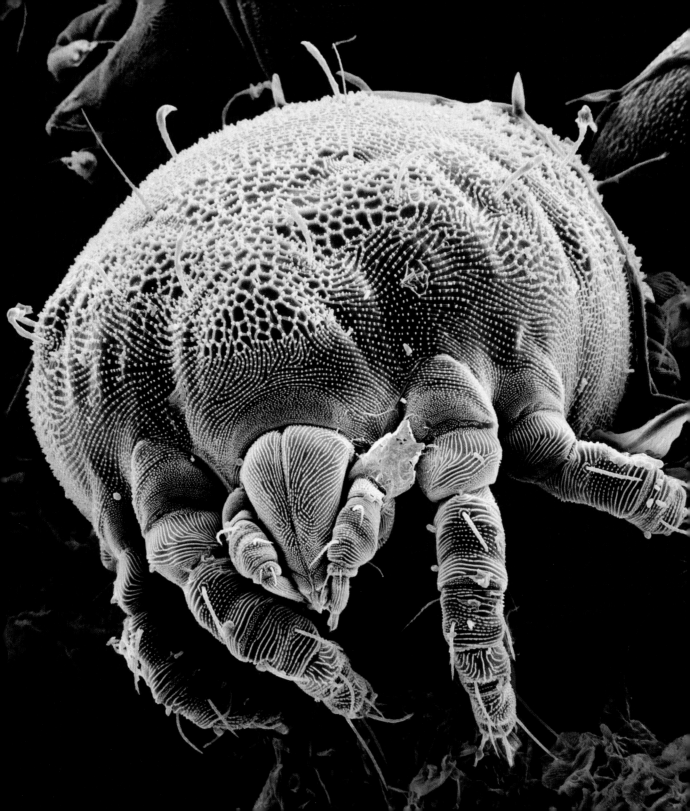

Separation of Conjoined Twins

Johannes Fatio (1649–1691), **Chang Bunker** (1811–1874), **Eng Bunker** (1811–1874)

The history of conjoined twins (CTs) and surgical attempts at their separation involves perplexing medical and ethical issues that challenge our everyday notions of personhood. Philosopher Christine Overall writes, "Moreover, we human beings do not merely inhabit our bodies, like a pilot in a ship, a ghost in a machine, or a divine soul in an earthly casement. We *are* our bodies." Ethicists continue to ponder the scenarios in which risky separations are performed.

CTs (once referred to as Siamese twins) are identical twins whose bodies become joined while developing in the womb. The mechanism of their formation continues to be researched, with the theory of fission suggesting that the fertilized egg undergoes only a partial split. According to the theory of fusion, the fertilized egg separates to generate two embryos that later fuse.

CTs may be fused at different locations of the body—for example, along the chest with the twins sharing a single heart, liver, or portion of the digestive system. As another example, the twins might share one head with a single face but with four ears and two bodies. Arguably the most famous CTs are Chang and Eng Bunker, who were joined at their torsos with a fused liver. In 1843, they married sisters, with Chang later producing ten children and Eng producing 11. If born today, Chang and Eng could have been successfully separated.

In 1689, Swiss surgeon Johannes Fatio performed the first successful separation of twins joined at the abdomen. Interestingly, in 945, a successful attempt was made in Constantinople to separate CTs after one of the boys died, but the surviving boy lived for only three days.

With modern surgical techniques and **CAT scans**, more complex surgeries can be performed, but various ethical concerns remain. In 2000, CTs were separated in Great Britain despite the religious objections of their parents. Before surgery, it was certain that the surgery would kill the weaker of the twins. However, if surgeons had not operated, both would have died.

SEE ALSO Abortion (70), Informed Consent (1947), Thalidomide Disaster (1962), CAT Scans (1967), and First Test-Tube Baby (1978).

Ectopagus (laterally conjoined) dicephalus dibrachius tripus twins, from Human Monstrosities (1891–1893) *by Barton Cooke Hirst (1861–1935) and George Arthur Piersol (1856–1924).*

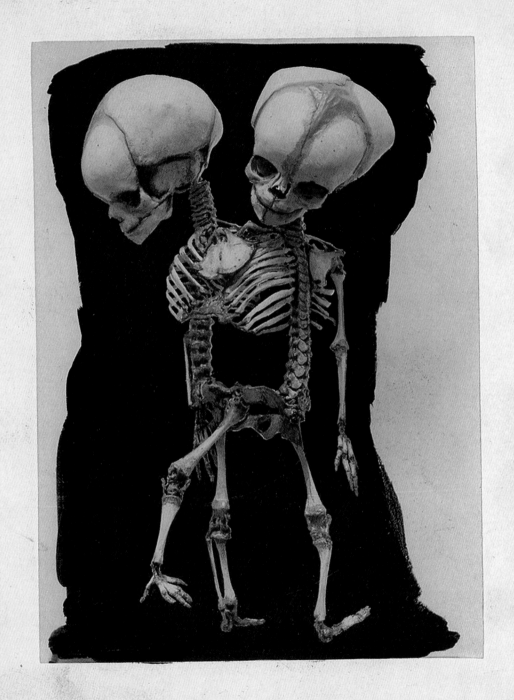

XXXIII   Ectopagno

Pulse Watch

Herophilus of Chalcedon (335 B.C.–280 B.C.), Sir John Floyer (1649–1734)

According to medical historian Logan Clendening, "No science attains maturity until it acquires methods of measurement. Clinical medicine could not advance until it acquired objective methods of determining or measuring the nature and extent of organic disease present in a patient's body." One very important medical observation includes the pulse, or periodic expansion of an artery caused by the pumping of blood via heart contractions. For a long time, accurate measurements were difficult, and early pocket watches did not include second hands.

Medical historian Denis Gibbs writes, "Sir John Floyer may justifiably be credited with the invention of the first efficient instrument of precision to merit application in clinical practice. . . . He also tabulated the vital signs of pulse and respiration rates, made under different conditions, in a form which found no equal for 150 years." Floyer, an English physician, was appalled that there was no easy or standard way for measuring pulses at a patient's bedside, so he invented the pulse watch, a portable instrument designed to run for exactly one minute. Floyer published *The Physician's Pulse Watch* in 1707, the same year that the watch—which now had a second hand and also a pushpin to stop the watch—became commercially available. The measurement of beats per minute eventually became a common measurement and a fundamental part of medical examinations, and portable watches became associated with physicians for more than 200 years.

Interest in the pulse dates back to ancient times. For example, the ancient Greek physician Herophilus attempted to quantify pulse rates using a water clock (a timepiece in which time is measured by the flow of liquid). Today, abnormal pulses can be used to indicate maladies such as dehydration, Stokes-Adams syndrome, and vessel blockages in people with diabetes or with atherosclerosis from high cholesterol.

Floyer was known for certain eccentricities and was a major proponent of cold bathing for health. He sometimes compelled his patients to bathe in very uncomfortable icy water.

SEE ALSO Digitalis (1785), Stethoscope (1816), Sphygmomanometer (1881), Electrocardiograph (1903), and Statins (1973).

Physician measuring a woman's pulse (c. 1665), oil on canvas, by Dutch artist Jan Steen (1626–1679).

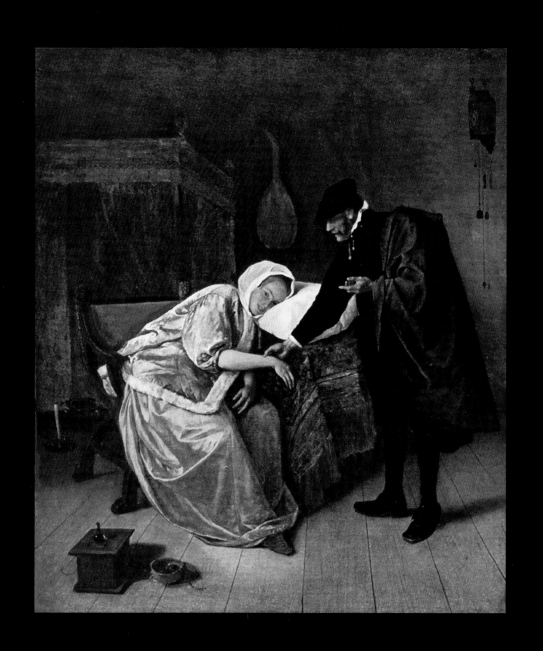

Mary Toft's Rabbits

Nathaniel St. André (1680–1776), **John Maubray** (1700–1732), **Mary Toft** (1701–1763)

Mary Toft was a young English woman with a peculiar passion—and an ordinary life that was changed forever when she gave birth to something not human. From that moment onward, she was propelled into a world she had never dreamed existed: a dark, alien, medical subculture flourishing in the courts of the king. She careened out of control, a pawn in the hands of the powerful, while forcing her contemporaries to question their most basic beliefs. Some of Toft's doctors were convinced her animal births were real. Decades later, priests still debated what had actually transpired, and even today we don't have all the answers.

In 1726, Mary Toft appeared to give birth to numerous rabbit parts (including a rabbit head) and other animal fragments. Prominent physicians of the day examined her and concluded the births were real, causing a national sensation. Later, when Toft confessed (under pressure) to secretly stashing animal parts within her, the careers of several famous but gullible surgeons were ruined.

Toft's story is important in this history of medicine because it reinforces the need for vigilance when presented with strange theories and potential hoaxes. The story also offers a glimpse at the outdated theory of maternal impressions, whereby a pregnant woman's emotions and longings were thought to physically transform her embryo. For example, London obstetrician John Maubray suggested to pregnant women that they must not play with "dogs, squirrels, and apes" because this might cause their children to be born resembling these creatures. Toft's story also touched on basic anxieties about having deformed children, of being deceived, and of being helpless pawns in the hands of uncaring physicians. Her story revealed the chilling gullibility of "great" people in whom we place trust. Many educated people were convinced by Toft's claims because eminent men—like Nathaniel St. André, surgeon to the royal household of George I— believed her after witnessing the rabbit births.

SEE ALSO Burning of Dr. Wertt (1522), Obstetrical Forceps (1580), Hunter's *Gravid Uterus* (1774), and Modern Midwifery (1925).

Credulity, Superstition, and Fanaticism (1762) by English artist William Hogarth (1697–1764). Mary Toft is on the floor giving birth to rabbits, which are hopping beneath her dress. Next to her is the nail-vomiting Boy of Bilston, who perpetrated a hoax to convince people he was bewitched.

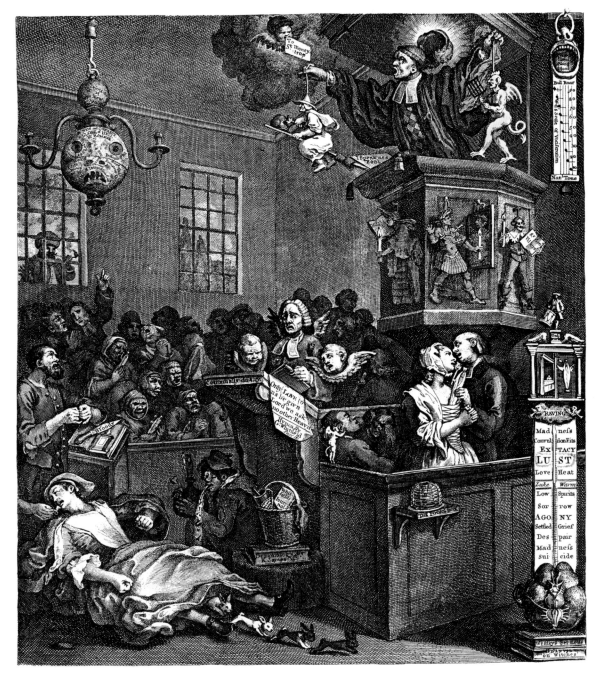

CREDULITY, SUPERSTITION, and FANATICISM.

A MEDLEY.

Believe not every Spirit, but try the Spirits whether they are of God: because many false Prophets are gone out into the World.

1. John. Ch. 4. V. 1.

Design'd and Engrav'd by Wm. Hogarth.

Publish'd as the Act directs March ye 15th 1762.

Cheselden's *Osteographia*

Jacob Schijnvoet (1685–1733), **William Cheselden** (1688–1752), **Gerard van der Gucht** (1696–1776)

Art historians Martin Kemp and Marina Wallace write, "The portrayal of the human body, however ostensibly neutral or technical the illustration, always involves a series of choices, and invariably brings into play strong sensations. Historical images of the dissected body range from the most flamboyant of the multicolored waxes, in which dissected figures assume the roles of expressive actors . . . in their own timeless drama, to the remorselessly sober woodcuts in Henry Gray's famous *Anatomy*. All the images exhibit what an art historian would call 'style.'"

One of the most intriguing examples of anatomy "with style" is *Osteographia, or the Anatomy of Bones*, one of the first books to give a comprehensive and careful depiction of the human skeletal system. *Osteographia* was created by English anatomist and surgeon William Cheselden and published in 1733.

Humanities professor Allister Neher writes, "Creating a naturalistic representation of a complex object like a skull is a matter of artifice and convention. The principal trick is to render the three-dimensional world of experience—alive with light, color and texture—into the two-dimensional world of black and white depiction. It is a testimony to the skills of an artist if this can be accomplished without the viewer commenting on the loss."

To help make his drawings accurate, Cheselden employed a camera obscura, an optical device that projects an image of the subject onto a surface. In fact, the frontispiece for *Osteographia* shows a scientist peering into a huge, dark, boxlike structure that is used to reproduce the skeletal subject with color and perspective preserved. Cheselden's artists, Gerard van der Gucht and Jacob Schijnvoet, then used this projection for creating the drawings.

Cheselden wrote, "The actions of all the sceletons [*sic*] . . . as well as the attitudes of every bone, were my own choice: and where particular parts needed to be more distinctly expressed on account of the anatomy, there I always [indicated that] where the anatomist does not take this care, he will scarce have his work well performed."

SEE ALSO Leonardo's Anatomical Drawings (1510), *De Humani Corporis Fabrica* (1543), Eustachi's Rescued Masterpieces (1552), Drawings of Pietro da Cortona (1618), Albinus's *Tables of the Human Body* (1747), Hunter's *Gravid Uterus* (1774), Anatomy Act of 1832 (1832), and *Gray's Anatomy* (1858).

Figure from Osteographia, or the Anatomy of Bones *(1733), by William Cheselden.*

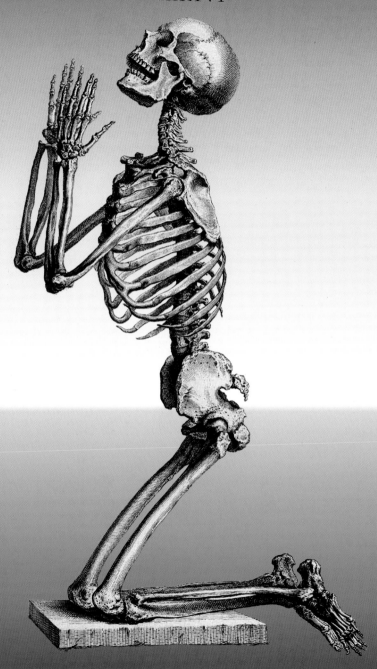

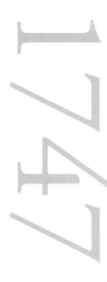

Albinus's *Tables of the Human Body*

Jan Wandelaar (1690–1759), **Bernhard Siegfried Albinus** (1697–1770)

Historian Andrew Cunningham writes, "It was the intention of Bernhard Siegfried Albinus . . . to produce the most beautiful anatomical tables ever seen, and . . . his obsessive perfectionism and overwhelming concern with accuracy in portrayal created many problems and delays. . . . He wanted to portray the 'ideal' human body. . . . No project of anatomical illustration can have had more time, thought, labor, artistry and money spent upon it."

Albinus was a prodigy. He began his medical studies at the age of 12 at Leiden University in the Netherlands, receiving his medical degree in 1719 without sitting through examinations. He was awarded a professorship of anatomy at age 24 and soon became famous as one of the most skilled teachers of anatomy in Europe. He is best known for his monumental illustrated work *Tabulae sceleti et musculorum corporis humani (Tables of the Skeleton and Muscles of the Human Body)*, which was first published in Leiden in 1747. While creating *Tables*, Albinus worked constantly with the artist Jan Wandelaar. According to Albinus, Wandelaar was "instructed, directed, and was entirely ruled by me, as if he were a tool in my hands, and I made the figures myself." Facing each engraving in *Tables* was a page labeling all the anatomical features of interest.

In order to ensure the accuracy of *Tables*, Albinus and Wandelaar placed nets in front of the specimens. The nets formed a grid pattern to guide the drawing. Albinus also held the skeletons in lifelike poses using cords and had a man stand naked in the same positions in order to make visual comparisons. Wandelaar added various landscape backgrounds to enhance the "three-dimensional reality" of the works.

The historian Charles Singer writes that the illustrations, "with their finely wrought ornamental backgrounds, were intended for artists as well as for physicians, and no finer work of their type has ever been executed." Historian Londa Schiebinger writes that "Albinus produced the definitive illustrations of the human skeleton, which remained unsurpassed for a least three quarters of a century."

SEE ALSO Leonardo's Anatomical Drawings (1510), *De Humani Corporis Fabrica* (1543), Eustachi's Rescued Masterpieces (1552), Drawings of Pietro da Cortona (1618), Cheselden's *Osteographia* (1733), Hunter's *Gravid Uterus* (1774), Anatomy Act of 1832 (1832), and *Gray's Anatomy* (1858).

Albinus's skeletal figure drawn in front of a rhinoceros, sketched by Wandelaar, from the first living rhinoceros in Europe, which came to the Amsterdam zoo in 1741.

TAB IV.

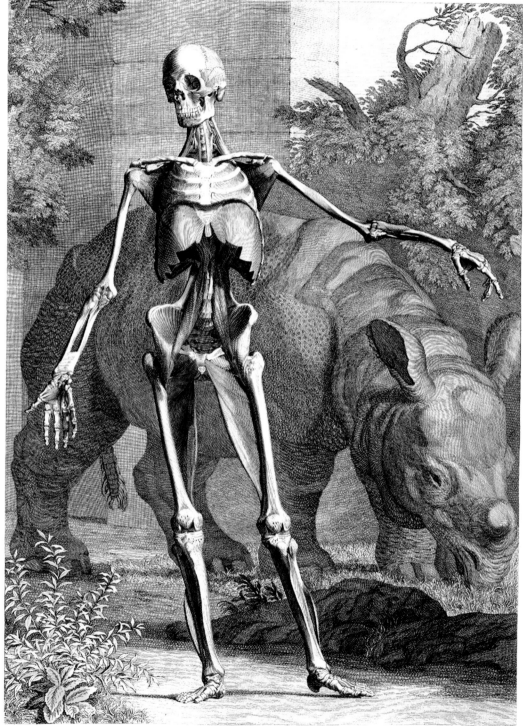

C. Grignion Sculp.   Impensis I. & P. Knapton Londini. 1747.

A Treatise on Scurvy

Sir James Lancaster (1554–1618), James Lind (1716–1794)

"Scurvy was responsible for more deaths at sea than storms, shipwreck, combat, and all other disease combined," writes historian Stephen Bown. "Historians have conservatively estimated that more than two million sailors perished from scurvy during the Age of Sail—a time period that began with Columbus's voyages . . . and ended with the development of steam power . . . on ships in the mid-nineteenth century."

Today, we know that scurvy is a disease resulting from a deficiency of vitamin C, required for the synthesis of collagen found in connective tissues. Scurvy symptoms include bleeding gums, weakness, and the opening of old wounds. Scurvy was once common among sailors and soldiers whose journeys left them without access to fruits and vegetables for long periods of time. In 1601, the English navigator Sir James Lancaster wrote that lemons helped to prevent scurvy, and today we know that this fruit is high in vitamin C. Alas, practical approaches involving lemons were often overlooked, either due to cost or uncertainty about the efficacy of fruits. Note that American Indians used teas made from pine bark and needles to treat scurvy, but European explorers were often not prepared to learn from "heathen savages."

The famous scurvy experiment of Scottish naval physician James Lind is notable because it is one of the first clinical trials ever conducted to discover a cure for scurvy. As described in his 1753 *A Treatise on Scurvy*, Lind divided sailors with scurvy into six groups, letting them access different foods. Only the sailors who ate lemons and oranges recovered rapidly. Unfortunately, he failed to recommend a precise treatment for the malady, and his work was largely ignored. Not until around 1795 was lemon juice routinely issued to sailors, effectively eliminating the disease from the British fleet.

Bown concludes, "The defeat of scurvy was one of the great medical and socio-military advances of the era, a discovery on par with the accurate calculation of longitude at sea, the creation of the **smallpox vaccine**, or the development of steam power."

SEE ALSO "Analytic" Vitamin Discovery (1906), Banishing Rickets (1922), Liver Therapy (1926), and Randomized Controlled Trials (1948).

Vintage map from 1746. More than two million sailors perished from scurvy during the Age of Sail, when international trade and naval warfare were dominated by sailing ships.

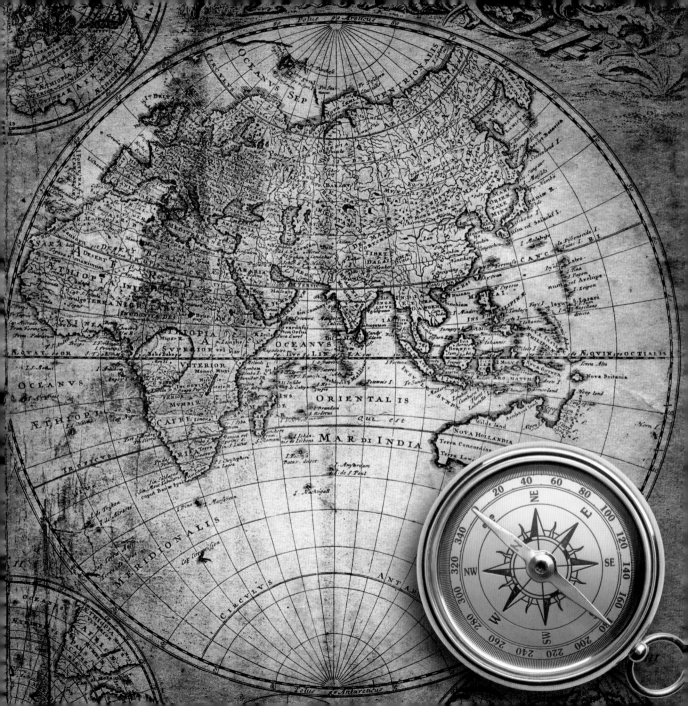

Autopsy

Frederick II of Hohenstaufen (1194–1250), **Giovanni Battista Morgagni** (1682–1771), **Carl von Rokitansky** (1804–1878), **Rudolf Ludwig Karl Virchow** (1821–1902)

"After my death, I wish you to do an autopsy," Napoleon Bonaparte said to his physician. "Make a detailed report to my son. Indicate to him what remedies or mode of life he can pursue that will prevent his suffering. . . . This is very important, for my father died . . . with symptoms very much like mine." Napoleon had been experiencing vomiting and fever, and his autopsy revealed stomach **cancer**.

An autopsy is a medical procedure involving a careful examination of a corpse, often to determine the cause of death. One of the earliest and most famous laws authorizing human dissection in Europe is credited to Frederick II, emperor of the Holy Roman Empire, in 1240. Italian anatomist Giovanni Morgagni became well known for his autopsies that correlated symptoms with organic changes, and he published hundreds of reports in his 1761 *De sedibus et causis morborum per anatomen indagatis (On the Seats and Causes of Disease, Investigated by Anatomy)*, which included descriptions of coronary artery disease, pneumonia, and various cancers. The Bohemian physician Carl von Rokitansky performed many thousands of autopsies using a definite protocol, making autopsy a separate branch of medicine. German pathologist Rudolf Virchow emphasized the importance of the microscope to study autopsy tissues.

Today, a physician makes a large incision along the front of the body, and many of the organs may initially be removed together as one large mass. Major blood vessels are opened and inspected. Stomach and intestinal contents can sometimes give an indication of the time of death. A Stryker electric saw is used to open the skull and expose the brain. Specialized techniques may be used that include electron microscopy, radiology, and toxicology (to check for poisons).

Although autopsies have often revealed diagnostic errors and unexpected findings as to the cause of death since around 1960, the number of autopsies performed in Western countries has been greatly declining, perhaps partly due to physicians' fear of malpractice lawsuits. The incidence of autopsies varies according to nationality and religion—Judaism and Islam generally do not encourage widespread use of autopsies.

SEE ALSO *De Humani Corporis Fabrica* (1543), Morgagni's "Cries of Suffering Organs" (1761), Anatomy Act of 1832 (1832), Cryonics (1962), and Peptic Ulcers and Bacteria (1984).

The Anatomy Lesson of Dr. Nicolaes Tulp *(1632), oil on canvas, by Dutch painter Rembrandt van Rijn (1606–1669). Nicolaes Tulp (1593–1674) was a Dutch surgeon and mayor of Amsterdam.*

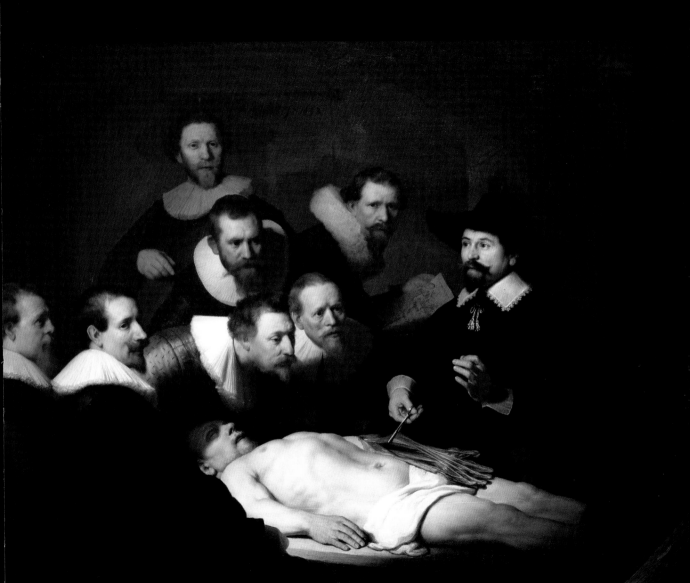

Causes of Cancer

Bernardino Ramazzini (1633–1714), John Hill (1707–1775), Sir Percivall Pott (1714–1788), Heinrich Wilhelm Gottfried von Waldeyer-Hartz (1836–1921), Katsusaburo Yamagiwa (1863–1930)

Journalist John Bloom writes, "If the body's cells represent a kind of Plato's republic of somatic harmony—[the cells] each doing a specific job in precise proportion to every other cell—then cancer cells represent guerilla soldiers bent on a coup d'état." Cancer refers to a group of diseases in which cells exhibit uncontrolled growth and sometimes metastasis (spreading to other areas of the body). Cancers are caused by abnormalities in the genetic material of cells and have many possible causes, including carcinogens (e.g., tobacco smoke, sunlight, or viruses) and random errors in **DNA** replication.

Among the earliest documented cases of probable cancer are described in an Egyptian papyrus, c. 1600 B.C., involving eight cases of tumors in the breast. These tumors were treated by cauterization using a hot device called "the fire drill" (see entry **"Edwin Smith Surgical Papyrus"**).

In 1713, Italian physician Bernardino Ramazzini reported on the virtual absence of cervical cancer in nuns when compared with married woman, speculating that sexual intercourse may increase cancer risk. The first paper describing a relationship between use of tobacco snuff and nasal cancer was published by English physician John Hill in 1761, after his startling discovery that his patients were all snuff users. He suggested, more generally, that substances in the environment may promote cancer. In 1775, another English physician, Percivall Pott, attributed high incidences of cancer of the scrotum among chimney sweeps to their contact with coal soot. He even recorded the cancer of a young boy who had been an apprentice to a chimney sweep. Finally, in 1915, Japanese researcher Katsusaburo Yamagiwa showed that frequent painting of rabbits' skins with coal tar did indeed induce cancer.

Note that in the 1860s, the German anatomist Wilhelm von Waldeyer-Hartz classified various kinds of cancer cells and suggested that cancer begins in a single cell and may spread through the blood or **lymphatic system**. Today, we know that tumor-suppressor genes, which normally inhibit uncontrolled cell division, may be inactivated by genetic changes associated with cancers.

SEE ALSO Edwin Smith Surgical Papyrus (1600 B.C.), Lymphatic System (1652), Cell Division (1855), Discovery of Viruses (1892), Radiation Therapy (1903), Pap Smear Test (1928), Cancer Chemotherapy (1946), Mammography (1949), HeLa Cells (1951), Tobacco Smoking and Cancer (1951), DNA Structure (1953), Oncogenes (1976), Epigenetics (1983), and Telomerase (1984).

Two views of Clara Jacobi, a Dutch woman who had a tumor removed from her neck in 1689.

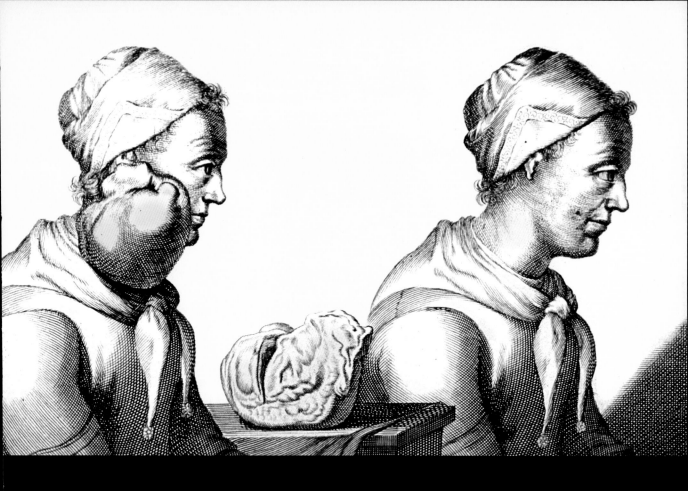

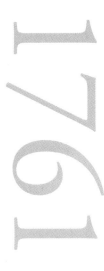

Morgagni's "Cries of Suffering Organs"

Andreas Vesalius (1514–1564), **Gabriele Falloppio** (1523–1562), **Giovanni Battista Morgagni** (1682–1771), **Marie François Xavier Bichat** (1771–1802), **Rudolf Ludwig Karl Virchow** (1821–1902)

"The idea that symptoms of disease, from colds to **cancer**, arise from changes in organs and tissues of the body seems commonplace if not banal," writes author John G. Simmons. "But the systematic correlation of the clinical history of disease with structural changes seen at **autopsy** was once a novel concept." With the 1761 publication of Italian anatomist Giovanni Morgagni's monumental work, *De sedibus et causis morborum per anatomen indagatis (On the Seats and Causes of Disease)*, Morgagni became the father of modern anatomical pathology, the diagnosis of disease based on examination of bodies, organs, and tissues. For Morgagni, disease symptoms were the "cries of suffering organs."

Although other researchers such as Andreas Vesalius and Gabriele Falloppio had performed extensive anatomical studies, Morgagni's work was notable in its accurate and systematic examinations of diseased organs and parts. *De sedibus*, published when Morgagni was 79 years old, records roughly 650 dissections. During clinical practice, Morgagni made careful observations of a patient's illness and then attempted to identify the underlying causes upon autopsy. In conducting his research, he essentially debunked the ancient humoral theory of diseases (see entry "**Hippocratic Oath**"), which posited an imbalance in bodily fluids as the root of disease. *De sedibus* identifies pathologies such as hepatic cirrhosis (a chronic degenerative disease in which normal liver cells are damaged and replaced by scar tissue), syphilitic lesions of the brain, stomach cancers and ulcers, and diseases of heart valves. Morgagni also observed that a lesion on one side of the brain, causing a stroke, led to paralysis of the other side of the body.

So immersed was Morgagni in his work that in old age he remarked, "I have passed my life amidst books and cadavers." Later, French anatomist Marie Bichat contributed to the field of pathology by identifying many kinds of body tissues and the effect of diseases on tissues. In the 1800s, the German pathologist Rudolf Virchow contributed to cellular pathology and was the first to recognize the effect of leukemia on blood cells.

SEE ALSO Hippocratic Oath (400 B.C.), *De Humani Corporis Fabrica* (1543), Autopsy (1761), and Artificial Heart Valves (1952).

Frontispiece and title page of Giovanni Morgagni's De sedibus.

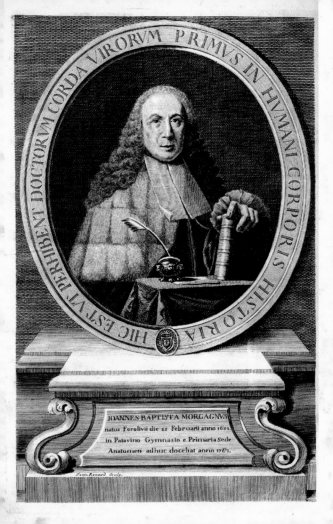

HIC EST VT PERHIBENT DOCTORVM CORDA VIRORVM PRIMVS IN HVMANI CORPORIS HISTORIA

JOANNES BAPTISTA MORGAGNVS
natus Forolivii die 25 Februarii anno 1682
in Patavino Gymnasio e Primaria Sede
Anatomen adhuc docebat anno 1767.

Joan. Renard Sculp.

JO. BAPTISTÆ
MORGAGNI
P. P. P. P.
DE SEDIBUS, ET CAUSIS
MORBORUM
PER ANATOMEN INDAGATIS
LIBRI QUINQUE.

DISSECTIONES, ET ANIMADVERSIONES, NUNC PRIMUM EDITAS,
COMPLECTUNTUR PROPEMODUM INNUMERAS, MEDICIS,
CHIRURGIS, ANATOMICIS PROFUTURAS.

Multiplex præfixus est Index rerum, & nominum
accuratissimus.

TOMUS PRIMUS
DUOS PRIORES CONTINENS LIBROS.
EDITIO SECUNDA
Ab Auctore recognita, atque a mendis omnibus expurgata.

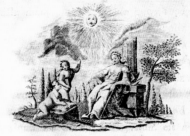

PATAVII,
MDCCLXV.
SUMPTIBUS REMONDINIANIS.
SUPERIORUM PERMISSU, AC PRIVILEGIO.

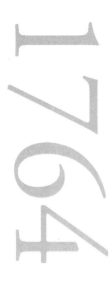

Cerebrospinal Fluid

Emanuel Swedenborg (1688–1772), **Domenico Felice Antonio Cotugno** (1736–1822)

Cerebrospinal fluid (CSF) is the clear, colorless fluid that fills the brain's ventricles, the four cavities in the brain that are also connected to the central canal of the spinal cord. Additionally, CSF surrounds the brain and spinal cord, providing lubrication and a cushion against shock. Produced in the ventricles (e.g., by cells in the ventricle's choroid plexus), it carries waste products away from the brain and spinal cord into the bloodstream. The continual production of CSF at a rate of about 500 milliliters (17 ounces) per day means that all of it is replaced roughly every seven hours.

Physicians can examine the CSF by inserting a needle into the spine's lumbar region of the lower back. A cloudy CSF may indicate meningitis, an inflammation of the lining of the brain or spinal cord. The causes of meningitis (e.g., bacteria, viruses, or fungi) are sometimes distinguishable by further studying the color and levels of protein, glucose, and white blood cells. The presence of blood in CSF may suggest a hemorrhage in or around the brain, and the presence of certain proteins may be suggestive of **Alzheimer's disease**. The CSF can also be used for diagnosing possible brain tumors, syphilis, and multiple sclerosis (a disease of the lining of the nerve cells).

In 1736, CSF was identified by the Swedish mystic Emanuel Swedenborg as a "spirituous lymph" and a "highly gifted juice." In 1764, Italian physician Domenico Cotugno described the CSF found within the ventricles and bathing the brain and spinal cord and that he believed was continually renewed. In honor of his work, CSF was once referred to as Liquor Cotunnii. Prior to Cotugno's research, a number of physicians erroneously believed that the brain's ventricles were filled with vapor, which sometimes condensed into water due to the rapidly decreasing temperatures in cadavers prior to examination. Many anatomists of the past had not even observed CSF because, prior to dissection, the head was brutally severed from the body—an act that emptied both the spine and skull of their fluids.

SEE ALSO Cranial Nerves Classified (1664), Cerebellum Function (1809), Modern Brain Surgery (1879), Alzheimer's Disease (1906), and Searches for the Soul (1907).

Brain ventricles (yellow), from Andreas Vesalius's De Humani Corporis Fabrica (1543). In Vesalius's day, some physicians believed that brain ventricles were reservoirs of both the soul and the spirits responsible for motor and sensory activity of the body.

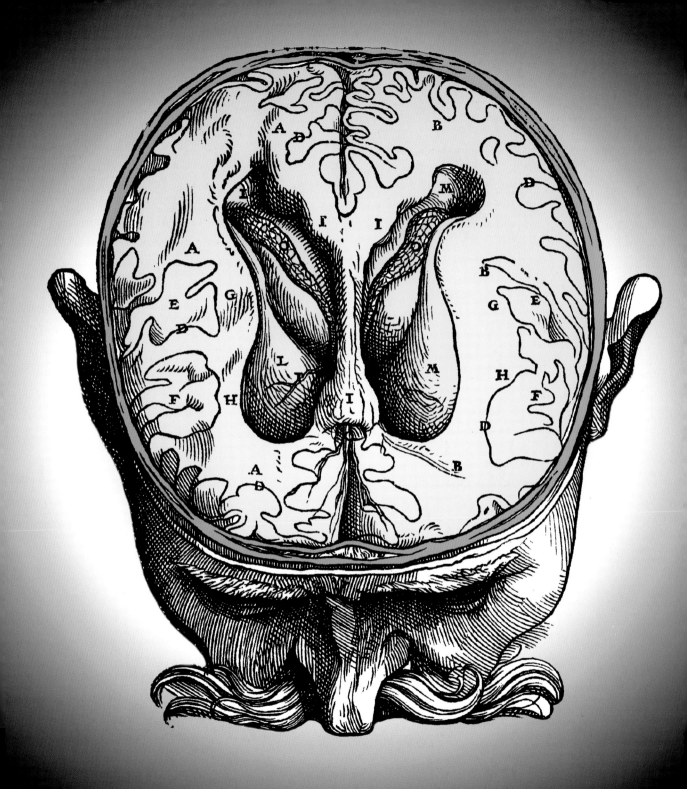

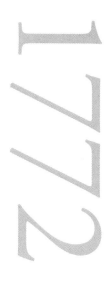
1772

Exploring the Labyrinth

Antonio Scarpa (1752–1832)

Anatomist David Bainbridge writes, "The first person to find his way around the [ear's] labyrinth . . . was by all accounts an arrogant, sarcastic, domineering, rude, vindictive, artist-anatomist-genius named Antonio Scarpa." Physician by the age of 18, this Italian anatomist later presided over the anatomy department of the University of Pavia for more than 50 years. He is best remembered today for his 1772 publication describing his delicate dissections of the mazelike structures of the inner ear. The fluid inside the ear's labyrinth is sometimes referred to as Scarpa's fluid in his honor. Oddly enough, upon Scarpa's death, his assistant chopped off his head and placed it on display. Scarpa's head is still exhibited in the university museum today.

The ear may be considered in three parts. The outer ear includes the pinna, or earlobe. The middle ear is filled with air and includes the tympanic membrane, or eardrum. The inner ear has organs needed for balance and hearing. A complex set of fluid-filled bony tubes contains a set of membranous tubes. This bony labyrinth has three sections: (1) the spiral cochlea, which has hair cells that vibrate and convey sounds to the auditory nerve; (2) the semicircular canals, which assist with balance; and (3) the vestibule, which connects the cochlea and semicircular canals and which contains additional structures that help assist with balance. The term *vestibular system* refers to the semicircular canals and the vestibule. The movement of fluid in the three semicircular canals in each ear corresponds to rotations of the head, and hair cells convert such movement to nerve signals.

Otolithic organs in the vestibule help to sense accelerations in body movement. Otoliths (crystals of calcium carbonate) in the organs are displaced by the acceleration, which deflects hair cells and produces sensory signals. In the normal cochlea, high frequencies produce maximal vibrations at the start of the spiral coil, and low frequencies stimulate the distant end of the cochlea. Note that labyrinthitis (inflammation of the labyrinth) can cause dizziness and nausea.

SEE ALSO Eustachi's Rescued Masterpieces (1552), Hearing Aids (1899), and Cochlear Implants (1977).

Cross section of inner ear showing the spiral cochlea and the semicircular canals, three looping, interconnected tubes.

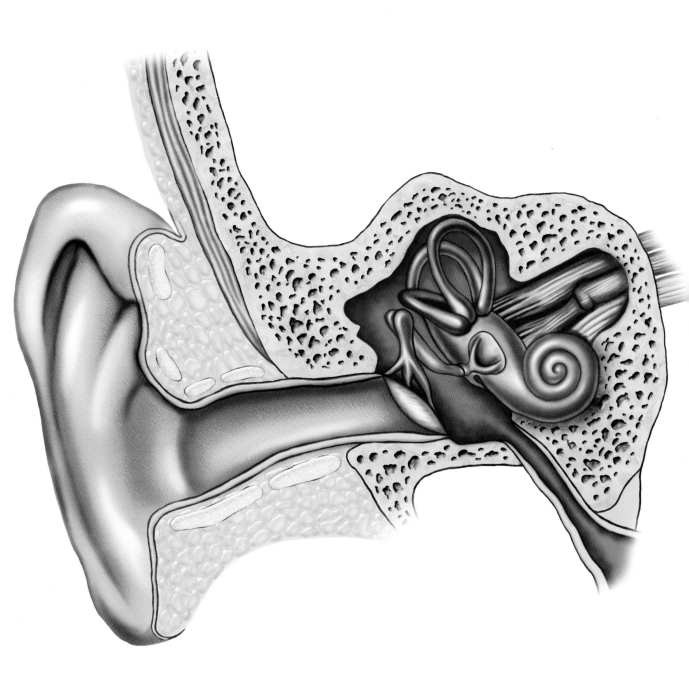

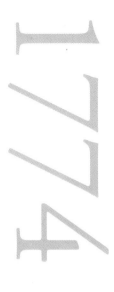

Hunter's *Gravid Uterus*

William Hunter (1718–1783), **Jan van Rymsdyk** (1730–1790), **Charlotte of Mecklenburg-Strelitz** (1744–1818)

Scottish anatomist and obstetrician William Hunter wrote, "Anatomy is the only solid foundation of medicine; it is to the physician and surgeon what geometry is to the astronomer. It discovers and ascertains truth, [and] overturns superstition and vulgar error."

In 1764, Hunter became physician to Queen Charlotte, wife of King George III. George III and Charlotte had 15 children, 13 of whom survived to adulthood.

Hunter's midwifery practice soon became the largest in London, and his greatest work was *Anatomia uteri umani gravidi (The Anatomy of the Human Gravid Uterus Exhibited in Figures)*, published in 1774. The plates were engraved by Dutch-born medical artist Jan van Rymsdyk and elucidate the anatomy of the pregnant woman and the fetus at various stages of development.

Hunter describes the genesis of his work when, in 1751, he acquired his first female corpse: "A woman died suddenly, when very near the end of her pregnancy; the body was procured before any sensible putrefaction had begun; the season of the year was favorable to dissection. . . . Every part was examined in the most public manner, and the truth was thereby well authenticated." In the previous century, the fetus was sometimes depicted as a tiny adult form floating in space. However, Hunter's depictions provided what he called a "universal language" that gave viewers a special and accurate glimpse into human development.

Hunter understood that the public might be shocked and concerned about the source of his anatomical dissections, and in 1783 he wrote to his anatomy students, "In a country where . . . anatomists are not legally supplied with dead bodies, particular care should be taken to avoid giving offense to the populace. . . . Therefore, it is to be hoped that you will be upon your guard and out of doors speak with caution of what may be passing here especially with respect to dead bodies."

SEE ALSO Leonardo's Anatomical Drawings (1510), Mary Toft's Rabbits (1726), Hysterectomy (1813), Anatomy Act of 1832 (1832), Cesarean Section (1882), and Modern Midwifery (1925).

A drawing from William Hunter's The Anatomy of the Human Gravid Uterus Exhibited in Figures *(1774).*

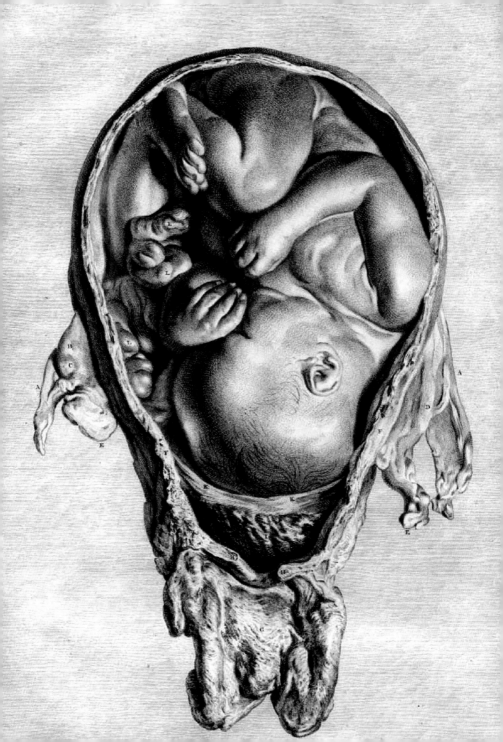

Hospitals

Pandukabhaya (reigned 437 B.C.–367 B.C.), Ashoka (304 B.C.–232 B.C.), Johann Peter Frank (1745–1821)

Surgeon Richard Selzer writes, "A hospital is only a building until you hear the slate hooves of dreams galloping upon its roof. You listen then and know that here is no mere pile of stone and precisely cut timber but an inner space full of pain and relief. Such a place invites mankind to heroism."

Today, the term *hospital* usually refers to an institution that provides health care using specialized staff and equipment, funded by the public sector, corporations, charities, and other means. Historically, hospitals were often funded by religious orders and charitable leaders. In ancient Egypt and Greece, various temples functioned as centers of medical advice and healing. King Pandukabhaya of Sri Lanka (c. 400 B.C.) ordered the construction of "lying-in" homes and hospitals. King Ashoka (c. 250 B.C.) founded several hospitals with physicians and **nurses** in India. During the sixth and seventh centuries, the Academy of Gundishapur in the Persian Empire became one of the first teaching hospitals, with numerous students supervised by physicians. In 325 A.D., the First Council of Nicaea suggested that the Church provide care for the poor and sick through hospitals to be built in every cathedral town. In the early hospitals, the goal was not only to ameliorate suffering and save lives but also to save souls.

The Vienna General Hospital (VGH) opened in 1784, becoming the world's largest hospital, with more than 2,000 beds. The VGH was divided into sections for medicine, surgery, venereal concerns, and contagious diseases. It also had a lying-in facility, a tower for the insane, and a section for abandoned children. German physician Johann Frank was an important figure in the history of hospitals, encouraging hospitals to keep accurate statistical records. His *Complete System of Medical Policy*, first published in 1779, concerned hygiene and public health. He was director of the VGH in 1795, where he attempted to combat the spread of infections between patients. The oldest public hospital in the United States is Bellevue Hospital in New York City, founded in 1736.

SEE ALSO Ambulance (1792), Nursing (1854), Halstedian Surgery (1904), Flexner Report and Medical Education (1910), and Do Not Resuscitate (1991).

In 1679, Louis XIV of France (1638–1715) initiated a project to build Les Invalides, a hospital and home for aged and sick soldiers. The hospital includes a church, which emphasizes the historically close connection between hospitals and religion.

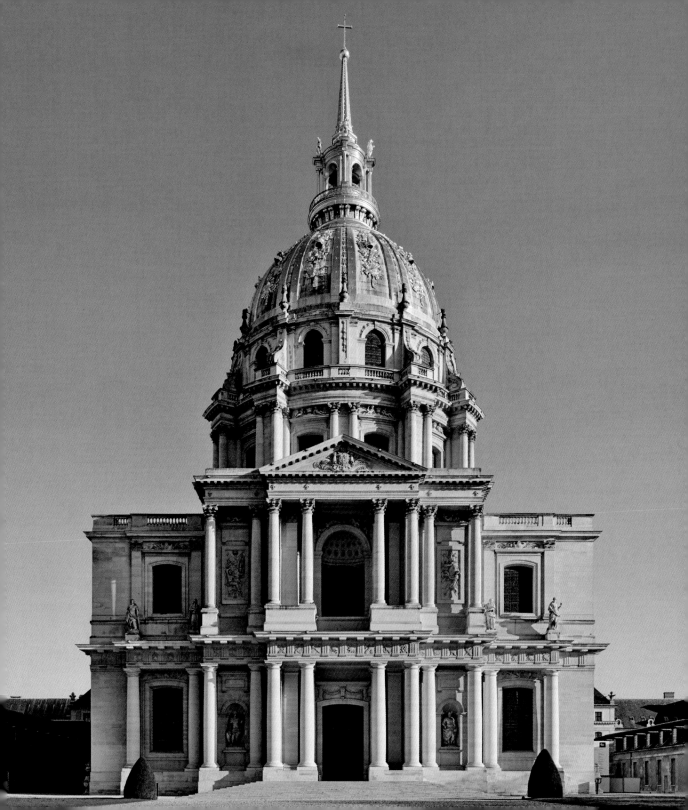

Lavoisier's Respiration

Antoine-Laurent de Lavoisier (1743–1794), Pierre-Simon, Marquis de Laplace (1749–1827)

Today, scientists understand that the process of respiration produces energy needed to power the body, and that this energy comes from the oxidation of substances like proteins and carbohydrates. The important relevant chemical reactions occur in tiny mitochondria within cells, which use oxygen during respiration. This oxygen is acquired by the lungs and conveyed to the tissues by hemoglobin in red blood cells. Eventually, the body expels carbon dioxide through the lungs.

One of the early links among respiration, body heat, perspiration, and food was established by French chemist Antoine Lavoisier, who wrote that the "animal machine" is governed principally by respiration, which creates body heat, and by perspiration and digestion, the latter of which "restores to the blood what it has lost through respiration and perspiration."

In 1784, Lavoisier and the mathematician-astronomer Simon de Laplace invented an apparatus for measuring the production of heat and carbon dioxide produced by live guinea pigs. Lavoisier found that certain amounts of heat and "fixed air" (known today as carbon dioxide) are produced by animals as they convert the oxygen in the air to carbon dioxide. He reasoned that respiration consumes and generates the same gases produced in combustion, for example, when a candle burns and consumes oxygen. In the body, the fuels of respiration are replenished by food.

Lavoisier also showed that the human body consumed more oxygen when exercising than when at rest, and he even suggested that it might be possible to determine the energetic costs of virtually any human activity, such as "giving a speech or playing a musical instrument. One might even evaluate the mechanical energy spent by a philosopher who is thinking."

Sadly, Lavoisier lost his head to the guillotine during the French Revolution. According to the scientist C. S. Minot, "Compared with the growth of science, the shifting of governments are minor events. Until it is clearly realized that the gravest crime of the French Revolution was not the execution of the king, but of Lavoisier, there is no right measure of values."

SEE ALSO Al-Nafis's Pulmonary Circulation (1242), Spirometry (1846), and Mitochondrial Diseases (1962).

Portrait of Antoine Lavoisier, his wife and chemist Marie-Anne Pierrette Paulze, and various scientific equipment (1788), by French painter Jacques-Louis David.

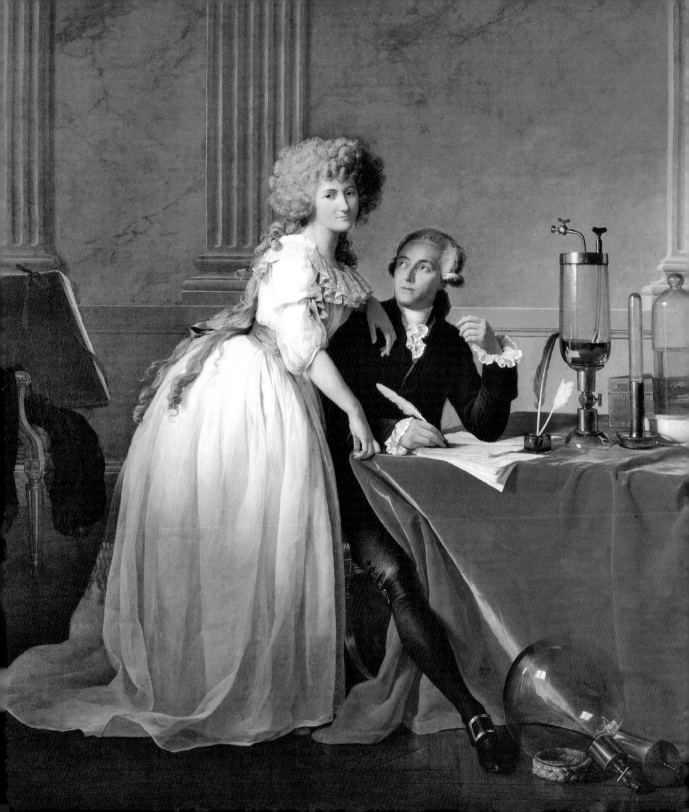

Digitalis

William Withering (1741–1799)

Physician and historian Ralph Major wrote in the 1930s, "Digitalis is without question the most valuable cardiac drug ever discovered and one of the most valuable drugs in the entire pharmacopoeia." *Digitalis purpurea*, also called purple foxglove, is a flowering plant native to most of Europe. For centuries, foxglove leaves were known to have a variety of effects on the human body. English botanist and physician William Withering became famous for his careful tests of the plant in the treatment of dropsy, a swelling of the body and accumulation of fluids due to congestive heart failure (CHF). CHF results from the inability of the heart to supply sufficient blood flow and is often caused by malfunctioning heart valves.

Withering first learned of the use of digitalis (which later became the name of the active ingredient) from an old woman who practiced as a folk herbalist. Her concoction consisted of 20 different ingredients that seemed helpful for treating dropsy. Withering determined that digitalis was the important component. In 1785 he published *An Account of the Foxglove and Some of Its Medical Uses*, in which he discussed his trials on patients, along with remarkable beneficial effects and warnings about lethal toxicity at high doses. The main toxins in digitalis are digitoxin and digoxin. However, at appropriate doses, these "toxins" increase intracellular calcium levels, increase the force of heart muscle contractions, and are useful as antiarrhythmic agents to control the heart rate. Blood-flow through the kidneys is improved, and accumulated fluids are voided through the bladder.

Author H. Panda writes, "His thorough, controlled experimentation not only gave the world a major heart medicine (capable of slowing and strengthening the heartbeat, improving circulation, and moving out excess fluid), but served as a model to put pharmacognosy (the science of natural product drugs) back on its feet. Through the efforts of Withering, pharmacognosy regained an impetus given to it by **Dioscorides** more than 1,700 years earlier."

SEE ALSO Dioscorides's *De Materia Medica* (70), Pulse Watch (1707), Aspirin (1899), Defibrillator (1899), Truth Serum (1922), Blalock-Taussig Shunt (1944), Artificial Heart Valves (1952), and Artificial Pacemaker for Heart (1958).

Digitalis purpurea *(common foxglove).*

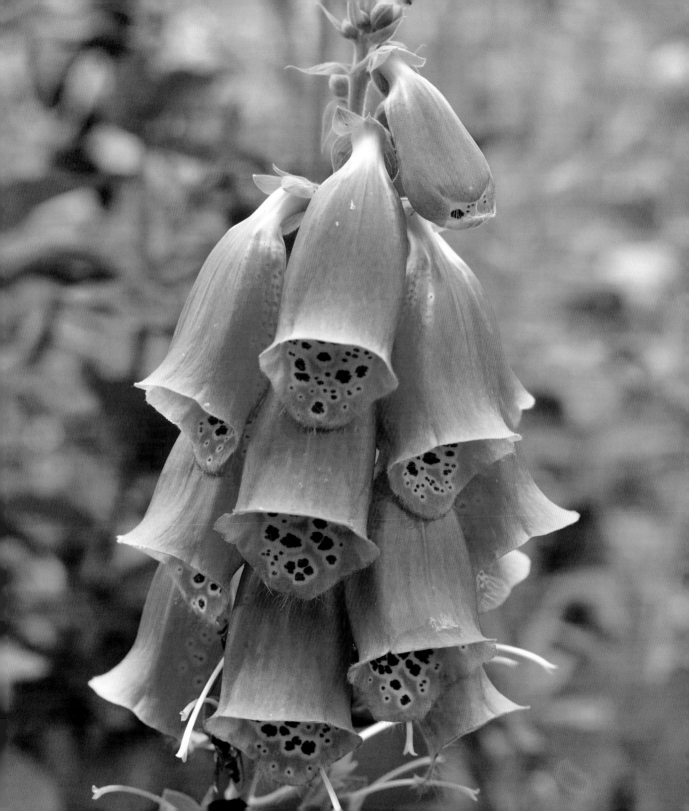

Ambulance

Isabella I (1451–1504), Dominique Jean Larrey (1766–1842)

The concept of an ambulance—a means of transporting the sick or injured to a place of medical care—has its roots in antiquity, with stretchers, hammocks, chariots, and carts. Around 1487, Queen Isabella I of Spain authorized the construction of special bedded wagons with awnings to carry wounded soldiers to tents where they could receive care. Another important stage in the history of the ambulance started around 1792 in France. Physician Ryan Bell writes, "War and carnage inspired the best in humanity to ameliorate the worst when Napoleonic surgeon Dominique Larrey matched his genius for healing against his generation's appetite for war, in the process organizing the first recognizably modern ambulance service." Larrey helped to develop *ambulances volantes* ("flying ambulances") in two forms: a light, two-wheeled covered vehicle with space for two patients, and a heavier, four-wheeled version that held two to four people, drawn by four horses and designed for use on rough terrain. The ambulances had removable litters and carried water, food, bandages, and other equipment. The term *ambulance* comes from the Latin word *ambulare*, meaning "to walk or move."

During the American Civil War, ambulances were initially rare and often driven by civilian drunkards and thieves! The first known ambulance service for U.S. **hospitals** was implemented in 1865 at the Commercial Hospital in Cincinnati, Ohio. These horse-drawn American ambulances carried equipment such as splints, morphine, brandy, and stomach pumps. The first motor-powered ambulances went into action in 1899 at the Michael Reese Hospital in Chicago. In the 1950s, the U.S. military pioneered the use of helicopter ambulances during the Korean War.

Today, the term *ambulance* refers to a wide range of vehicles and even bicycle-controlled conveyances. In the United States, important information, such as estimated time of arrival, may be exchanged with the receiving hospital using two-way radios or other means. On battlefields, military ambulances are often heavily armored. Around 2004, Israel modified several of its Merkava battle tanks to contain ambulance features with various life-support systems.

SEE ALSO Hospitals (1784), Snow Anesthesia (1812), Nursing (1854), Red Cross (1863), and Cardiopulmonary Resuscitation (1956).

Ipswich Ambulance Depot (c. 1900), Queensland, Australia. A. E. Roberts Carriage Works built vehicles and equipment for the Ipswich Ambulance Transport Brigade Hospital. (The Queensland Museum contains many negatives and prints from the era.)

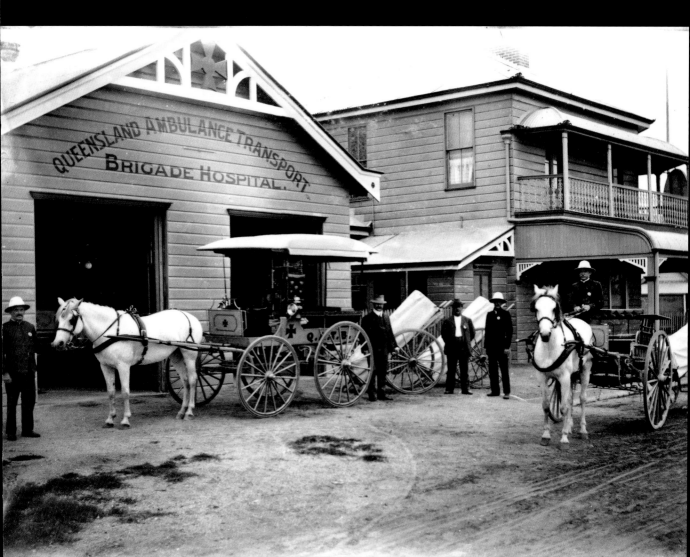

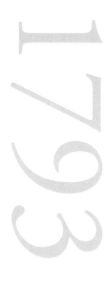

Unchaining the Lunatics

William Tuke (1732–1822), Philippe Pinel (1745–1826), Jean-Baptiste Pussin (1745–1811), Vincenzo Chiarugi (1759–1820)

In his 1801 book *A Treatise on Insanity*, the French physician Philippe Pinel wrote of the horrific treatment of the mentally ill housed in French asylums: "The blood of maniacs is sometimes so lavishly spilled, and with so little discernment, as to render it doubtful whether the patient or his physician has the best claim to the appellation of madman." In 1793, when Pinel became the superintendent of the Bicêtre **Hospital**, he argued that the mentally ill should be viewed as suffering from a disease and should not be punished for supposed demonic possession or sinful behavior. His idea that patients should be treated with kindness was revolutionary at a time when asylum patients were beaten, chained, starved, bled, blistered, whirled in chairs, made to vomit, and sometimes even displayed like zoo animals.

Pinel learned much from Jean-Baptiste Pussin, a hospital superintendent who was interested in treating asylum inmates with greater kindness. Starting around 1793, Pussin and Pinel removed the chains from several inmates at the Bicêtre asylum, carefully watched them, and saw improvement in many of them. Pinel forbade harsh punishments and insisted on better food, occupational therapy, and maintaining careful patient case histories. He also sought intelligent and kind asylum personnel who could work more effectively with the insane. As a result of this approach, inmate deaths decreased dramatically, and the number of released inmates increased. In 1795, he became director of the largest asylum in Europe at the Salpêtrière Hospital, which housed thousands of insane women. Here, he successfully instituted similar reforms and later came to be known as one of the founders of psychiatry. Pinel referred to his humane approach as *traitement moral*, which emphasized that compassionate psychological treatment should be tried before physical approaches.

Other early asylum reformers include the British Quaker William Tuke, who in 1792 created a retreat for the mentally ill, and Italian physician Vincenzo Chiarugi, who in 1788 headed a hospital in Florence in which humane treatment was encouraged.

SEE ALSO *De Praestigiis Daemonum* (1563), Psychoanalysis (1899), Electroconvulsive Therapy (1938), Transorbital Lobotomy (1946), Antipsychotics (1950), and Cognitive Behavioral Therapy (1963).

Once known as the Buffalo State Asylum for the Insane, this New York facility was designed in 1870 by architect Henry Hobson Richardson. Patients were segregated by sex. The wards housed mental patients until the mid-1970s.

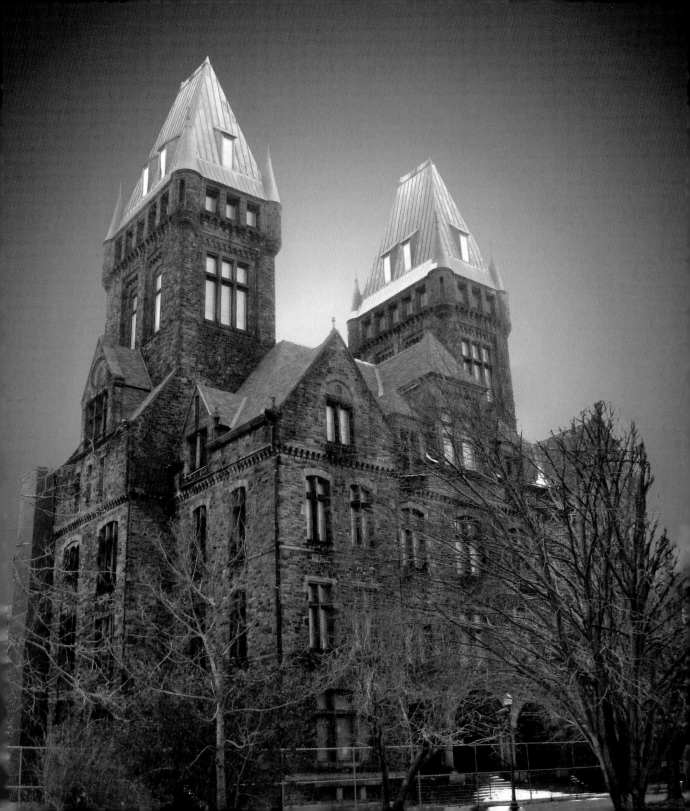

Alternative Medicine

Christian Friedrich Samuel Hahnemann (1755–1843), **Daniel David Palmer** (1845–1913)

Many people make use of complementary or alternative medicine (CAM), which includes medical practices that are not presently considered part of conventional medicine. The term *complementary* is used when such treatments are employed together with conventional medicine, and *alternative* is used when the treatments are employed in place of conventional medicine.

The National Center for Complementary and Alternative Medicine is a U.S. government agency dedicated to the scientific study of CAM, and the agency cites numerous examples of CAM, including **acupuncture**, **Ayurvedic medicine**, **chiropractic**, herbalism, Traditional Chinese Medicine, meditation, yoga, biofeedback, hypnosis, and homeopathy. For example, chiropractors often manipulate the spinal column to alleviate "neural dysfunctions," and homeopaths may use extremely diluted preparations of substances to treat symptoms, believing that when a substance in large doses causes certain symptoms, in small doses it can alleviate those same symptoms.

This entry is dated to 1796, the date when German physician Samuel Hahnemann proposed the concept of homeopathy. Chiropractic was founded in 1895 by American Daniel Palmer, who suggested that physical manipulation of the spine could cure disease. While the benefits of many CAMs may be due to the **placebo effect**, it is interesting to note that, until recently, the entire history of medical treatment was essentially the history of the placebo effect, with many ancient treatments that seem odd to us today. Some individuals may choose CAM due to fear of surgery or the side effects of drugs. The downside of some CAMs is that they have not been rigorously tested and may lead some people to forgo more effective mainstream treatments.

The physician Allan Rosenfield writes, "In many parts of the world, where medicines are not readily available or affordable, the public continues to rely on medicines used traditionally in their cultures. At the same time, affluent consumers in the industrialized world are spending their own money on [CAM]. . . .The scale of this is so sizeable that it constitutes a public health phenomenon in itself."

SEE ALSO Ayurvedic Medicine (2000 B.C.), Paracelsus Burns Medical Books (1527), Acupuncture *Compendium* (1601), Osteopathy (1892), D.D. Palmer and Chiropractic (1895), and Placebo Effect (1955).

Moxibustion is a traditional Chinese medicine technique that involves the burning of the mugwort herb. Sometimes, a cone-shaped moxa is placed on the skin and burned, or a heated moxa stick may be held next to the skin. Ginseng (shown in the foreground) has been used medicinally for centuries.

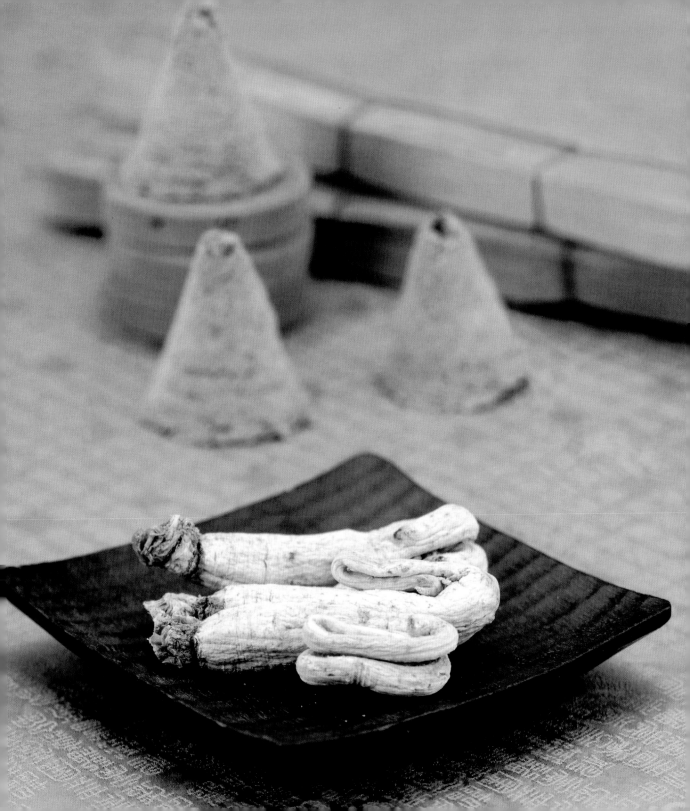

Phrenology

Franz Joseph Gall (1758–1828), Johann Gaspar Spurzheim (1776–1832)

In 1796, German neuroanatomist Franz Joseph Gall posited that the brain was composed of a set of 27 organs and that each organ was associated with a mental ability or personality trait. Although we now know that different areas of the brain are in fact specialized for different functions (see entry "**Cerebral Localization**"), Gall made the error of claiming that the relative sizes and activities of the 27 hypothetical organs could be inferred from the size of the overlying areas and bumps of the skull.

During the 1820s through the 1840s, many people took phrenology seriously, and the concept permeated novels and popular culture. People consulted phrenologists when making decisions related to job hiring, the future of a child, and the suitability of marriage partners! Even Queen Victoria had her children's heads analyzed. Simply by feeling the bumps and contours of the head, a trained phrenologist was thought to be able to infer characteristics related to the 27 "organs," which included "love of one's offspring," "affection and friendship," "pride," "the sense of language and speech," "religiosity," "a sense of numbers," and so forth.

Gall made his assignments to the regions of the skull based on examinations of skulls of people at the "extremes" of society, such as writers, poets, criminals, and lunatics. To help him with his correlations, he collected more than 300 skulls. For example, "destructiveness" was localized above the ear, in part because a prominence was located in a student who tortured animals and in an apothecary who became an executioner. Curiously, he believed that 19 of the 27 faculties could be demonstrated in animals.

The German physician Johann Spurzheim sensationalized phrenology in the United States through his lectures, making Gall's theory more acceptable by "removing" the "murder" and "theft" organs and adding several more phrenological zones. Although phrenology is viewed today as pseudoscience, it played a role in the history of medicine, focusing attention on the valid idea of specialization of brain regions, later demonstrated by neurosurgeons.

SEE ALSO Cerebellum Function (1809), Cerebral Localization (1861), Osteopathy (1892), Psychoanalysis (1899), and Transorbital Lobotomy (1946).

Phrenology diagram, from People's Cyclopedia of Universal Knowledge *(1883).*

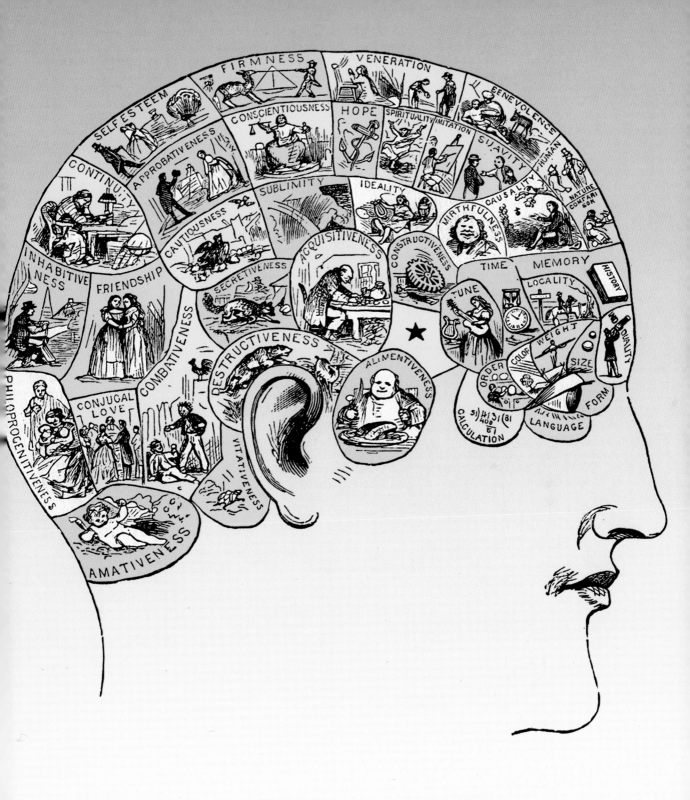

Smallpox Vaccination

Edward Anthony Jenner (1749–1823)

"Smallpox is a disease that terrified people for thousands of years," writes medical historian Robert Mulcahy. "During the 1700s, this disease took approximately 400,000 lives each year in Europe alone and left hundreds of thousands more living with scarred and disfigured faces. The smallpox virus could spread through a town like wildfire, bringing high fever and a blistering rash to everyone who caught it. Half of those who contracted the disease would die within weeks—and there was no cure."

Smallpox is a contagious viral disease that has devastated populations since the dawn of humanity. Smallpox skin lesions have even been found on the faces of ancient Egyptian mummies (c. 1100 B.C.). When Europeans introduced the disease to the New World, smallpox became instrumental in the fall of the Aztec and Incan empires.

For many years, English physician Edward Jenner had heard tales that dairymaids were protected from smallpox after they had been afflicted with cowpox, a similar disease that affects cows but is not fatal for humans. In 1796, he removed material from a dairymaid's cowpox lesions and transferred it into two scratches he made in the skin of an eight-year-old boy. The boy developed a minor fever and discomfort but soon was completely recovered. Later, Jenner inoculated the boy with material from a smallpox lesion, and no disease developed in the boy. In 1798, Jenner published additional findings in *An Inquiry into the Causes and Effects of the Variolae Vaccinae*. He called the procedure vaccination—which stems from *vacca*, the Latin word for cow—and began to send cowpox vaccine samples to anyone who requested them.

Jenner was not the first to vaccinate against smallpox. However, his work is considered among the first *scientific* attempts to control infectious disease. Physician Stefan Riedel writes that it was Jenner's "relentless promotion and devoted research of vaccination that changed the way medicine was practiced." Eventually, the smallpox vaccination was used throughout the world. By 1979 the world was essentially free of smallpox, and routine vaccination was no longer needed.

SEE ALSO Antitoxins (1890), Discovery of Viruses (1892), Cause of Yellow Fever (1937), Polio Vaccine (1955), and Structure of Antibodies (1959).

An 1802 cartoon by British satirist James Gillray, depicting the early controversy surrounding Jenner's vaccination theory. Note the cows emerging from the people's bodies.

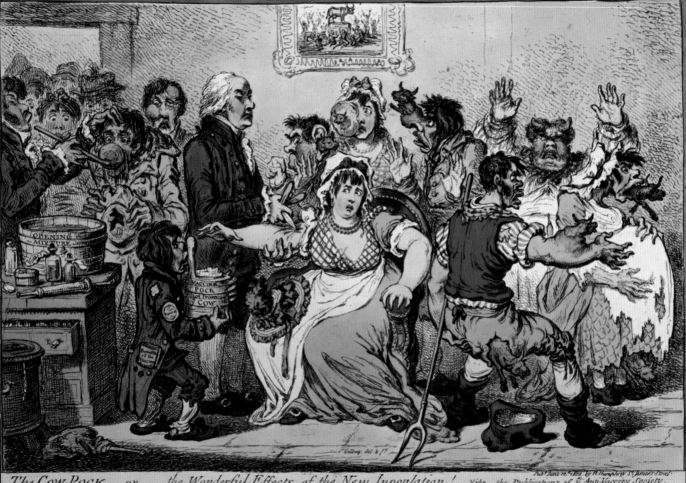

The Cow-Pock — or — the Wonderful Effects of the New Inoculation! — Vide. the Publications of ỹ Anti-Vaccine Society.

Cerebellum Function

Luigi Rolando (1773–1831), Marie Jean Pierre Flourens (1794–1867)

Whenever you see a ballet dancer, a martial artist, or a piano player, you should thank the cerebellum—that plum-size, heavily grooved part of the brain located below the large cerebral hemispheres and behind the brainstem. The cerebellum (Latin for "little brain") coordinates sensory input with muscular responses and helps the ballerina leap gracefully though the air without consciously thinking of all the small motion corrections and details needed to achieve her goal. In 1809, Italian anatomist Luigi Rolando observed that damage to the cerebellum of animals caused obvious disturbances to their movements. In 1824, French physiologist Jean Pierre Flourens performed additional experiments demonstrating that, although animals with damaged cerebellums can still move, their movements are awkward and uncoordinated. Flourens correctly suggested that the cerebellum coordinates motions but does not initiate or consciously plan the movements.

Today, we know that in addition to facilitating smooth, fine-tuned movements by integrating nerve signals from the **labyrinths** of the ears (which provide information on body orientation for balance) and from positional sensors in muscles, the cerebellum also plays a role in language processing and emotional responses. Anatomically, the organ includes a right and left hemisphere connected by the worm-shaped vermis. Remarkably, the organ contains more than 50 percent of the total number of neurons in the brain in the form of numerous small cerebellar granule cells. Because of the many folds of the cerebellum, only about a sixth of the surface is visible from outside the organ.

Recent research shows that patients with abnormal cerebellums or with cerebellar lesions can exhibit decreased verbal fluency, depression, autistic-like obsessive rituals, and difficulty understanding social cues. The cerebellum may serve to dampen oscillations in behaviors—shaping personality, mood, and intellect in addition to muscle motions.

SEE ALSO Cranial Nerves Classified (1664), Cerebrospinal Fluid (1764), Exploring the Labyrinth (1772), Cerebral Localization (1861), Neuron Doctrine (1891), and Pineal Body (1958).

The cerebellum is the smaller, heavily grooved part of the brain. It is located above the spinal column and below the large cerebral hemispheres.

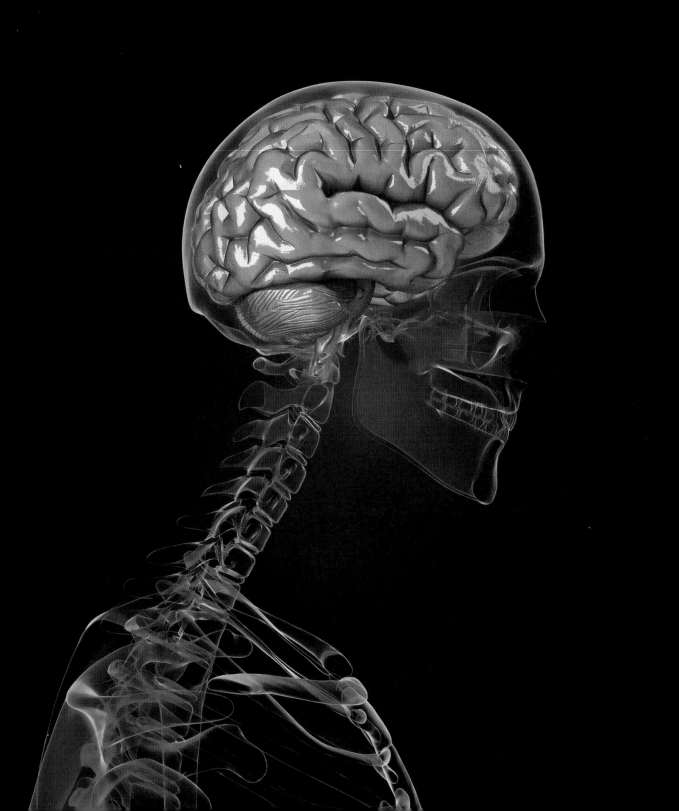

Bell-Magendie Law

Sir Charles Bell (1774–1842), François Magendie (1783–1855)

Neuroanatomist Marian Diamond writes, "The brain is a three-pound mass you can hold in your hand that can conceive of a universe a hundred billion light-years across." In humans, the brain, along with the spinal cord and nerves, comprise the nervous system. Sensory neurons (nerve cells) are activated by various stimuli, such as someone touching the skin. Motor neurons connect the nervous system to muscles and can be used to trigger muscle movements.

One important law in the history of medicine is the Bell Magendie Law, which states that sensory nerves enter the spinal cord dorsally—that is, from the back of the spinal cord. On the other hand, motor neurons exit the spinal cord ventrally (at the front, toward the belly). Scottish anatomist Charles Bell's privately circulated book *Idea of a New Anatomy of the Brain* (1811) contains a reference to experimental work on the motor functions of the ventral spinal nerves. Although considered one of the foundations of clinical neurology, it did not definitively establish the sensory functions of the dorsal nerves. In 1822, French physiologist François Magendie, working independently of Bell, discovered that the ventral root is associated with motor functions and that the dorsal root is sensory. By dissecting live mammals, he showed that he could systematically destroy certain nerves to elicit either paralysis or lack of sensation. An intense rivalry developed between Magendie and Bell with respect to who actually discovered the law that today bears both of their names.

Magendie's public vivisections (dissections of live animals) were shocking and led to the introduction of a bill banning animal cruelty in the United Kingdom. In one famous incident, Magendie dissected half the nerves of the face of a living greyhound after the dog was nailed through its ears and paws. The dog was then left alive overnight for further dissection the next day. Even those physicians who defended the use of animals in medical research suggested that Magendie was too uncaring with respect to animal subjects.

SEE ALSO Cranial Nerves Classified (1664), Neuron Doctrine (1891), and Neurotransmitters (1914).

View of the back of the spinal column, with nerves in green. Sensory nerves enter the spinal cord (central orange tube) from the back of the spinal cord, near a person's back. Motor neurons exit the spinal cord toward the front of a person.

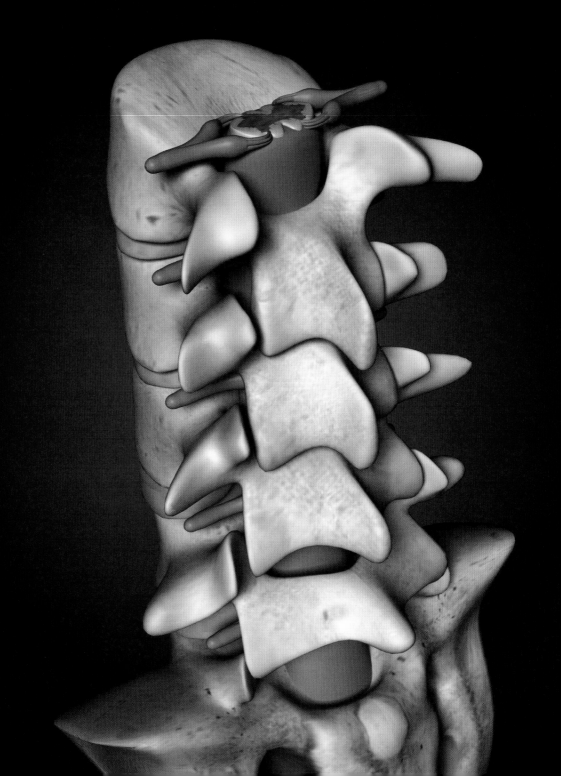

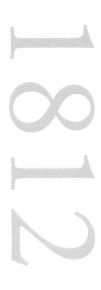

Snow Anesthesia

Hippocrates of Cos (460 B.C.–377 B.C.), **Abu 'Ali al-Husayn ibn 'Abd-Allah Ibn Sina (Avicenna)** (980–1037), **Dominique Jean Larrey** (1766–1842), **James Arnott** (1797–1883)

Divinum est opus sedare dolorem ("Divine is the work to subdue pain"): This ancient Latin aphorism for physicians is emblematic of the quest to control pain during surgery. As early as 2500 B.C., the ancient Egyptians sometimes used low temperatures to treat injuries and reduce inflammation. The Greek physician Hippocrates suggested that "swellings and pains in the joints . . . and sprains are generally improved by a copious infusion of cold water . . . for a moderate degree of numbness removes pain." Avicenna, the famous Islamic physician, used ice-cold water to numb the tooth and gum before surgery.

One of the most famous users of snow and ice for pain control was French surgeon Dominique Larrey, who also introduced a system of special horse-drawn **ambulances** and developed the concept of triage, in which injured soldiers were treated according to the severity of their wounds. In 1807, Larrey observed at the Battle of Eylau in Prussia that the pain of amputations was very much reduced when limbs were extremely cold. In 1812, during the Battle of Borodino against Russia, Larrey is said to have performed 200 amputations within a 24-hour period; he performed 300 more at the Battle of Berezina. Whenever possible, he used snow and ice to dull the pain.

One ardent supporter of cold anesthesia was the British surgeon James Arnott, who was concerned by some of the deaths caused by early experiments with ether and chloroform anesthesia. Arnott's approach involved a mixture of crushed ice and salt applied to the skin around the site of the operation. He wrote, "In all superficial operations . . . cold is superior to chloroform in the circumstances of safety, ease of application or the saving of time and trouble, and certainly of producing anesthesia [and preventing inflammation]."

This book's 1842 entry on **general anesthesia** discusses the use of various inhaled gases to provide relief from pain, and the 1884 entry on **cocaine** describes the use of local anesthetics to numb the eye during surgery.

SEE ALSO Ambulance (1792), General Anesthesia (1842), and Cocaine as Local Anesthetic (1884).

The Battle of Eylau (February 7–8, 1807), by Antoine-Jean Gros (1771–1835). Larrey observed that the pain of amputations was very much reduced when limbs were extremely cold.

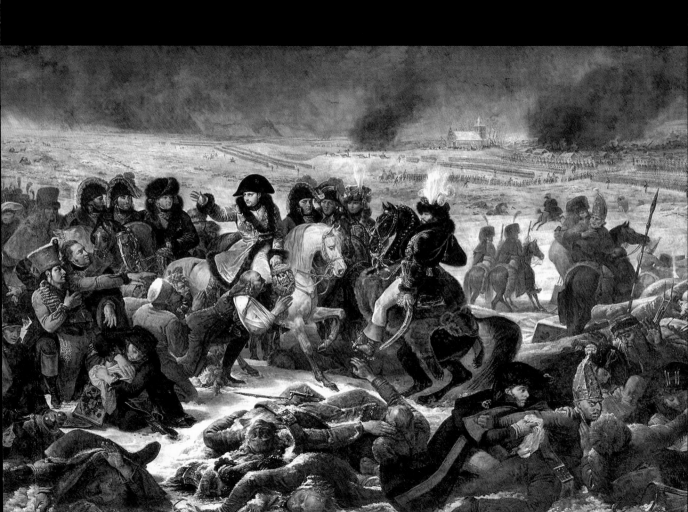

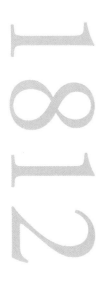

Women Medical Students

Dorothea Christiane Erxleben (née Leporin; 1715–1762), James Barry (1792–1865), Elizabeth Blackwell (1821–1910)

A 1957 questionnaire to U.S. male physicians elicited responses such as "I'd prefer a third-rate man to a first-rate woman doctor" and "Women were created to be wives." In antiquity, women sometimes had less difficulty practicing medicine. For example, in ancient Egypt, many female physicians existed, but the practice was gradually discouraged in the West, and by the Middle Ages women physicians were essentially nonexistent.

Consider the case of James Barry, military surgeon in the British Army who graduated from the University of Edinburgh in 1812. For more than 40 years, Barry served in garrisons across the British Empire, becoming well known as a zealous reformer who improved the health of soldiers and civilians. He was the first British surgeon to perform a successful **cesarean section** in Africa, saving both the child and mother. Upon his death in 1865, a maid who was asked to lay out the body discovered that Barry was a woman. Today, most historians feel that Barry was actually Margaret Ann Bulkley and had chosen to live as a man so that she would be able to pursue a career as a surgeon. Thus, Bulkley/Barry was the first woman in Britain to become a qualified medical doctor.

Elizabeth Blackwell was the first woman to become a doctor in the United States and the first woman to be accepted to and graduate from medical school in modern times (without pretending to be a man). When Blackwell had applied to medical school at Geneva College in New York, the faculty asked the students if she should be admitted. Thinking that her application was a hoax, they voted for admission and were shocked when Blackwell actually enrolled. She graduated in 1849. Banned from practice in most **hospitals**, she went to Paris to further her practical knowledge. In 1857, Blackwell cofounded the New York Infirmary for Indigent Women and Children. Perhaps less famous than Barry and Blackwell is Dorothea Erxleben, the first female medical doctor in Germany. She received her M.D. in 1754.

SEE ALSO Nursing (1854), Cesarean Section (1882), Flexner Report and Medical Education (1910), and Modern Midwifery (1925).

Elizabeth Blackwell was the first woman to become a physician in the United States. She graduated from the medical school at Geneva College in New York in 1849.

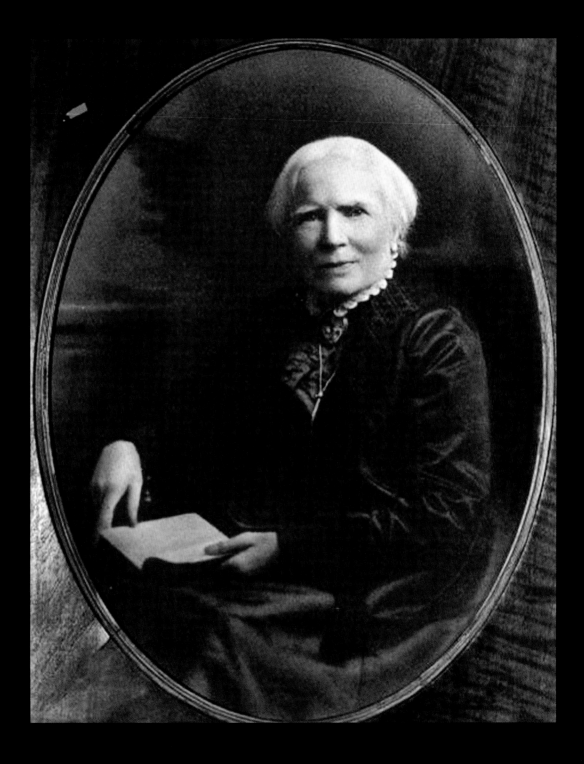

Hysterectomy

Ephraim McDowell (1771–1830), Konrad Johann Martin Langenbeck (1776–1851), Walter Burnham (1808–1883)

The path to routine, successful hysterectomies is long and fraught with misery, particularly in the days before **anesthesia** and antibiotics. A hysterectomy is the partial or total surgical removal of the uterus, the muscular organ in which the fetus develops prior to its travel through the cervix (the lower end of the uterus) and through the vagina during birth. Today, the hysterectomy is the most common gynecological surgical procedure and may be performed for such maladies as uterine **cancer** and severe endometriosis (growth of the uterine lining outside the uterus).

One notable event on the path to modern hysterectomies occurred in 1809 when American physician Ephraim McDowell operated on Jane Todd Crawford, who had a massive ovarian tumor that made it difficult for her to breathe. In order to receive her surgery, she rode by horse for 60 miles to McDowell's home, with her huge tumor resting on the pommel of her saddle. With no anesthesia, Crawford successfully operated on his kitchen table and removed a tumor that weighed 22.5 pounds (10.2 kilograms).

In 1813, German surgeon Konrad Langenbeck performed one of the earliest carefully planned hysterectomies through the vagina, but colleagues did not believe he had actually removed the uterus. When the patient died 26 years later, an **autopsy** revealed that the operation had indeed taken place.

In 1853, American surgeon Walter Burnham performed the first abdominal hysterectomy in which the patient survived. Burnham started what he thought would be an ovary removal for an ovarian cyst, but when he had cut open his patient and she began to vomit, he saw that the "tumor" that popped through the incision was not on the ovary but an enlarged fibroid uterus, which he had no choice but to remove.

Today, several approaches to hysterectomies may be considered, including removal through an abdominal incision, removal through the vagina (with or without **laparoscopic** assistance), and total laparoscopic hysterectomies (in which the uterus is removed through small openings made in the abdominal wall).

SEE ALSO Hunter's *Gravid Uterus* (1774), Cesarean Section (1882), Salpingectomy (1883), and Laparoscopic Surgery (1981).

The uterus, a muscular organ in which the fetus develops. In this figure, it is depicted as an orange-colored, bulbous object. Also shown are the fallopian tubes, emerging to the right and left of the uterus and leading to the ovaries, as well as the vagina, below the uterus.

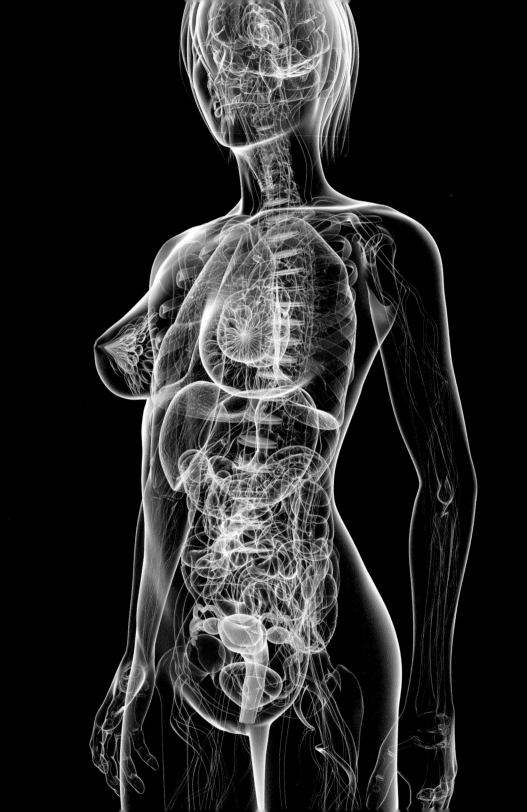

Stethoscope

René-Théophile-Hyacinthe Laennec (1781–1826)

Social historian Roy Porter writes, "By giving access to body noises—the sound of breathing, the blood gurgling around the heart—the stethoscope changed approaches to internal disease and hence doctor-patient relations. As last, the living body was no longer a closed book: pathology could now be done on the living."

In 1816, French physician René Laennec invented the stethoscope, which consisted of a wooden tube with a trumpetlike end that made contact with the chest. The air-filled cavity transmitted sounds from the patient's body to the physician's ear. In the 1940s, stethoscopes with two-sided chest-pieces became standard. One side of the chest-piece is a diaphragm (a plastic disc that closes the opening) made to vibrate through skin contact that produces acoustic pressure waves that travel through the air cavity of the stethoscope. The other side contains a bell-shaped endpiece that is better at transmitting low-frequency sounds. The diaphragm side actually tunes out low frequencies and is used to listen to lung sounds of higher frequencies than heart sounds. When using the bell side, the physician can vary the pressure of the bell on the skin to "tune" the skin vibration frequency in order to best reveal the heartbeat sounds. Many other refinements occurred over the years, involving improved amplification, noise reduction, and other characteristics that were optimized by application of simple physical principles (see "Notes and Further Reading").

In Laennec's day, a physician often placed his ear directly on the patient's chest or back. However, Laennec complained that this technique "is always inconvenient, both to the physician and the patient; in the case of females, it is not only indelicate, but often impractical." Later, an extra-long stethoscope was used to treat the very poor when physicians wanted to be farther away from their flea-ridden patients. Aside from inventing the device, Laennec carefully recorded how specific physical diseases (e.g., pneumonia, tuberculosis, and bronchitis) corresponded to the sounds heard. Ironically, Laennec himself died at age 45 of tuberculosis, which his colleagues diagnosed using a stethoscope.

SEE ALSO Pulse Watch (1707), Spirometry (1846), Medical Thermometer (1866), Hearing Aids (1899), Electrocardiograph (1903), and Cochlear Implants (1977).

Modern stethoscope. Various acoustic experiments have been done to determine the effect on sound collection of chest-piece size and material.

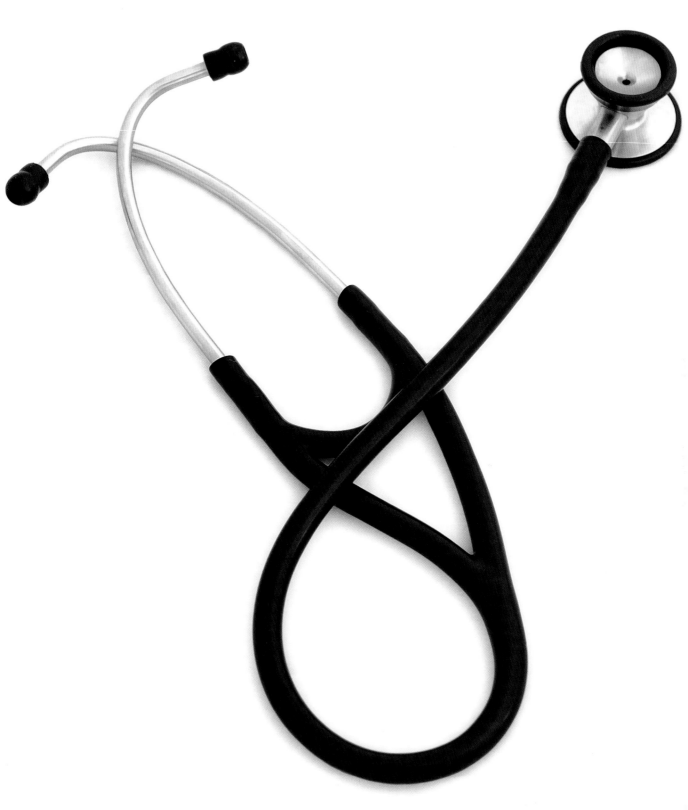

Ligation of the Abdominal Aorta

Astley Paston Cooper (1768–1841), Rudolph Matas (1860–1957)

According to author Harold Ellis, English surgeon Astley Cooper is "the father of arterial surgery" and the first person in history to tie the "mother of all arteries," the abdominal aorta. The aorta stems from the heart's left ventricle, proceeds upward in an arch, and then extends down through the body to the abdomen, where it finally branches into two large arteries called the common iliac arteries.

In 1811, Cooper demonstrated in dogs that the lower part of the aorta, known as the abdominal aorta, could be ligated (tied up and constricted) without resulting in death. Apparently, sufficient blood could reach the hind limbs through other arterial channels. In 1817, Charles Huston suffered from a huge, leaking iliac artery aneurysm (swelling) in his left groin, and he bled profusely. In order to save Huston's life, Cooper attempted to ligate the abdominal aorta about an inch before it branched into the iliac arteries. Without removing the patient from bed, Cooper cut into Huston's abdomen near the umbilicus (navel, or belly button), passed his finger along the aorta, and turned to his onlookers, saying, "Gentlemen, I have the pleasure of informing you that the aorta is now hooked upon my finger." He passed his finger between the aorta and the spine and, while avoiding bowel loops, ligated the aorta.

Alas, about 40 hours after the operation, Huston died. Although the right leg remained healthy-looking, the tissue on the left leg exhibited gangrene (tissue death). Finally, in 1923, American surgeon Rudolph Matas successfully treated an aortic aneurysm by ligating the aorta. The patient survived for more than a year before dying of unrelated complications of tuberculosis.

Aortic aneurysms may result from a weakness in the wall of the aorta at any location, but abdominal aortic aneurysms are the most common. Aneurysms may swell and eventually rupture, causing rapid death if not treated. One form of modern treatment involves the insertion of a stent (tube) within the aorta for the length of the swelling.

SEE ALSO Paré's "Rational Surgery" (1545), Vascular Suturing (1902), Blalock-Taussig Shunt (1944), and Angioplasty (1964).

Schematic depiction of an abdominal aorta that has developed an aneurysm (swelling), just above the location where the aorta bifurcates (splits) into two large arteries, called the common iliac arteries.

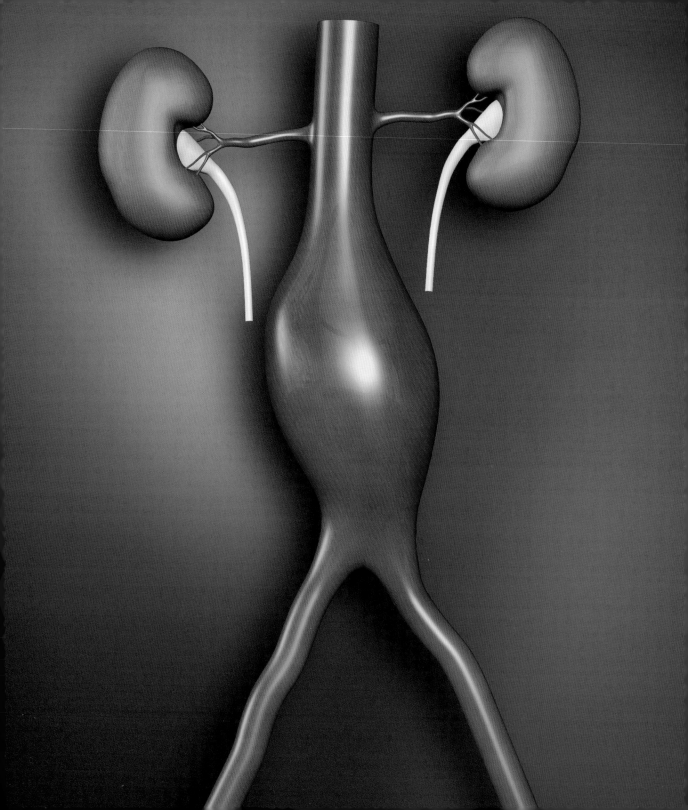

Leech Therapy

François-Joseph-Victor Broussais (1772–1838), John Brown (1810–1882)

The medical use of leeches to remove blood from the body has been around for millennia in Europe and Asia, but often for reasons that would be considered unscientific today, such as for restoring balance in the body's humors (fluids). In Europe, the exuberant use of leeches reached a high during what I refer to as the Broussaisian age, when French physician François Broussais suggested that almost all diseases were caused by inflammation and that virtually any disease could be aided by leeching. The practice of leeching became so extravagant that some physicians of the Broussaisian age referred to his practice as vampirism. It was not uncommon to use many dozens of leeches in a single session, and several *million* leeches were used each year in France, England, and Germany. In 1825, one representative pleaded with the French parliament to stop the madness, saying that the physicians use leeches to drive farmers "to their graves" and that the leeches "made more blood flow than the most pitiless conqueror."

By 1828, roughly 100 million leeches were used annually in France. Demand outstripped supply. Leech prices skyrocketed. Leech farms were everywhere, as leeches were used to "cure" everything from obesity and hemorrhoids to mental illness. Even the famous Scottish physician John Brown treated his own sore throat by applying six leeches to his neck and 12 leeches behind the ear.

Despite the obvious leech madness of the Broussaisian age, starting around the 1980s, medical leeches (e.g., *Hirudo medicinalis*) have been used successfully after reconstructive surgery, including ear or finger reattachment operations, to relieve venous congestion, which results when arterial blood pools at a site because veins have not had time to regrow. The leech's mouth is applied to the skin so that its saliva can supply anticoagulants (e.g., hirudin), vasodilators (blood vessel wideners), and **anesthetics**. The leech removes about five milliliters (one teaspoon) of blood, and after the leech is removed, blood continues to ooze beneficially for a day or two. Pooling and pressure are reduced, allowing time for veins to rebuild.

SEE ALSO Bloodletting (1500 B.C.), Barber Pole (1210), Heparin (1916), and Maggot Therapy (1929).

*Bloodsucking leeches (*Hirudo medicinalis*) on woman's neck.*

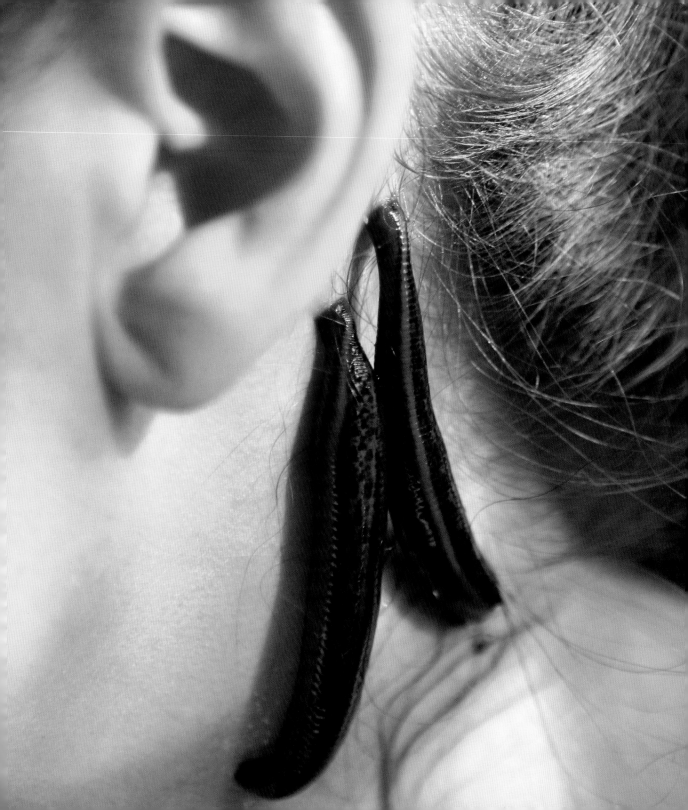

Blood Transfusion

James Blundell (1791–1878), Karl Landsteiner (1868–1943)

"The history of blood transfusion is a fascinating story and is marked by alternating periods of intense enthusiasm and periods of disillusionment, more so than the introduction of any other therapeutic measure," writes the surgeon Raymond Hurt. "Its full potential was not achieved until the discovery of blood groups and introduction of a satisfactory anticoagulant."

Blood transfusion often refers to the transfer of blood, or blood components, from one person to another in order to combat blood loss during trauma or surgery. Transfusions of blood may also be required during the treatment of various diseases such as hemophilia and **sickle-cell anemia**.

Various animal-to-animal blood transfusions, as well as animal-to-human transfusions, had been attempted in the 1600s in Europe. However, the English obstetrician James Blundell is credited with the first *successful* transfusion of blood from one human to another. Not only did he begin to place the art of transfusion on a scientific basis, he reawakened interest in a procedure that was generally quite unsafe. In 1818, Blundell had used several donors to transfuse a man dying from stomach **cancer**, but the man died about two days later. In 1829, through the use of a syringe, he transfused blood from a husband to his wife, who was bleeding heavily after giving birth. She happily survived, representing the first successful documented transfusion.

Blundell soon came to realize that many transfusions led to kidney damage and death. It was not until around 1900 that Austrian physician Karl Landsteiner discovered three blood groups—A, B, and O—and found that transfusion between people with the same blood group usually led to safe transfusions. A fourth blood type, AB, was discovered shortly thereafter. The development of electrical refrigeration led to the first "blood banks" in the mid-1930s. After the Rh blood factor was discovered in 1939, dangerous blood-transfusion reactions became rare. (See "Vasculature Suturing" for additional history about tranfusions.)

Transfusions have sometimes been limited due to prejudice. For example, in the 1950s, Louisiana made it a crime for physicians to give a white person "black blood" without obtaining prior permission.

SEE ALSO Intravenous Saline Solutions (1832), Red Cross (1863), Vascular Suturing (1902), Heparin (1916), and Cause of Sickle-Cell Anemia (1949).

Hand-colored engraved image, The Transfusion of Blood—An Operation at the Hôpital de la Pitié *(1874), by Miranda, from* Harper's Weekly.

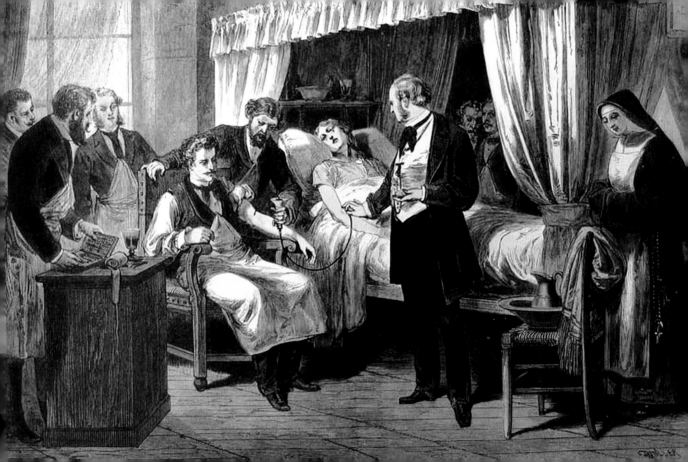

Medical Specialization

The biochemist and author Isaac Asimov wrote, "I believe that scientific knowledge has fractal properties, that no matter how much we learn, whatever is left, however small it may seem, is just as infinitely complex as the whole was to start with." In medicine, the explosion of information, procedures, and technologies is particularly apparent and requires the need for specialty areas of medical practice and education.

Medical historian George Weisz suggests that medical specialization—motivated partly by the quest for new medical knowledge, advances in education, new treatments, and dissemination of knowledge—began on a large scale in the great **hospitals** of Paris in the 1830s. Medical specialization rapidly expanded in Vienna beginning in the 1850s. In the United States, specialization slowly grew after the American Civil War, driven by the rise of large cities, the interests of American physicians returning from European training, and new knowledge gained from experiences during the Civil War.

Today, a large range of medical specialties and subspecialties exists, with decreasing numbers of general practitioners. As an example, a physician may have the specialty of anesthesiology with a subspecialty of cardiothoracic anesthesiology or pediatric anesthesiology. As additional examples, consider that the American Board of Medical Specialties (ABMS) has Member Boards that certify physicians in more than 145 specialties and subspecialties, including boards for the specialty areas of Allergy and Immunology, Anesthesiology, Colon and Rectal Surgery, Dermatology, Emergency Medicine, Family Medicine, Internal Medicine, Medical Genetics, Neurological Surgery, Nuclear Medicine, Obstetrics and Gynecology, Ophthalmology, Orthopedic Surgery, Otolaryngology, Pathology, Pediatrics, Physical Medicine and Rehabilitation, Plastic Surgery, Preventive Medicine, Psychiatry and Neurology, Radiology, Surgery, Thoracic Surgery, and Urology.

Physicians who specialize in fields such as surgery, obstetrics and gynecology, and radiology generally earn greater incomes than nonspecialists, and recipients of such care benefit from the specialized knowledge of experts who continue to learn about treatments for specific diseases. On the downside, specialization adds to the cost of medical care.

SEE ALSO American Medical Association (1847), Halstedian Surgery (1904), and Flexner Report and Medical Education (1910).

Medical specialization began on a large scale in the great hospitals of Paris in the 1830s. Pictured here is Jean-Martin Charcot (1825–1893), one of the founders of modern neurology, with a "hysterical" patient at the Pitié-Salpêtrière Hospital, in an1887 painting by Pierre-André Brouille (1857–1914).

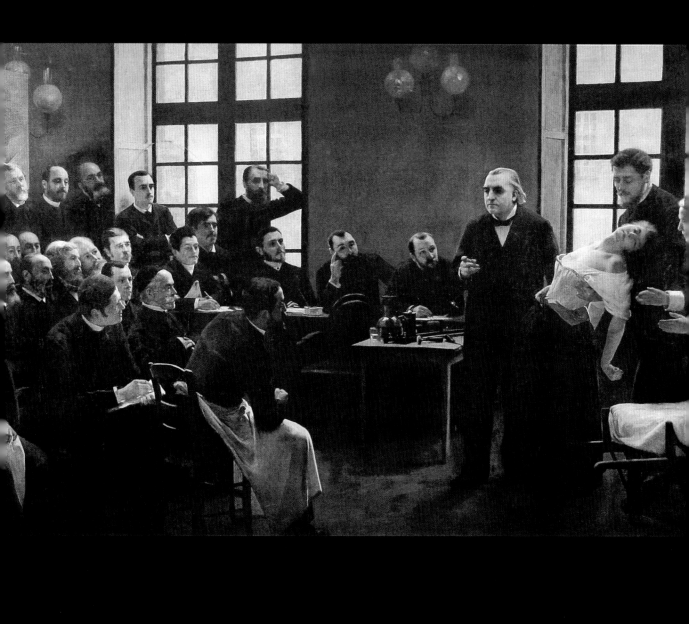

Anatomy Act of 1832

William Harvey (1578–1657), William Burke (1792–1829)

During the European Renaissance, scholars came to believe that dissection of human bodies was essential for furthering medical knowledge, and that simply relying on ancient medical texts was insufficient. In the sixteenth and seventeenth centuries, Italy led the world in anatomical learning. However, by the 1800s, London and Edinburgh were among the "hot spots" for anatomical and medical breakthroughs.

In order to become seasoned dissectors and anatomists, surgeons of the time seemed to be able to suppress normal emotional responses for their human brethren. For example, English physician William Harvey, famous for his elucidation of blood circulation, participated in dissections of both his sister and his father. In the early 1800s, the appetite for corpses was so great in England that anatomists frequently collaborated with grave robbers to secure needed specimens. Prior to 1832 in England, only the corpses of executed murderers could be legally used for dissection. The Anatomy Act of 1832, a United Kingdom Act of Parliament, allowed physicians legal access to corpses that relatives did not claim, and it became easy to obtain corpses of poor people who died in workhouses—places where people unable to support themselves often stayed until death.

The Anatomy Act was motivated by the need for corpses to study and the growing anger at the "resurrectionists" who robbed graves for medical study. Also, the passage of the act was accelerated by the 1828 murders in Edinburgh by William Burke and William Hare, who strangled at least 16 live victims and then sold their corpses to anatomists.

After the Anatomy Act passed, riots broke out, and some medical school buildings were damaged. Many citizens felt that it was unfair to the poor, whose corpses were used without their consent. Before the act passed, dissection was a punishment for murderers, but it now seemed to be a punishment for poverty. Some religious individuals, who felt that the body should not be desecrated, buried loved ones in lead coffins to protect them until resurrection on Judgment Day.

SEE ALSO Leonardo's Anatomical Drawings (1510), *De Humani Corporis Fabrica* (1543), Eustachi's Rescued Masterpieces (1552), Drawings of Pietro da Cortona (1618), Circulatory System (1628), Cheselden's *Osteographia* (1733), Albinus's *Tables of the Human Body* (1747), Autopsy (1761), Hunter's *Gravid Uterus* (1774), and *Gray's Anatomy* (1858).

The Anatomy Act was motivated by the need for skeletons and cadavers and the growing anger at "resurrectionists," who robbed graves for medical study.

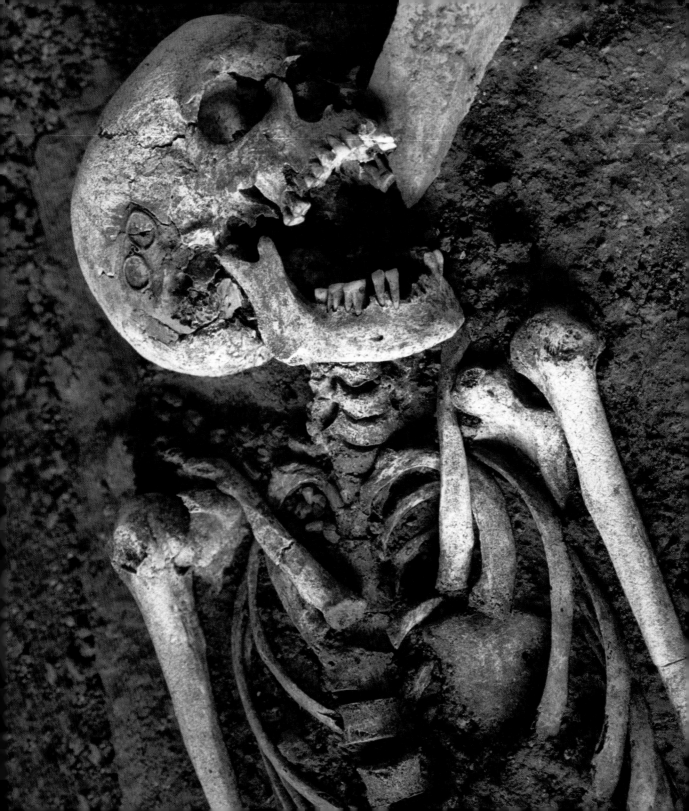

Intravenous Saline Solutions

Thomas Aitchison Latta (1790–1833), William Brooke O'Shaughnessy (1808–1889)

In 1832, the physician Thomas Latta of Leith, Scotland, became one of the first physicians to carry out intravenous ("into the vein") injections of saline solutions (salt water created with sodium chloride) in his attempts to save people suffering from dehydration due to cholera. Today, we know that cholera is caused by a bacterium, and the resulting severe diarrhea has killed many millions of people over the centuries. Latta's treatments were stimulated by Irish physician William O'Shaughnessy, who had suggested similar treatments for cholera patients.

Latta's first patient was an elderly woman who had "apparently reached the last moments of her earthly existence." Latta inserted a tube into a large vein in her upper arm and slowly injected saline solution. After some time, she began to breathe easier and "soon her sunken eyes, and fallen jaw, pale and cold, bearing the manifest imprint of death's signet, began to glow with returning animation; the pulse returned to the wrist." Within 30 minutes, after six pints of fluid had been injected, the woman said that she was "free from all uneasiness." Her arms and legs were warm. Latta felt that she was on the road to recovery and let a **hospital** surgeon take care of her. While Latta was away, the woman returned to vomiting and died within five hours. Latta suggested that she might have lived if the injections were continued. These kinds of saline injections were repeated on other patients, with a mixture of success and failure.

Alas, Latta died a year later, and his work was largely forgotten. Although Latta's ideas were mostly sound, success was probably hampered because of the lack of sterile procedures and because the injections were tried only on patients close to death and were not repeated sufficiently to replace fluids.

Today, intravenous saline solutions can save lives, and they are used to replace water and salt lost because of a person's inadequate fluid intake, trauma leading to bleeding, and illnesses such as cholera or norovirus infections, which cause dehydration through diarrhea and vomiting.

SEE ALSO Blood Transfusion (1829), Hypodermic Syringe (1853), and Broad Street Pump Handle (1854).

Thanks to Thomas Latta and other pioneering physicians, intravenous saline solutions saved lives of people afflicted with cholera. Shown here is a World War I poster from 1918, by American illustrator Boardman Robinson (1876–1952).

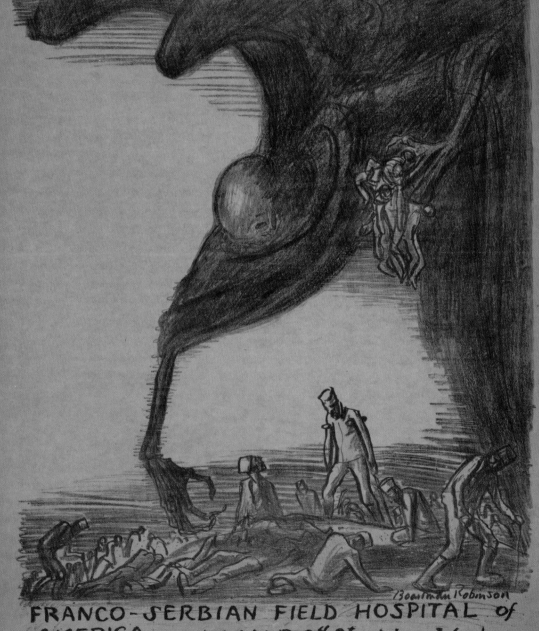

Observations of St. Martin's Stomach

William Hunter (1718–1783), **William Beaumont** (1785–1853), **Alexis St. Martin** (1794–1880)

For millennia, digestive processes and stomach functioning were mysteries. The great Scottish anatomist and physician William Hunter lamented, "Some . . . will have it that the stomach is a mill, others that it is a fermenting vat, others again that it is a stew pan."

One important episode in our understanding of the stomach occurred through sheer luck—when Alexis St. Martin, an employee of the American Fur Company, was accidentally shot in the stomach. The U.S. Army surgeon William Beaumont treated St. Martin, who survived with a permanent hole, or fistula, in his stomach, which allowed Beaumont to make many pioneering observations of the stomach in action. After St. Martin recovered, Beaumont hired him as a handyman so that he could continue his experiments on him. For example, Beaumont tied pieces of food to strings, inserted them into the stomach through the hole, and periodically removed the food to study the degree of digestion that had taken place. Beaumont also studied the effects of exercise, temperature, and even emotions on digestion. His experiments were published in 1833 in his book *Experiments and Observations on the Gastric Juice and the Physiology of Digestion*.

After St. Martin's death—58 years after his accident—family members were so determined to avoid further scrutiny by physicians that they intentionally let his body decompose before burial in a deep, unmarked grave. Beaumont is notable in that he pursued his careful study of digestion even while at an aging military **hospital** in the small frontier outpost of Prairie du Chien, Wisconsin. His research definitively established that digestion relied strongly on a chemical process, and he was the first American to become internationally recognized for physiological research.

Today, we understand that the stomach releases proteases—protein-digesting enzymes such as pepsin—along with hydrochloric acid, which destroys many bacteria and provides the acidic environment to facilitate the action of the proteases. The muscles of the stomach also churn the food. Various digestive-system hormones control the stomach secretions and movements.

SEE ALSO Brunner's Glands (1679) and Peptic Ulcers and Bacteria (1984).

Diagram of the stomach from the classic work Gray's Anatomy *(1918 edition), by Henry Gray. Also indicated is the celiac artery, the first major branch of the abdominal aorta, which supplies blood to the liver, stomach, and other organs.*

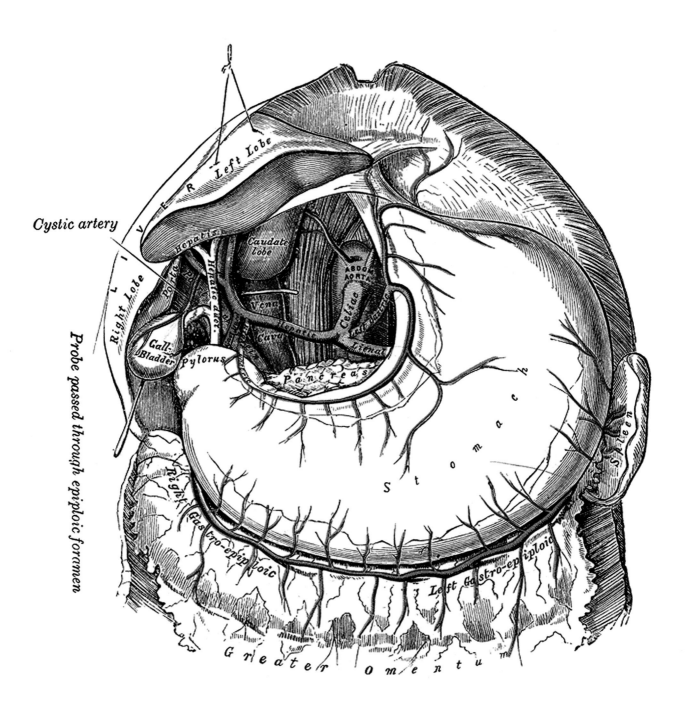

Cystic artery

Probe passed through epiploic foramen

L I V E R Left Lobe

Right Lobe

Hepatic Artery

Porta

Hepatic duct

Caudate Lobe

ABDOM AORTA

Vena

Hepatic

Cava

Celiac

Renal

Gall-Bladder

Pylorus

Pancreas

S t o m a c h

Spleen

Right Gastro-epiploic

Left Gastro-epiploic

G r e a t e r   o m e n t u m

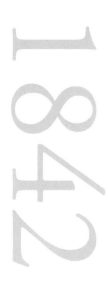

General Anesthesia

Frances Burney (1752–1840), **Johann Friedrich Dieffenbach** (1795–1847), **Crawford Williamson Long** (1815–1878), **Horace Wells** (1815–1848), **William Thomas Green Morton** (1819–1868)

In our modern world, we are likely to forget the horrifying realities of surgery before anesthesia. Fanny Burney, a famous nineteenth-century novelist and playwright, recounts the mastectomy she endured with only a glass of wine for the pain. Seven males held her down as the surgery began. She writes, "When the dreadful steel was plunged into the breast—cutting through veins-arteries-flesh-nerves—I needed no injunction not to restrain my cries. I began a scream that lasted unintermittently during the whole time of the incision. . . . Oh Heaven!—I then felt the knife racking against the breast bone—scraping it! This was performed while I yet remained in utterly speechless torture."

General anesthesia is a state of unconsciousness induced by drugs, allowing a patient to undergo surgery without pain. Early forms of anesthesia date back to prehistoric times in the form of opium. Inca shamans used coca leaves to locally numb a site on the body. However, the discovery of general anesthesia suitable for modern operations is often attributed to three Americans: physician Crawford W. Long and dentists Horace Wells and William Morton. In 1842, Long removed a neck cyst while the patient inhaled ether, an anesthetic gas. In 1844, Wells extracted many teeth using nitrous oxide, commonly known as laughing gas. Morton is famous for his public demonstration of the use of ether in 1846 to assist a surgeon in removing a tumor from a patient's jaw, and newspapers carried the story. In 1847, chloroform was also used, but it had higher risks than ether. Safer and more effective drugs are used today.

After Morton's demonstrations, the use of anesthetics began to spread rapidly. In 1847, Johann Friedrich Dieffenbach, a pioneer in plastic surgery, wrote, "The wonderful dream that pain has been taken away from us has become reality. Pain, the highest consciousness of our earthly existence, the most distinct sensation of the imperfection of our body, must now bow before the power of the human mind, before the power of ether vapor."

SEE ALSO Snow Anesthesia (1812) and Cocaine as Local Anesthetic (1884).

Three medical gases on a surgical room machine. Nitrous oxide (N_2O) is sometimes used as a carrier gas in a 2:1 ratio with oxygen for more powerful general anesthesia drugs, such as desflurane or sevoflurane.

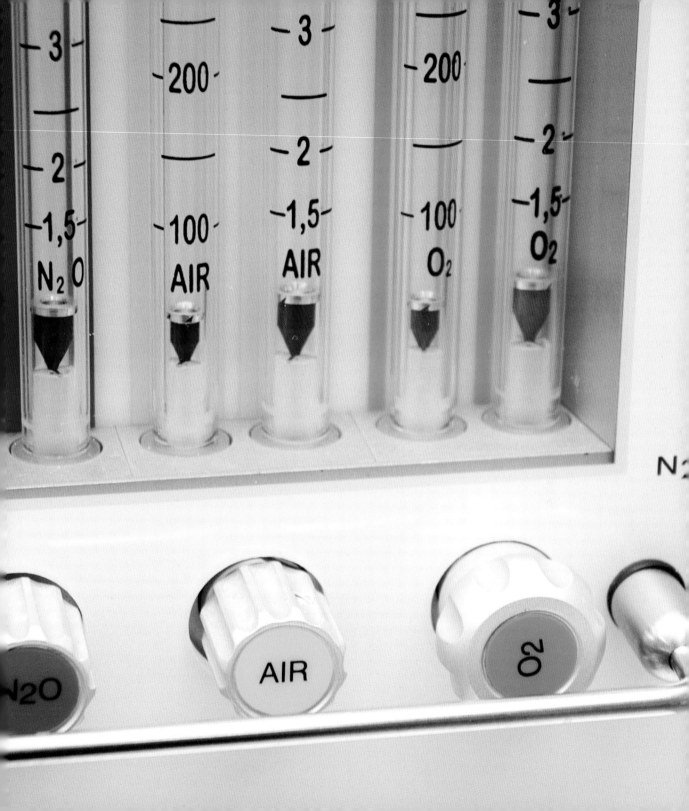

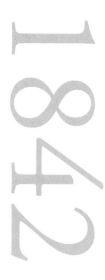

The Sanitary Condition of the Labouring Population of Great Britain

Sir Edwin Chadwick (1800–1890), **Charles-Edward Amory Winslow** (1877–1957)

In 1920, Charles-Edward Winslow, an American bacteriologist and public health expert, defined public health as "the science and art of preventing disease, prolonging life and promoting health through the organized efforts and informed choices of society, organizations (public and private), communities, and individuals." For example, over the years, public health officials have focused on preventing diseases through vaccination, hand washing, the building of sewers, the **chlorination of water**, and garbage collection. During the 1900s, public health initiatives significantly improved average life expectancy in many nations.

One early influential advocate of public health in the West was the English social reformer Edwin Chadwick, who published, at his own expense, *The Sanitary Condition of the Labouring Population of Great Britain* in 1842. In this document, Chadwick wrote, "The annual loss of life from filth and bad ventilation is greater than the loss from death or wounds in any wars in which the country has been engaged in modern times." He also noted that the average age of death in the laboring populations that lived in squalid, overcrowded conditions was often less than half that of professional men.

Chadwick was the primary architect of sanitary reform in Britain, and he requested that the government invest in measures that were desperately needed to improve drainage, housing conditions, and the water supply in order to prevent early deaths of working men, while also fostering economic growth. In 1848, Parliament passed a Public Health Act that provided for the formation of a Central Board of Health, which created local boards to facilitate street cleaning, garbage collection, and sewage removal. Chadwick also advocated for removal of storm water and sewage through the use of separate systems.

Chadwick faced initial resistance from individuals who wanted neither a centralized government nor the cost of his public-works projects. Some even believed that the health of the poor was primarily a matter of fate or lax moral habits rather than from environmental causes that could be addressed.

SEE ALSO Sewage Systems (600 B.C.), Semmelweis's Hand Washing (1847), Broad Street Pump Handle (1854), Meat Inspection Act of 1906 (1906), Imprisonment of Typhoid Mary (1907), and Chlorination of Water (1910).

Modern water treatment plants may use circular clarifiers to remove suspended solids. This improves water safety because germs and toxic material can adhere to particles. Sludge scrapers, attached to a rotating arm, can scrape the sludge toward a central hopper.

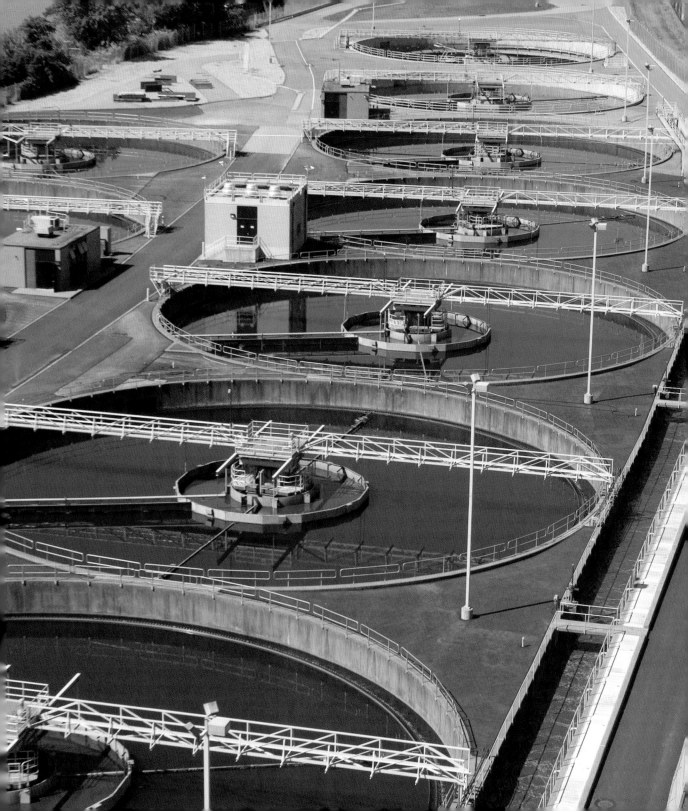

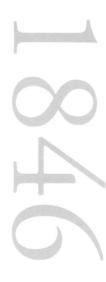

Panum's "Measles on the Faroe Islands"

Abu 'Ali al-Husayn ibn 'Abd-Allah Ibn Sina (Avicenna) (980–1037),
William Budd (1811–1880), John Snow (1813–1858), Peter Ludvig Panum
(1820–1885)

Long before the actual causes of diseases were understood in terms of bacteria and other microorganisms, the field of epidemiology had its early beginnings. Epidemiology is the study of factors that affect the health of populations. For example, the Persian physician Avicenna discussed in *The Canon of Medicine* (c. 1025) the contagious spreading of sexually transmitted diseases and tuberculosis, as well as the utility of quarantine to limit the spread of certain diseases. Among the most famous epidemiologists of the 1800s were Danish physiologist Peter Panum (who studied the spread of measles), John Snow (the spread of cholera), and English physician William Budd (the spread of typhoid fever).

Panum's study was of paramount importance, being among the first extensive contributions to the modern field of epidemiology. In 1846, the Danish government asked 26-year-old Panum to study the spread of measles in the Faroe Islands, located in the mists of the North Atlantic Ocean. Today, measles (characterized in part by a skin rash) is preventable by vaccinations, but in Panum's time it was often deadly. In 1846, measles had not caused death in the Faroe Islands for 65 years, but suddenly more than 6,000 of the 7,782 inhabitants fell victim to measles. Coastal valleys separated the various populations of the islands, so the history of the disease in each small settlement could be studied in isolation from those in the others. By studying the various villages, Panum determined that the incubation period for measles was about two weeks. He also supplied evidence of long-lasting immunity by interviewing old people who had been infected many years earlier, none of whom contracted measles in 1846. Panum was convinced that measles was spread by infectious agents via contaminated articles or by close human contact.

Panum's prominent place in the history of medicine rests upon his meticulous field studies, "Observations Made During the Epidemic of Measles on the Faroe Islands in 1846," which was an early seed in the nascent field of epidemiology.

SEE ALSO Avicenna's *Canon of Medicine* (1025), *The Sanitary Condition of the Labouring Population of Great Britain* (1842), Broad Street Pump Handle (1854), Germ Theory of Disease (1862), Cause of Bubonic Plague (1894), and Imprisonment of Typhoid Mary (1907).

One of the many natural harbors in the Faroe Islands. The populations of the islands were separated by coastal valleys, creating isolated communities in which the history of measles could be studied.

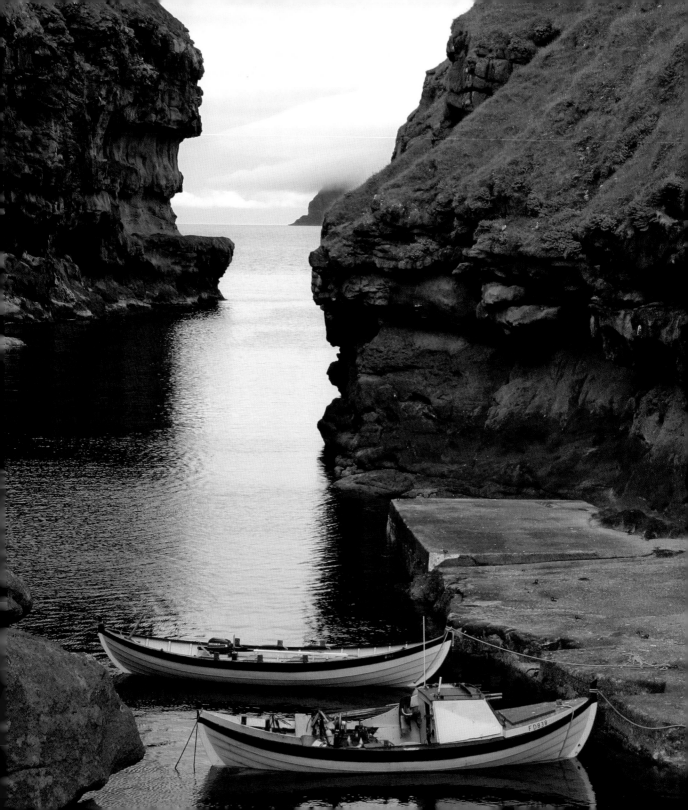

Spirometry

John Hutchinson (1811–1861)

There's an old Sanskrit proverb much adored by modern-day meditators: "For breath is life, and if you breathe well you will live long on earth." Similarly, scientists have long been intrigued with measuring respiration and lung capacity to assess human health. In 1846, British surgeon John Hutchinson, who was interested in diagnosing tuberculosis, published an article on the lung capacity of more than 2,000 individuals, and he came to the conclusion that the volume of air that can be forcibly exhaled from fully inflated lungs is a useful indicator of risk of premature death (a finding confirmed in numerous modern studies). He also found that lung capacity generally diminishes with age in adults.

In order to make measurements, Hutchinson invented a spirometer that made use of a calibrated bell shape submerged in water that captured air exhaled into a tube. He assessed a wide variety of subjects, ranging from wrestlers and dwarfs to corpses. He tested the corpses using bellows to force as much air as possible into the lungs and then measured the volume of air expelled during the elastic recoil of the lungs and chest.

Today, physicians use modern versions of the Hutchinson spirometer to measure lung function and test the volume and speed of air that can be exhaled after a subject takes the deepest possible breath and exhales as hard as possible. Graphical traces of exhaled air volume through time (e.g., forced exhalation for a period of six seconds) are helpful in assessing conditions such as lung **cancer**, heart attack, COPD (chronic obstructive pulmonary disease, in which the airways become narrowed, for example, as a result of chronic bronchitis and emphysema), asthma, cystic fibrosis (associated with lung disease resulting from mucus-clogging of the airways), and pulmonary fibrosis (formation of excess fibrous connective tissue in the lungs).

Hutchinson was not the first to study human lung capacity, but his thousands of clinical measurements made with his new device justify his being considered the inventor of spirometry.

SEE ALSO Lavoisier's Respiration (1784), Stethoscope (1816), Iron Lung (1928), Tobacco Smoking and Cancer (1951), Heart-Lung Machine (1953), and Lung Transplant (1963).

An "incentive" spirometer, used to encourage deep breathing after major surgery. Using the device, a patient attempts to breathe as deeply as possible and assesses progress by examining the gauge.

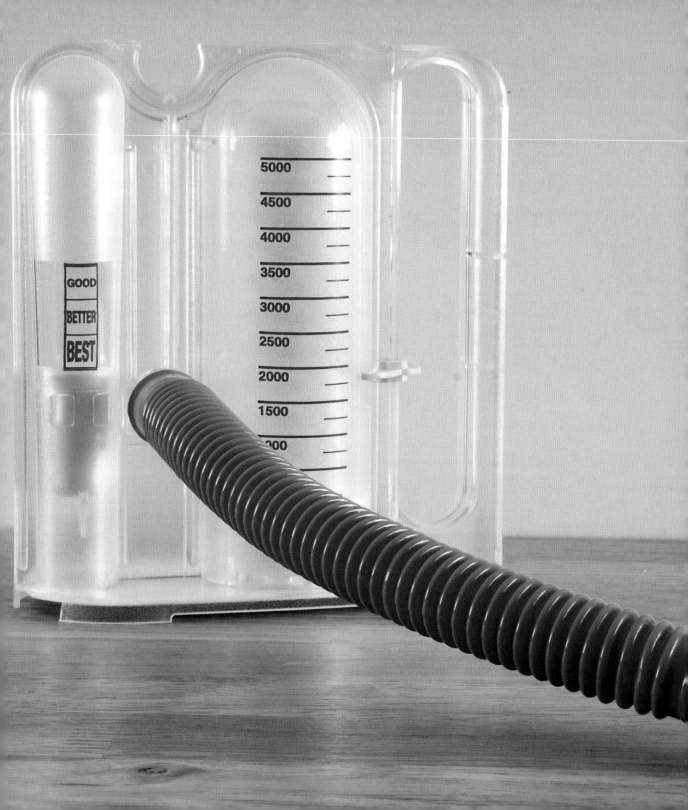

American Medical Association

Nathan Smith Davis Sr. (1817–1904)

The American Medical Association (AMA), founded in 1847, is the largest and oldest association of physicians and medical students in the United States. The AMA also publishes the prestigious *Journal of the American Medical Association (JAMA)*, established in 1883. New York physician Nathan Davis was instrumental in establishing the AMA and was the first editor of *JAMA*.

The AMA arose during a time when some physicians grew concerned with the varying quality of medical education in America, which was not regulated on a national level (see entry "**Flexner Report and Medical Education**"). In addition to raising medical education standards, the AMA also combated medical fraud, unscientific practices, and the ubiquitous **patent medicines** that were sold with infective or dangerous secret ingredients. The AMA also encouraged the sharing of information in order to raise the standards of medical training. In 1848, the AMA recommended that medical colleges and **hospitals** cooperate to provide students with greater experience. Today, it publishes a list of Physician Specialty Codes that provide a standard in the United States for identifying physician specialties.

Since its inception, the AMA has played a prominent role in public health policy. In 1920, the association condemned any national health insurance policy, fearing that the government would interfere with the doctor-patient relationship and that physicians would not be fairly compensated for their treatments if a compulsory insurance system were established. In 1936, the AMA recommended enriching milk with vitamin D and suggested that salt be iodized to prevent hypothyroid disease. Later, it promoted **fluoridation** of drinking water and encouraged the use of the Sabin oral vaccine against polio. The AMA supported the passage of vehicle seatbelt laws and suggested that alcoholism be treated as an illness. Starting around 1985, it called for limits on tobacco advertising and supported laws that banned smoking on public transportation. The AMA has also supported changes in medical malpractice laws to limit damage awards and has condemned physician-assisted suicides.

SEE ALSO Medical Specialization (1830), Health Insurance (1883), Patent Medicines (1906), Flexner Report and Medical Education (1910), Fluoridated Toothpaste (1914), Banishing Rickets (1922), Tobacco Smoking and Cancer (1951), and Polio Vaccine (1955).

In 1849, the AMA established a board to analyze possible quack remedies, such as this "snake oil" for "man and beast," and to educate the public about possible dangers of such remedies.

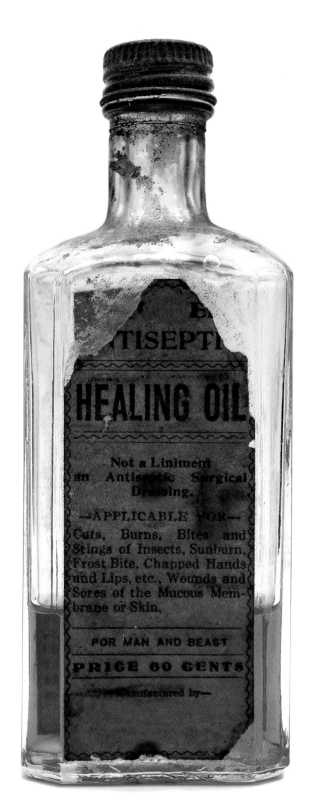

1847

Semmelweis's Hand Washing

Ignaz Philipp Semmelweis (1818–1865), **Louis Pasteur** (1822–1895), **Sir Joseph Lister** (1827–1912)

Authors K. Codell Carter and Barbara Carter write, "Medical advances are purchased by two kinds of sacrifice: the sacrifice of researchers trying to understand disease and the sacrifice of patients who die or are killed in the process. [One] particular advance was purchased, in part, by the sacrifice of hundreds of thousands of young women who died, following childbirth, of a terrible disease known as childbed fever—a disease that was rampant in the charity maternity clinics of the early nineteenth century."

Although several physicians had suggested the value of cleanliness in preventing infection even before microorganisms were discovered as causes of disease, the individual most famous for early systematic studies of disinfection was the Hungarian obstetrician Ignaz Semmelweis. Semmelweis noticed that the Vienna **hospital** in which he worked had a much higher rate of maternal mortality due to childbed fever than a similar hospital. He also noted that only in his hospital did physicians routinely study cadavers before examining patients.

Childbed fever, also known as puerperal fever, is a form of bacteria-caused sepsis informally referred to as blood poisoning. Semmelweis also noticed that puerperal fever was rare among women who gave birth in the streets, and he surmised that infectious substances (e.g., particles of some kind) were being passed from cadavers to the women. After instructing hospital staff to always wash their hands in a chlorinated disinfecting solution before treating women, the number of deaths plummeted dramatically.

Alas, despite his amazing results, many of the physicians of the time did not accept his findings, perhaps in part because this would have been admitting that they were the unwitting cause of so much death. Additionally, many physicians of the time blamed such diseases on miasma, a kind of toxic atmosphere. In the end, Semmelweis went mad and was involuntarily confined to an insane asylum, where he was beaten to death by guards. After his death, however, he was vindicated by the germ studies of French microbiologist Louis Pasteur and innovations in **antiseptic** surgery by British surgeon Joseph Lister.

SEE ALSO Sewage Systems (600 B.C.), *The Sanitary Condition of the Labouring Population of Great Britain* (1842), Broad Street Pump Handle (1854), Germ Theory of Disease (1862), Antiseptics (1865), Latex Surgical Gloves (1890), and Chlorination of Water (1910).

Today, when surgeons scrub their hands before an operation, it is common to use a sterile brush, chlorhexidine or iodine wash, and a tap that can be turned on and off without hand intervention.

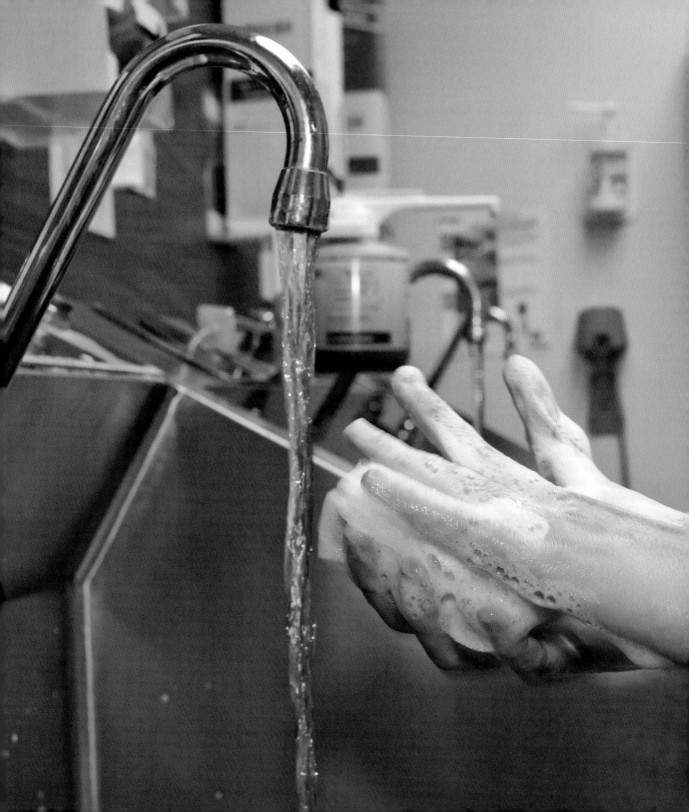

Appendectomy

Claudius Aymand (1660–1740), **Henry Hancock** (1809–1880)

According to medical journalist Naomi Craft, "Although appendicitis was first described in the sixteenth century, having been identified during postmortem examinations, it was not until two centuries later that doctors learned how to correctly diagnose it in a living patient. Remedies have varied from treatment with **leeches, bloodletting**, and enemas to constant horseback riding or laying a newly killed and cut-open puppy across the patient. Not surprisingly, patients in such cases usually died."

The vermiform appendix is the wormlike closed tube that is attached to the large intestine near the junction between the large and small intestines. Appendicitis, an inflammation of the appendix, causes severe abdominal pain; if left untreated, the appendix can rupture, spread infection, and cause death. An appendectomy is the surgical removal of the appendix, usually to cure appendicitis. Appendicitis may result from an obstruction within the appendix, causing the appendix to become filled with mucus. In addition to pain in the lower right of the body, the patient may exhibit an elevated white blood cell count.

In 1735, French surgeon Claudius Aymand performed the first recorded successful appendectomy on an eleven-year-old boy who had an inguinal hernia. Once Aymand was looking inside the boy, he noticed the inflamed appendix. The boy was fully conscious during the surgery and made a full recovery. English surgeon Henry Hancock is credited with being the first to intentionally operate on a patient with appendicitis and successfully remove an appendix. In 1848, he used chloroform **anesthesia** during the operation on the thirty-year-old woman, and he recommended surgery for all early-stage cases of appendicitis. In 1961, a Soviet surgeon had to remove his own appendix while in Antarctica.

Today, the appendix can be removed by cutting open the abdominal wall or through **laparoscopic surgery** using a snakelike tube inserted through small holes into the body. It is thought that the appendix may harbor bacteria that are beneficial for the function of the large intestine. Additionally, the appendix contains infection-fighting lymphoid cells, suggesting it may aid in the body's immune functioning.

SEE ALSO Zoo Within Us (1683), Salpingectomy (1883), Self-Surgery (1961), Laparoscopic Surgery (1981), and Small Bowel Transplant (1987).

Schematic representation of the wormlike appendix, pointing downward from the large intestine (lower left).

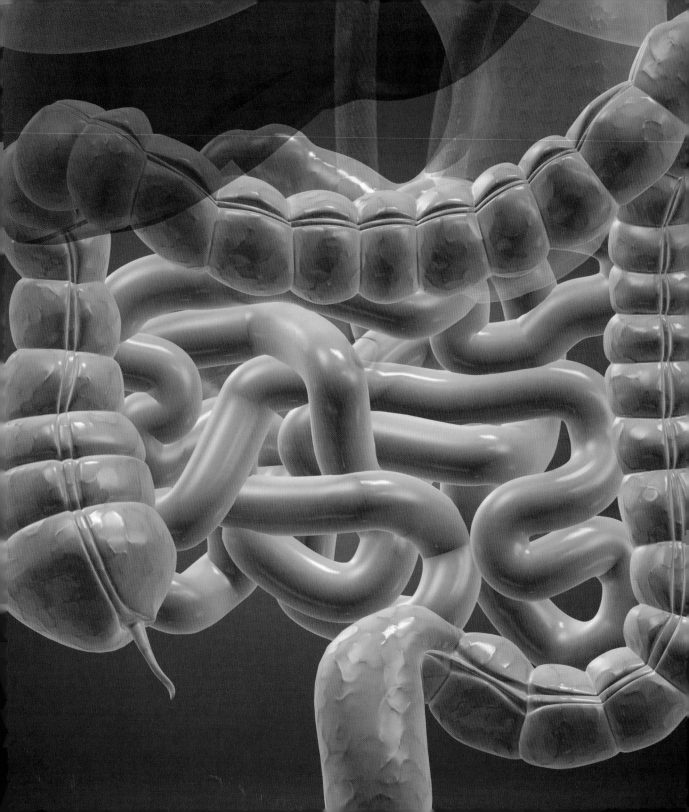

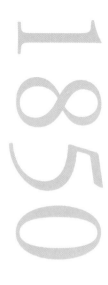

Ophthalmoscope

Hermann Ludwig Ferdinand von Helmholtz (1821–1894), **Friedrich Wilhelm Ernst Albrecht von Graefe** (1828–1870)

In 1850, German physician and physicist Hermann von Helmholtz created an ophthalmoscope—a device that enables physicians to view the back of the interior of the eye, including the retina, along with the vitreous humor, which is the clear gel that fills much of the eyeball. American ophthalmologist Edward Loring wrote in the opening of his *Text-Book of Ophthalmology* in 1892, two years before the death of Hermann von Helmholtz, "In the whole history of medicine, there is no more beautiful episode than the invention of the ophthalmoscope, and physiology has few greater triumphs."

Using simple optical principles, von Helmholtz understood that in order to optimally see into a patient's eye, he needed to shine a light into the eye and position his own eye along the path in which light rays entered and reflected from the patient's eye. To accomplish this, he positioned a lamp at his side and faced the patient. Next, a set of glass plates, positioned between himself and the patient, acted as a partial mirror and reflected the light into the patient's eye while also allowing reflected light from the patient's eye to pass through the glass to von Helmholtz's eye. Finally, he added a concave lens to better focus the light so that he could clearly see the retina, with all of its intricate structures and blood vessels. Not only did this provide information about the eye's health, but it also provided clues as to the state of the blood vessels in general. Since von Helmholtz's time, ophthalmoscopes have become more sophisticated, with electric-light sources and various focusing lenses.

According to the physician John Gray, when the pioneering German ophthalmologist Albrecht von Graefe first peered inside "the living eye, with its optic disc and blood vessels, his face flushed with excitement, and he cried, 'Helmholtz has unfolded to us a new world! What remains to be discovered!'"

SEE ALSO Glass Eye (2800 B.C.), Eye Surgery (600 B.C.), Eyeglasses (1284), Sphygmomanometer (1881), and Corneal Transplant (1905).

An ophthalmogram, an image of the eye's fundus (the interior surface of the back of the eye) that includes the retina (light-sensitive tissue). The optic disc is the bright red and yellow area and the region where the optic nerve connects to the retina.

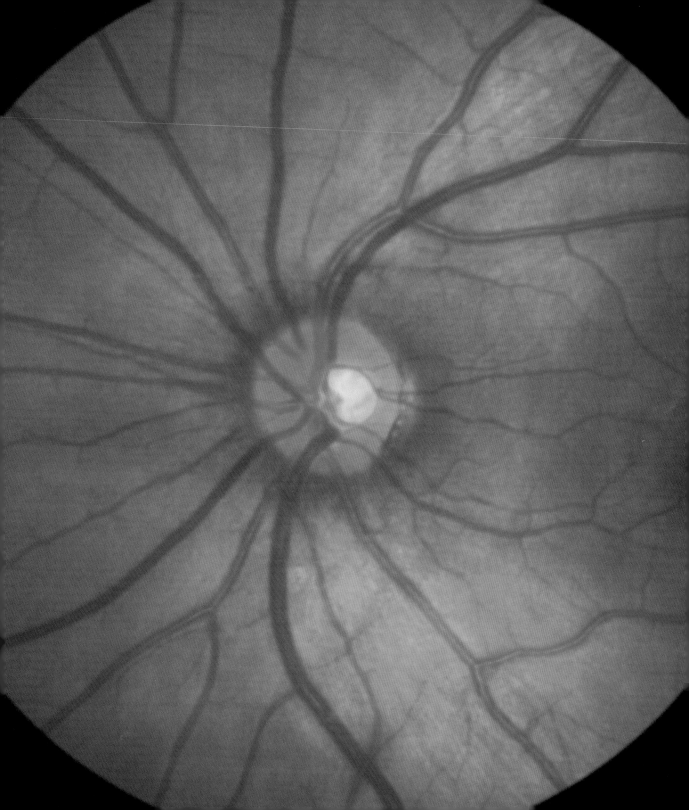

Plaster of Paris Casts

Antonius Mathijsen (1805–1878), **Nikolay Ivanovich Pirogov** (1810–1881)

In the best-selling novel *Harry Potter and the Sorcerer's Stone*, Madam Pomfrey, a magical healer who is in charge of the Hogwarts hospital wing, uses a bone-healing spell that almost instantly binds and repairs broken bones in a student's wrist. If only it were this easy for ordinary folk to heal bone fractures!

For thousands of years, healers have attempted to stabilize limbs to allow bones to rejoin after a break. For example, the ancient Egyptians used wooden splints wrapped in linen. Ancient Hindus used bamboo splints, and ancient Arabian physicians combined lime (from seashells) and egg whites to stiffen bandages. In medieval Europe, broken bones were sometimes treated by people known as bonesetters, who repositioned broken bones with their hands, often had no formal medical training, and were often veterinarians or blacksmiths.

A great advance in bone healing was made in 1851 when Dutch army surgeon Antonius Mathijsen used plaster of Paris to stabilize broken bones. Plaster of Paris, with the chemical name calcium sulfate hemihydrate, can be created by heating gypsum, a soft mineral. Plaster of Paris is named after the large gypsum deposits near the French capital. When water is added to the resultant powder, heat is generated and a strong material is created. Mathijsen used bandages impregnated with plaster of Paris to form strong casts around limbs. By wetting the bandages and then wrapping them around the affected part, he created a form-fitting rigid "splint" to hold bones in place as they healed. Russian physician Nikolay Pirogov was aware of Mathijsen's work and was first to use plaster of Paris casts to treat mass casualties during the Crimean War (1853–1856). Pirogov soaked coarse cloths in plaster of Paris just before application to limbs.

Plaster of Paris casts were commonly used until around the early 1980s, when lighter fiberglass casts replaced them in developed nations. The actual healing of the bone fracture involves cells known as fibroblasts (for collagen creation), chondroblasts (for cartilage creation), and osteoblasts (for bone creation).

SEE ALSO Edwin Smith Surgical Papyrus (1600 B.C.), Band-Aid Bandage (1920), Banishing Rickets (1922), Bone Marrow Transplant (1956), and Hip Replacement (1958).

Casts are applied to a patient from the 163rd Infantry, a casualty of a Japanese landmine explosion during World War II. The orthopedic table is made from a Japanese pipe, ammunition rods, and a piece from the windshield of a jeep.

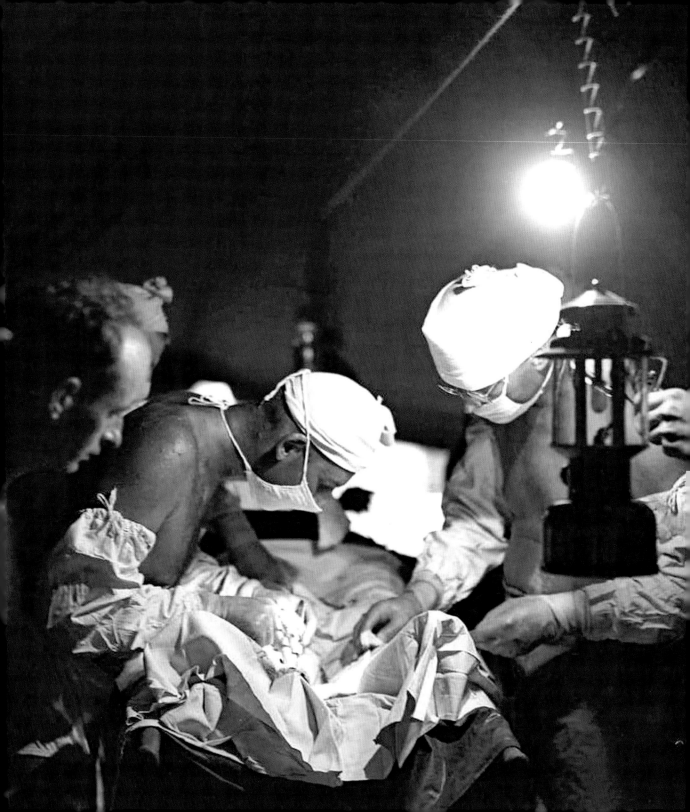

Hypodermic Syringe

Charles Gabriel Pravaz (1791–1853), Alexander Wood (1817–1884), William Stewart Halsted (1852–1922)

A syringe consists of a piston in a cylinder. When the piston is raised or lowered, liquid flows in and out of the syringe. Before the hypodermic (hollow) needle was invented, syringes could still be used to inject fluids into natural openings of the body or into openings cut by physicians. *Hypo* is Greek for "under," and "dermic" refers to skin. The Muslim surgeon Ammar ibn Ali of Mosul (c. 1000 A.D.) used a syringe and suction to extract soft cataracts from the eye.

In 1853, the French surgeon Charles Pravaz was among the first to use a hypodermic syringe with a hollow needle sufficiently fine to pierce the skin for injections. This instrument was made of silver and expelled liquid using a screwlike mechanism rather than the plunger we are familiar with today.

The Scottish physician Alexander Wood developed a similar instrument and was the first to inject a patient with the painkiller morphine. Ironically, Wood's wife, the first known intravenous morphine addict, died from an overdose delivered by her husband's invention. The use of injected morphine spread among the rich, and jeweled syringe cases were manufactured so that sophisticated ladies might carry their adored devices with them.

Despite the countless number of drug addicts through time, the syringe became an astounding medical breakthrough. Physicians can inject **anesthetics** and vaccines. Dentists inject anesthetics for dental procedures. Syringes with short needles are used to inject insulin. Today, hypodermic needles are disposable, thus avoiding the need to sterilize them for subsequent use.

The American surgeon William Halsted was among the first to use syringes to block nerves, for example, during inguinal hernia operations. During 1885 and 1886, he performed more than 2,000 different surgical interventions using regional anesthesia. Authors A. Martin Duce and F. Lopez Hernández write, "Halsted's discovery became a crucial turning point in the field of surgery. Most of all, it freed patients from pain during surgical intervention and allowed surgeons to explore techniques beyond the threshold of human endurance."

SEE ALSO Eye Surgery (600 B.C.), Abortion (70), Intravenous Saline Solutions (1832), and Cocaine as Local Anesthetic (1884).

A hypodermic syringe. Movement of the piston causes liquid to flow into or out of the syringe.

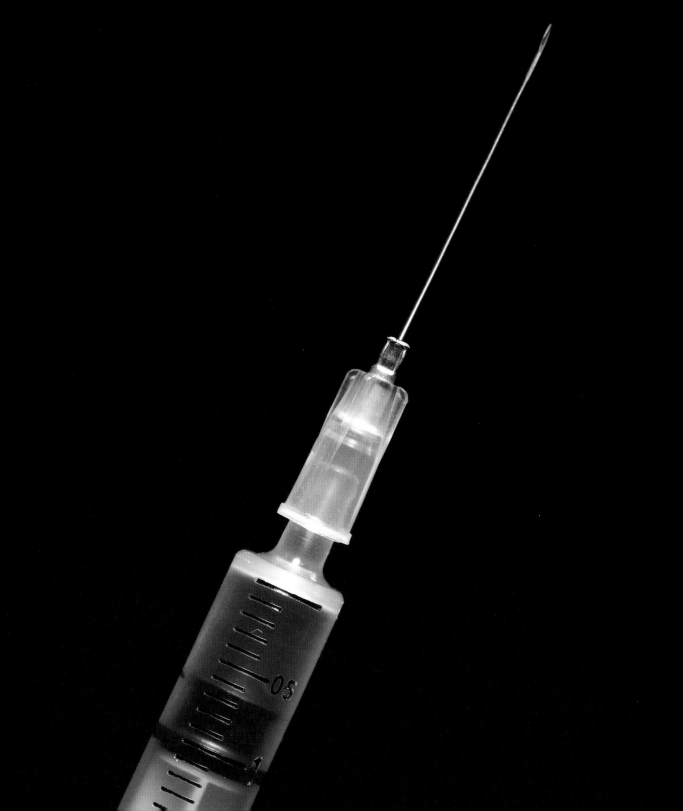

Broad Street Pump Handle

John Snow (1813–1858)

"A new and terrifying disease struck England in October of 1831 and quickly spread across the kingdom," writes science journalist Sharon Guynup. "Over the next two years, thousands died from this mysterious illness, so virulent that a person could be in good health at dawn and be buried at dusk. Citizens lived in terror, sealing their doors and windows at night against the feared 'night air.'"

The disease was cholera, which we today know is caused by the bacterium *Vibrio cholerae*, usually acquired by drinking water or eating food that has been in contact with human feces. The resulting severe diarrhea has killed many millions of people over the centuries.

When the 1854 cholera outbreak struck England, British physician John Snow argued that the disease was not airborne, even though many physicians of the time believed that the disease was contracted by breathing unhealthy air, or miasma. Snow decided to draw a map of the locations of cholera deaths, and he found unusual clusters of high mortality rates. For example, about 500 people died in ten days near the intersection of Broad Street and Cambridge Street, near a particular water source. Before making his map, Snow had already encouraged city officials to remove the water pump handle to disable the Broad Street pump, and cholera cases almost completely disappeared in this area of the city.

Snow, one of the key figures in the history of epidemiology (which includes the study of the spread of diseases), admitted that the epidemic was already declining by the time the pump handle was removed, perhaps partly due to flight of the population after the outbreak. Nevertheless, the removal of the pump handle at Broad Street has become a famous symbol for how simple measures and visionary medical thinking may have a dramatic effect on the spread of diseases. It was later determined that the Broad Street contamination occurred from an old cesspit that leaked fecal bacteria into the well. Snow also compared mortality from cholera among users of two water companies and showed that mortality was 14 times higher among people served by the more impure source.

SEE ALSO Sewage Systems (600 B.C.), Intravenous Saline Solutions (1832), Panum's "Measles on the Faroe Islands" (1846), and Imprisonment of Typhoid Mary (1907).

Once in the small intestine, V. cholerae *bacteria, artistically depicted here, start to produce the flagellin protein that makes flagella, the rotating whiplike tails that propel bacteria through the mucus of the small intestine.*

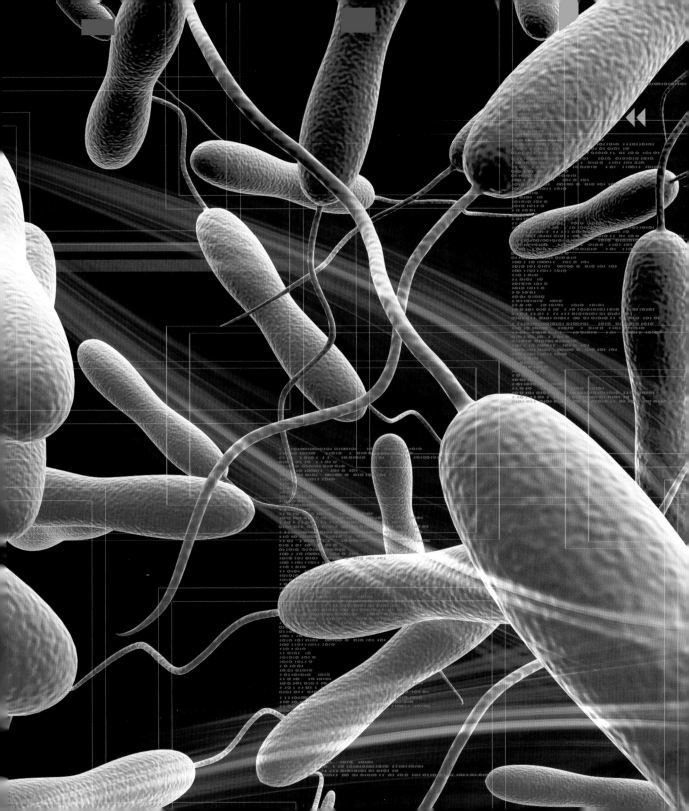

Nursing

Mary Jane Seacole (1805–1881), **Florence Nightingale** (1820–1910), **Clarissa Harlowe "Clara" Barton** (1821–1912), **Clara Louise Maass** (1876–1901), **Margaret Higgins Sanger Slee** (1879–1966), **Helen Fairchild** (1885–1918), **Virginia Henderson** (1897–1996)

According to the respected American nurse Virginia Henderson, "The unique function of the nurse is to assist the individual, sick or well, in the performance of those activities contributing to health or its recovery (or to peaceful death) that he would perform unaided if he had the necessary strength, will, or knowledge." Although the general concept of nurses originated centuries ago, including Catholic monks who cared for the sick during the European Dark Ages, several women have served as symbols for the modern nursing profession.

The English nurse and author Florence Nightingale became well known for her nursing activities during the Crimean War, when, in 1854, she traveled to Turkey, along with 38 women volunteer nurses, to care for wounded British soldiers who suffered in deplorable conditions amid lice, sewage, and rats. She came to realize that poor sanitation was the cause of many deaths and led a campaign for stricter sanitary conditions. In 1860, she laid the foundation for professional nursing with the establishment of her nursing school at St Thomas' Hospital in London.

The Jamaican nurse Mary Seacole is another prominent woman who became concerned about the suffering of soldiers in the Crimea. She journeyed to England with letters of recommendation from physicians in Jamaica and applied to the British War Office for their support in assisting the army in the Crimea. She was continually rejected, partly because of prejudice against mixed-race women. Seacole subsequently funded her own 3,000-mile trek to the Crimea, where she built a hotel in which the wounded could convalesce. Today, nurses practice in settings including homes, **hospitals**, and schools. Nurses also may specialize in fields such as mental health, pediatric nursing, and geriatric nursing. Other icons of American nursing include Clara Barton (founder of the American Red Cross), Margaret Sanger (birth-control activist), Helen Fairchild (who served in the American Expeditionary Force during World War I), and Clara Maass (who gave her life in medical experiments to study **yellow fever**).

SEE ALSO Hospitals (1784), Ambulance (1792), Women Medical Students (1812), *The Sanitary Condition of the Labouring Population of Great Britain* (1842), Red Cross (1863), Modern Midwifery (1925), and Cause of Yellow Fever (1937).

U.S Navy recruiting poster from World War II showing a Navy nurse and a hospital ship, by artist John Falter.

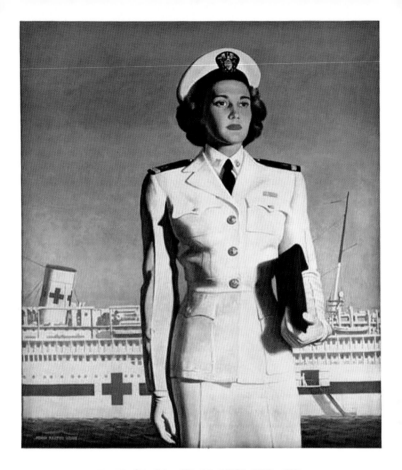

WANTED
MORE NAVY NURSES
Be a commissioned officer in the U. S. Navy

For information write: The Surgeon General, Navy Dept., Washington, D. C.

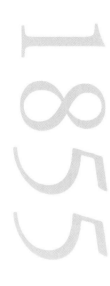

Cell Division

Matthias Jakob Schleiden (1804–1881), Theodor Schwann (1810–1882), Rudolf Ludwig Karl Virchow (1821–1902)

Based on his observations and theories, German physician Rudolf Virchow emphasized that diseases could be studied not only by observing a patient's symptoms but by realizing that all pathology (disease diagnosis) is ultimately a study of cells. Rather than focusing on the entire body, he helped to launch the field of cellular pathology by considering that certain cells or groups of cells can become sick.

In 1855, he popularized the famous aphorism *omnis cellula e cellula*, which means that every cell derives from a preexisting cell. This suggestion was a rejection of the theory of spontaneous generation, which posited that cells and organisms could arise from inanimate matter. Virchow's microscopic studies revealed cells dividing into two equal parts, which contributed to the cell theory, the other tenets of which posited that all living things are made of one cell or more, and that cells are the basic units of life. Other famous contributors to the cell theory were German physiologist Theodor Schwann and German botanist Matthias Jakob Schleiden. One of Virchow's famous phrases was "The task of science is to stake out the limits of the knowable, and to center consciousness within them."

As well as describing cell division, Virchow was the first to accurately identify leukemia cells in blood **cancer**. Despite these accomplishments, he rejected the notion that bacteria can cause disease, as well as the value of cleanliness in preventing infection (see entry "**Semmelweis's Hand Washing**"). He also rejected the **germ theory** of Pasteur, believing that diseased tissues were caused by a malfunctioning of cells and not from an invasion of a foreign microbe.

Science writer John G. Simmons notes, "With the cellular hypothesis, Virchow expanded the research horizons of biochemistry and physiology and had great influence in the broader field of biology, where the cell doctrine eventually evolved in molecular biology, as genetics evolved and reproduction became better understood." Today, we know that cancers result from uncontrolled cell divisions and that skin cells that heal a wound are created from preexisting, dividing skin cells.

SEE ALSO Causes of Cancer (1761), Semmelweis's Hand Washing (1847), Germ Theory of Disease (1862), HeLa Cells (1951), and Oncogenes (1976).

Artistic representation of a zygote after two cell-division steps. The zygote is the initial cell formed when a new organism is produced by the union of a sperm and an egg.

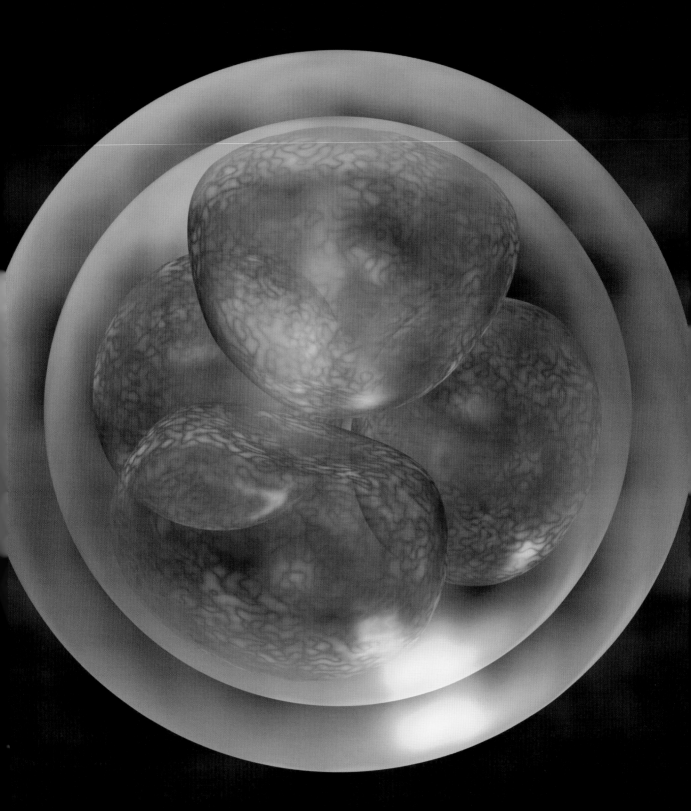

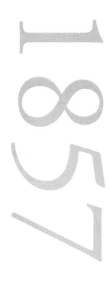

Treatment of Epilepsy

Charles Locock (1799–1875), **Sir Thomas Smith Clouston** (1840–1915)

Epilepsy is a neurological disorder characterized by seizures associated with sudden changes in the electrical activity of the brain that generate unusual movements, behaviors, emotions, and sensations. In ancient cultures, epilepsy was sometimes associated with possession by spirits, attack by demons, witchcraft, or prophetic experiences that were said to place individuals in touch with God.

Today, epilepsy can often be controlled through medication or surgery, such as the removal of a brain lesion that is causing abnormal electrical activity. Certain forms of epilepsy are triggered by external stimuli, such as flashing lights. In severe forms of epilepsy, removal of the cortex of an entire cerebral hemisphere may be the only means of decreasing the frequency and intensity of seizures. Other possible treatments involve electrical devices that stimulate the vagus nerve in the neck or structures deep in the brain.

Genetic mutations have been linked to some forms of epilepsy. Epilepsy may arise from improper brain "wiring" and/or an imbalance in nerve-signaling chemicals. The evaluation and diagnosis of epilepsy makes use of many of the medical scans discussed in this book, including **EEG**, **MRI**, **CAT**, and **PET** scans.

In 1857, British physician Charles Locock observed the anticonvulsant properties of potassium bromide (KBr), a simple salt. He understood that KBr calmed sexual desire and believed (incorrectly) that this was directly related to his successful application of KBr for treating seizures. Around 1868, Scottish psychiatrist Thomas Clouston conducted clinical trials to establish the correct dosage, and he showed that patients had a reduced number of seizures while receiving KBr. By the mid-1870s, more than two and a half tons of KBr were consumed each year at the National **Hospital** in London. Thus, KBr can be regarded as the first effective medicine for epilepsy. A better drug was not found until 1912, when phenobarbital (a barbiturate, or central-nervous-system depressant) was brought to market. KBr is still used to treat epilepsy in dogs and cats—and humans in some countries. Today, more than 20 different drugs are used to treat epilepsy, with varying benefits and side effects.

SEE ALSO Trepanation (6500 B.C.), Neuron Doctrine (1891), Neurotransmitters (1914), Human Electroencephalogram (1924), CAT Scans (1967), Positron Emission Tomography (PET) (1973), and Magnetic Resonance Imaging (MRI) (1977).

Saint Valentine, depicted in a ceiling fresco (1740), Unterleiterbach, Germany. Note the demons fleeing the child, who may have infantile spasm, a form of seizure exhibited in an epilepsy syndrome of infancy.

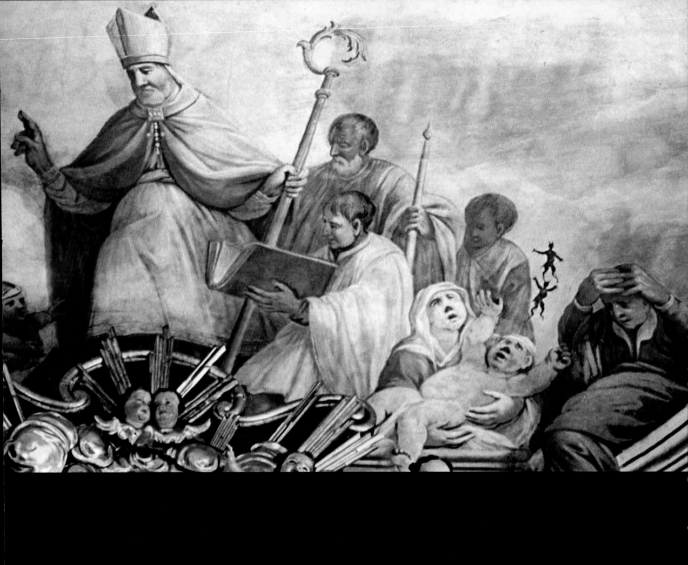

Gray's Anatomy

Henry Gray (1827–1861), Henry Vandyke Carter (1831–1897), Harry Sinclair Lewis (1885–1951)

American author Sinclair Lewis wrote in his 1925 novel *Arrowsmith* that three texts were crucial to a physician's education: the Bible, the works of Shakespeare, and *Gray's Anatomy*. Indeed, no medical book has achieved the fame and longevity of Henry Gray's anatomy text, first published in 1858 under the title *Anatomy: Descriptive and Surgical* and officially abbreviated to *Gray's Anatomy* in 1938.

Gray's Anatomy was published just three years after Gray approached the anatomist and artist Henry Carter to render the exquisite drawings and to perform dissections together. The first color illustrations appeared in the 1887 edition. Although the book was an instant bestseller and the drawings were largely responsible for the fame of *Gray's Anatomy*, Carter never received any royalties. Sadly, Gray contracted smallpox and died at age 34, just prior to the publication of the second edition. The book has since gone through many editions and has never been out of print.

Today's readers should remember that *Gray's Anatomy* was written in a time before **anesthesia** and antibiotics, and before electric lights could illuminate the dissected specimens. Britain's **Anatomy Act of 1832** had allowed physicians legal access to corpses that relatives did not claim, and it became easy to obtain corpses of people who died in public housing for the poor.

Buy yourself an old copy of *Gray's Anatomy*. Examine the illustrations; notice the fine lines re-creating the muscle striations. The names of anatomical parts are carefully lettered and placed near the parts of interest, so that the student can absorb the necessary information at a glance. No one knows the names of the poor men, women, and at least one child whose organs have lain exposed for countless readers. The next time you open *Gray's Anatomy*, trail your fingers lovingly over the ridges, foramina, and fossae and think of the individuals whose deaths provided so much insight for the living.

SEE ALSO *Leonardo's Anatomical Drawings* (1510), *De Humani Corporis Fabrica* (1543), Eustachi's Rescued Masterpieces (1552), Drawings of Pietro da Cortona (1618), Cheselden's *Osteographia* (1733), Albinus's *Tables of the Human Body* (1747), Hunter's *Gravid Uterus* (1774), and Anatomy Act of 1832 (1832).

An illustration of the internal carotid and vertebral arteries from Henry Gray's Anatomy of the Human Body (1918 edition).

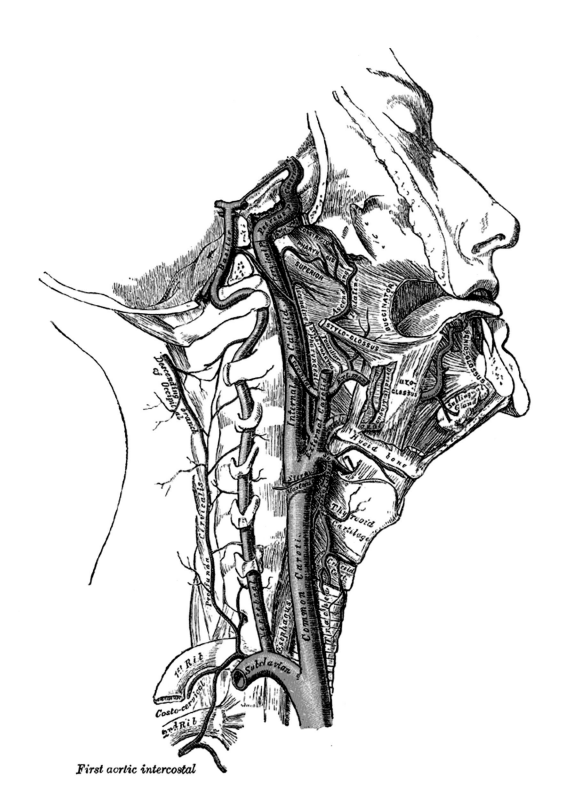

First aortic intercostal

Cerebral Localization

Hippocrates of Cos (460 B.C.–377 B.C.), **Galen of Pergamon** (129–199), **Franz Joseph Gall** (1758–1828), **Pierre Paul Broca** (1824–1880), **Gustav Theodor Fritsch** (1838–1927), **Eduard Hitzig** (1839–1907), **Wilder Graves Penfield** (1891–1976), **Herbert Henri Jasper** (1906–1999)

The ancient Greek physician Hippocrates was aware that the brain comprised the physical material underlying thoughts and emotions, and the Greek physician Galen declared, "Where the origin of the nerves is, there is the command of the soul." However, it wasn't until the 1800s that advanced research was performed with respect to cerebral localization—that is, the idea that different areas of the brain are specialized for different functions.

In 1796, German neuroanatomist Franz Joseph Gall conjectured that the brain should be considered as a mosaic of suborgans, each specialized to deal with various mental faculties, such as language, music, and so forth. However, he made the mistake of promoting the idea that the relative size and efficiency of these various suborgans could be inferred from the size of the overlying areas and bumps of the skull (see entry "**Phrenology**").

In 1861, French physician Pierre Broca discovered a particular region of the brain used for speech production. His findings were based on examination of two patients who had lost the ability to speak after injury to a particular region located on the frontal part of the left hemisphere of the brain, which today we refer to as Broca's area. Interestingly, gradual destruction of Broca's area by, for example, a brain tumor can sometimes preserve significant speech functionality, which suggests that speech function can shift to nearby areas in the brain.

Additional important evidence for cerebral localization was provided around 1870 from German researchers Gustav Fritsch and Eduard Hitzig, whose experiments on dogs showed that local body movement could be elicited by electrical stimulation of specific brain areas. In the 1940s, Canadian researchers Wilder Penfield and Herbert Jasper continued investigations involving electrical stimulation of a brain hemisphere's motor cortex, which produced contractions on the *opposite* side of the human body. They also created detailed functional maps of the brain's motor areas (which control voluntary muscle movement) and sensory areas.

SEE ALSO Trepanation (6500 B.C.), Cranial Nerves Classified (1664), Phrenology (1796), Cerebellum Function (1809), Modern Brain Surgery (1879), Prosopagnosia (1947), and Pineal Body (1958).

The cerebral cortex includes the frontal lobe (red), parietal lobe (yellow), occipital lobe (green), and temporal lobe (blue-green). The frontal lobe is responsible for "executive functions" such as planning and abstract thinking. The cerebellum (purple) is the region at the bottom.

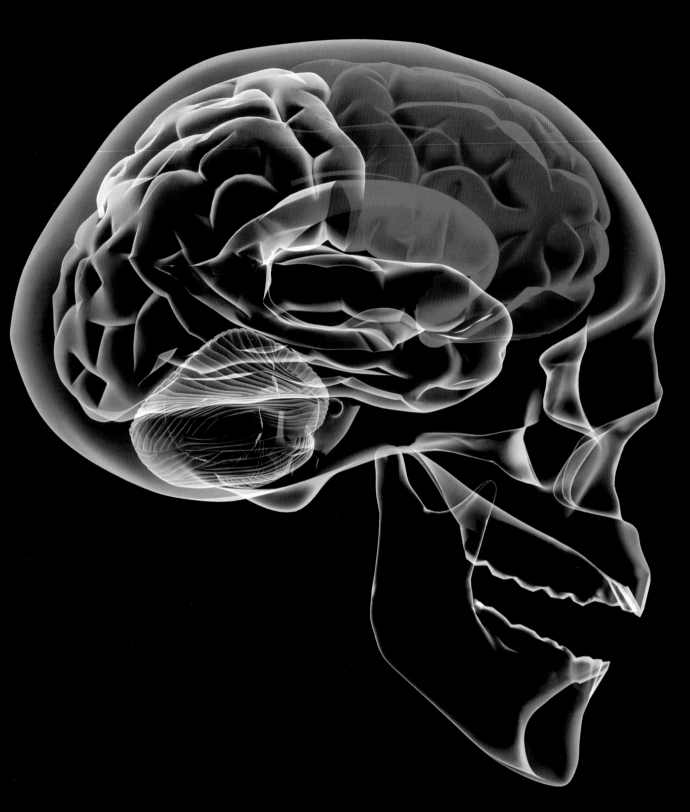

Germ Theory of Disease

Marcus Terentius Varro (116 B.C.–27 B.C.), Louis Pasteur (1822–1895)

To our modern minds, it is obvious that germs cause disease. We **chlorinate** our drinking water, use antibiotic ointments, and hope our doctors wash their hands. We are fortunate that the French chemist and microbiologist Louis Pasteur conducted his pioneering research into the causes and preventions of disease—and for experiments that supported the germ theory of disease, which suggests that microorganisms are the cause of many diseases.

In one famous experiment, conducted in 1862, Pasteur demonstrated that the growth of bacteria in sterilized nutrient broths is not due to spontaneous generation— a theory that suggests that life often arises from inanimate matter. For example, no organisms grew in flasks that contained a long, thin, twisting neck that made it extremely unlikely for dust, spores, and other particles to enter the broth. Only when Pasteur's flasks were broken open did organisms begin to grow in the medium. If spontaneous generation were valid, the broth in the curved-neck flasks would have eventually become infected because the germs would have spontaneously generated.

During his career, Pasteur studied fermentation in wines and diseases in sheep and silkworms. He created a vaccination for rabies. He showed that pasteurization (heating of a beverage to a specific temperature for a period of time) diminished microbial growth in food. In his studies of anthrax, he showed that even extremely diluted solutions of bacteria from infected animal blood could kill animals if the bacteria were allowed to multiply in the culture medium before injection into animals.

Pasteur was far from the first individual to suggest that invisible creatures caused diseases. Even the Roman scholar Marcus Terentius Varro published in 36 B.C. a warning for people living too close to swamps, "because there are bred certain minute creatures which cannot be seen by the eyes, which float in the air and enter the body through the mouth and nose and there cause serious diseases." However, the breadth of Pasteur's scientific experiments into microbial causes of disease revolutionized medicine and public health.

SEE ALSO *Micrographia* (1665), Panum's "Measles on the Faroe Islands" (1846), Semmelweis's Hand Washing (1847), Broad Street Pump Handle (1854), Cell Division (1855), Antiseptics (1865), and Chlorination of Water (1910).

Color-enhanced scanning electron micrograph showing Salmonella typhimurium *(red) invading cultured human cells (courtesy of Rocky Mountain Laboratories, NIAID, and NIH).* Salmonella *causes illnesses such as typhoid fever and food-borne illnesses.*

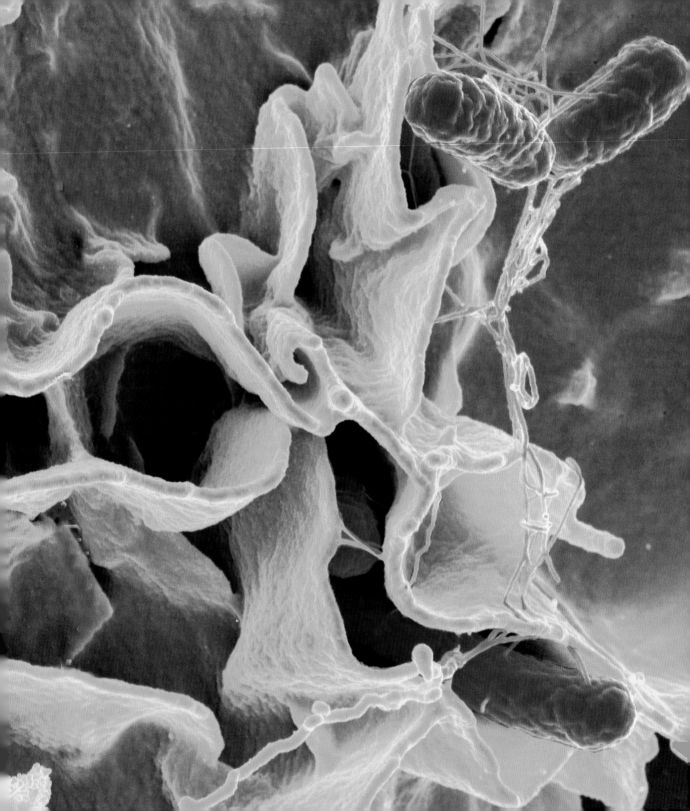

Red Cross

Clarissa Harlowe "Clara" Barton (1821–1912), Jean Henri Dunant (1828–1910)

Today's International Red Cross and Red Crescent Movement owes its existence to the Swiss social activist Henri Dunant, who was appalled by the horrors he had witnessed at the 1859 Battle of Solferino in Italy. In one day, 30,000 lay dead and thousands more wounded. Dunant tried the best he could to organize help and acquire bandages.

Dunant began to travel throughout Europe to gain support for an international aid society that could provide help to the wounded on all sides of a battle. From this early work evolved several organizations. In 1863, Dunant himself was involved with the founding of the International Committee of the Red Cross (ICRC), a private institution based in Geneva, Switzerland, with a focus on the humane treatment of victims of armed conflicts. In 1901, Dunant was awarded the first Nobel Prize for peace, and the ICRC was awarded the Nobel Peace Prize on three occasions.

The International Federation of Red Cross and Red Crescent Societies (IFRC) was founded in 1919 and, today, coordinates activities among numerous national Red Cross and Red Crescent Societies. One such national society is the American Red Cross (ARC), which is involved in collecting, processing, and distributing blood and blood products; providing relief in disasters; helping the needy; comforting military members and their families; and offering health education programs. The ARC also participates in international relief efforts, aiding in the reduction of measles and **malaria** in Africa.

The ARC was founded in 1881 by American **nurse** Clara Barton and, today, is the largest supplier of blood to U.S. **hospitals**. The ARC also performs extensive blood testing to ensure that its blood products are free of viruses, in addition to leukoreduction (the removal of white blood cells to reduce possible complications of **blood transfusions**). The famous Red Cross and Red Crescent symbols—when placed on people, vehicles, and buildings—are meant to suggest neutrality and to provide protection from military attack.

SEE ALSO Hospitals (1784), Ambulance (1792), Blood Transfusion (1829), Nursing (1854), Cause of Malaria (1897), and Caduceus (1902).

The U.S. Army's Stryker medical evacuation vehicle can move quickly and evacuate patients while its crew of three medics provides basic medical care.

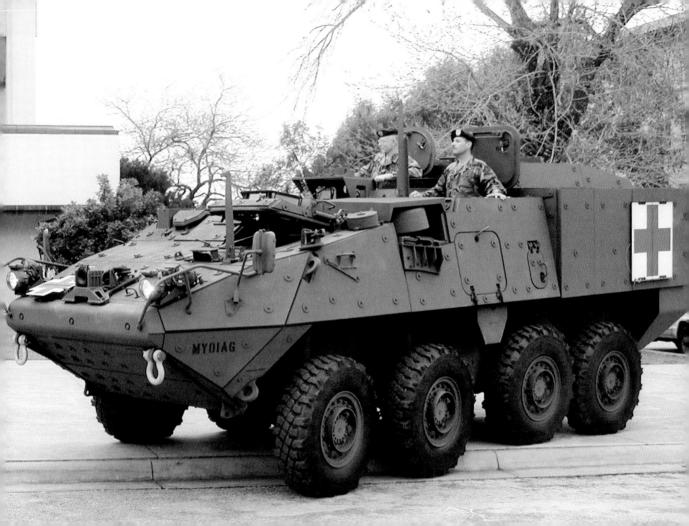

Dental Drill

Pierre Fauchard (1678–1761), **George Fellows Harrington** (1812–1895), **James Beall Morrison** (1829–1917), **George F. Green** (1932–1892)

In 1907, the author James Joyce wrote to his brother, "My mouth is full of decayed teeth and my soul of decayed ambitions." Indeed, we are lucky that the modern dental drill enables dentists to work fast and accurately, while inflicting less pain than ever before. Modern dental drills can rotate at 400,000 rpm (revolutions per minute), a high speed that reduces the jarring vibrations associated with slower drills of the past. Today's drills, often made of tungsten carbide, are used to remove decayed tooth material and to prepare the tooth for a dental filling.

Examples of ancient dental drills include ones made of flint 9,000 years ago by Stone Age people as well as drills developed by the Mayans more than 1,000 years ago. The Mayans used a jade tool, spun by the hand, to drill holes in teeth for placing jewels. However, since ancient times, dental drills were slow and clumsy, so tooth extraction was the most common treatment for cavities. In 1728, the French physician Pierre Fauchard, often referred to as the father of modern dentistry, used a drill that was spun by a moving bow with cords that rotated the drill bit.

In 1864, British dentist George Fellows Harrington invented the first motor-driven dental drill, which was much faster than earlier drills but also noisy and awkward to use. Like a clock, the drill was wound with a key and ran for two minutes per winding. In 1871, American dentist James Beall Morrison patented a foot-powered dental drill, which was an immediate success. The best hand-powered drills of his time might reach 100 rpm, but Morrison attained 2,000 rpm. In the early 1870s, American dentist George F. Green patented an electrical dental drill, but it depended on unreliable batteries and was too clumsy to generate much enthusiasm. Finally, in 1957, the first air-driven turbine drills became available, providing a speed of 3,000 rpm. Today, alternatives to drills include **laser**-ablation, particle-abrasion, and plasma-beam devices, as well as experimental robot-controlled drills.

SEE ALSO Fluoridated Toothpaste (1914), Robotic Surgery (2000).

Three dental handpieces. Various dental burrs (cutters) may be used to remove material.

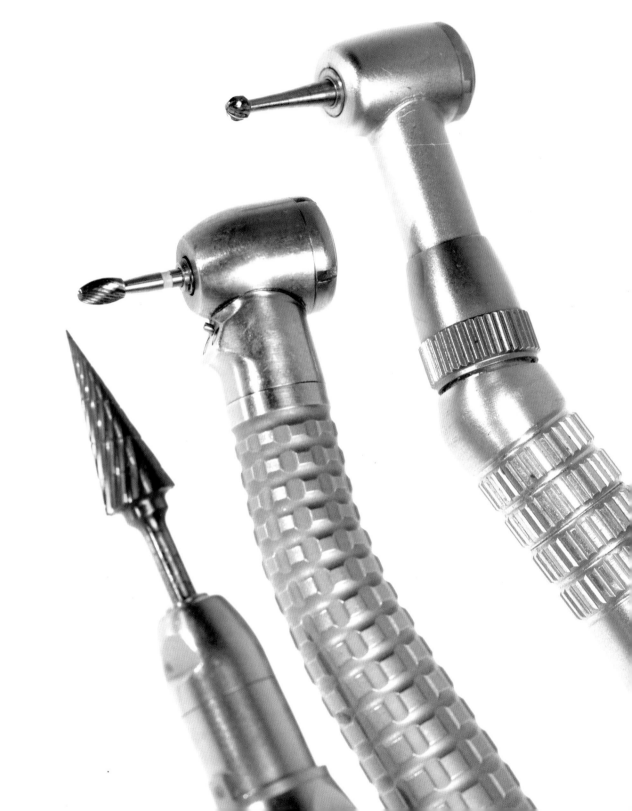

Antiseptics

William Henry (1775–1836), **Ignaz Philipp Semmelweis** (1818–1865), **Louis Pasteur** (1822–1895), **Joseph Lister** (1827–1912), **William Stewart Halsted** (1852–1922)

In 1907, the American physician Franklin C. Clark wrote, "Three notable events characterize the history of medicine, each of which in turn has completely revolutionized the practice of surgery." The first event involved the use of ligatures to stem the flow of blood during surgeries—for example, as performed by the French surgeon Ambroise Paré. The second involved methods for decreasing pain through general **anesthetics** such as ether, attributed to several Americans. The third concerned antiseptic surgery, which was promoted by British surgeon Joseph Lister. Lister's use of carbolic acid (now called phenol) as a means for sterilizing wounds and surgical instruments dramatically reduced postoperative infections.

Louis Pasteur's work on the **germ theory of disease** provided a stimulus for Lister to use carbolic acid in an attempt to destroy microorganisms. In 1865, he successfully treated a compound fracture of the leg, in which the bone juts through the skin, by dressing the leg with cloths dipped in carbolic acid solutions. Lister published his findings in the paper "Antiseptic Principle of the Practice of Surgery" in 1867.

Lister was not the first to suggest various forms of sterilization. For example, the British chemist William Henry advised sterilization of clothing through heating, and Hungarian obstetrician Ignaz Semmelweis advocated **hand washing** to prevent the spread of disease by physicians. Nevertheless, Lister's slopping of carbolic acid onto open wounds usually prevented the development of the horrific infections that so often occurred in **hospitals** of his time. His writings and talks convinced medical professionals of the need for using antiseptics.

Antiseptics are usually applied directly to the body surface. Modern methods for preventing infections focus more on the use of aseptic methods that involve sterilization to remove bacteria *before* they come near a patient (e.g., disinfection of equipment and the use of surgeons' masks). Antibiotic drugs are also used today to fight internal infections. In 1891, William Halsted pioneered the use of rubber gloves in surgery.

SEE ALSO Semmelweis's Hand Washing (1847), Germ Theory of Disease (1862), Latex Surgical Gloves (1890), and Maggot Therapy (1929).

Manuka honey has been shown to have antibacterial properties that assist in wound healing. Such honey is made by bees in New Zealand that feed on the manuka bush, Leptospermum scoparium.

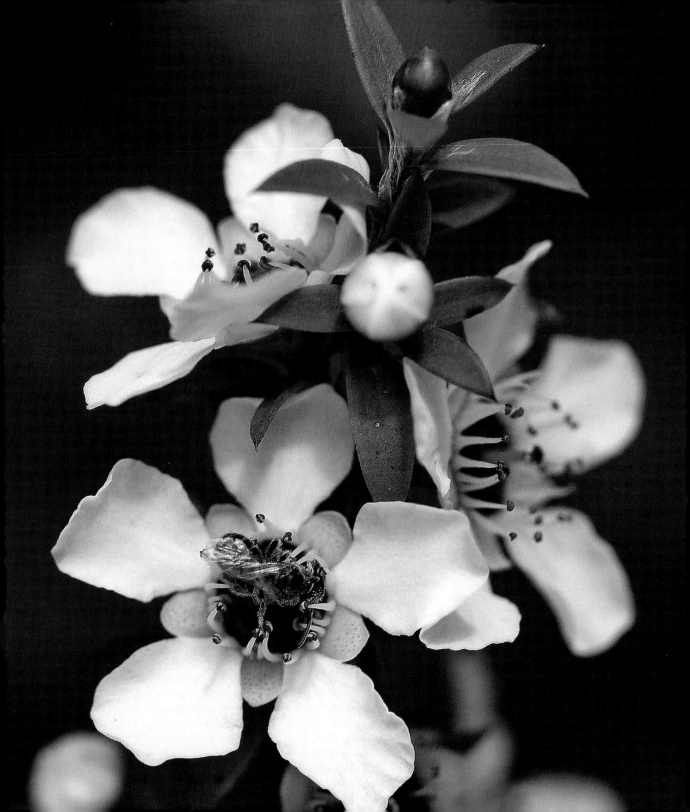

Mendel's Genetics

Gregor Johann Mendel (1822–1884)

The Austrian priest Gregor Mendel studied the inheritance of easily identifiable traits in pea plants, such as color or wrinkling, and showed that the inheritance could be understood in terms of mathematical laws and ratios. Although his work was not recognized in his lifetime, the laws that he discovered formed the foundation of genetics—the science of heredity and variation in organisms.

In 1865, Mendel reported on his studies of more than 20,000 pea plants, conducted over six years, which led him to formulate his laws of genetics. He observed that organisms inherit traits via discrete units that we now refer to as genes. This finding was in contrast to other popular theories of his time, such as an individual inheriting a smooth blend of traits from the parents, or an individual inheriting "acquired characteristics" from their parents (such as a son having large muscles simply because his father lifted weights).

As an example, consider that in peas, each plant has two alleles (versions) of each gene, and that the offspring inherit one allele from each parent. It is a matter of chance which gene from each parent is received. If the offspring receives a gene for a yellow seed together with a gene for a green seed, the yellow gene may dominate in the offspring, but the gene for green is still present and is transmitted to the plant's descendants in a consistent and predictable manner.

Today, medical geneticists aim to understand how genetic variations play a role in human health and disease. For example, the disease cystic fibrosis, which includes difficulty breathing among other symptoms, is caused by a mutation (change) in a single gene that affects membranes of cells. The ideas associated with Mendel's genetics eventually led to a better understanding of genes and chromosomes (composed of a **DNA** molecule containing many genes), along with the potential to cure many diseases and shape the evolution of the human species. Human genes have even been placed into bacteria to create large quantities of insulin for diabetic individuals.

SEE ALSO Chromosomal Theory of Inheritance (1902), Inborn Errors of Metabolism (1902), Genes and Sex Determination (1905), DNA Structure (1953), Mitochondrial Diseases (1962), Epigenetics (1983), Gene Therapy (1990), and Human Genome Project (2003).

Gregor Mendel studied the inheritance of easily identifiable traits in pea plants, such as color or wrinkling, and showed that inheritance could be understood in terms of simple mathematical ratios.

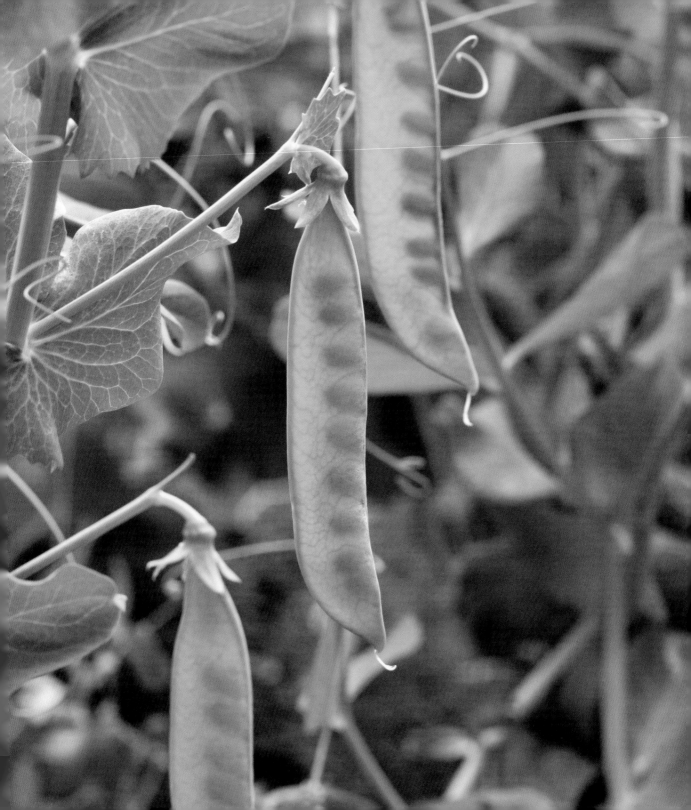

Medical Thermometer

**Santorio Santorio (1561–1636), Daniel Gabriel Fahrenheit (1686–1736),
Carl Reinhold August Wunderlich (1815–1877), Thomas Clifford Allbutt
(1836–1925), Thomas Maclagan (1838–1903)**

For centuries, caregivers placed the palms of their hands on the foreheads of sick people to detect fevers. Clinical thermometers were not widely used until the late 1800s to measure the temperature of the human body, with the sensing end of the thermometer placed in the mouth, armpit, or rectum. In mercury- or alcohol-containing thermometers, the liquid expands or contracts so that the length of the liquid column within the thermometer depends on the temperature. Mercury thermometers often employed a short constriction to prevent easy backflow, thus allowing the device to "store" the highest reading until the thermometer was shaken.

Around 1612, the Italian physician Santorio Santorio was among the first to add a numerical scale to thermometer-like devices, and he explained, "The patient grasps the bulb or breathes upon it into a hood, or takes the bulb into his mouth, so that we can tell if the patient be better or worse." Unfortunately, his devices were inaccurate because of the effects of varying air pressure on measurements.

German physicist Daniel Gabriel Fahrenheit invented the alcohol thermometer in 1709 and the mercury thermometer in 1714. Fahrenheit chose mercury because it expanded uniformly over an enormous range of temperatures, making it useful even beyond medicine.

Some early clinical thermometers were nearly a foot long (25 cm), which made them difficult to carry in a physician's bag and use on the patient. Measurements could require 20 minutes. We should be thankful to the English physician Thomas Clifford Allbutt, who, in 1866, finally invented a clinical thermometer that was only six inches (15 cm) long, which he said "could live habitually in my pocket, and be as constantly with me as a stethoscope."

One important milestone in the history of medical thermometers includes the work of German physician Carl Wunderlich, who published temperature information on 25,000 patients in 1868. That same year, Scottish physician Thomas Maclagan studied the temperatures of patients suffering from typhus, typhoid, and pneumonia.

Today, medical thermometers are often electronic devices that may employ infrared sensors to determine temperatures.

SEE ALSO Stethoscope (1816), Spirometry (1846), and Sphygmomanometer (1881).

Medical thermometer showing degrees in both Fahrenheit (top) and Celsius (bottom). A normal temperature is indicated.

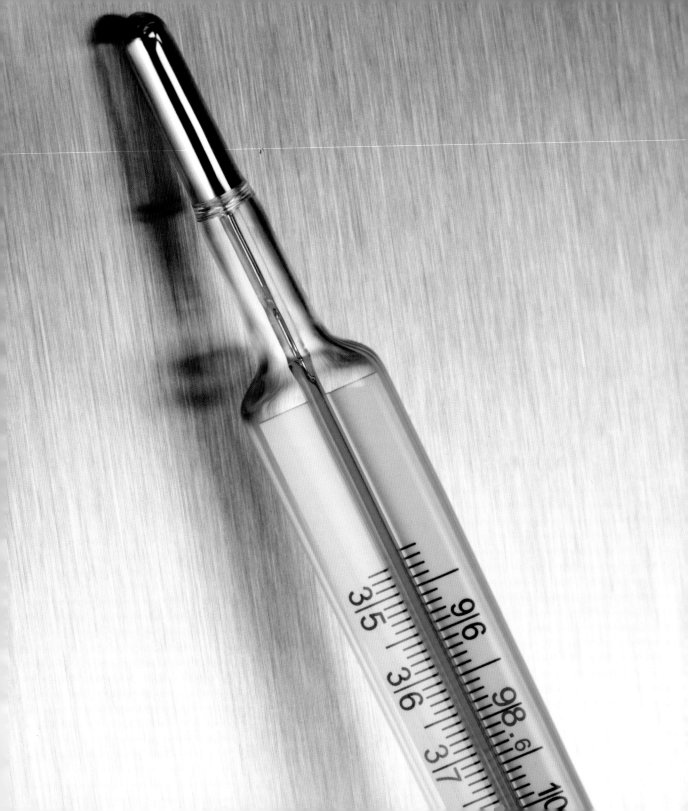

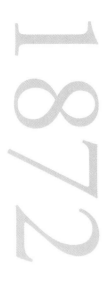

Thyroid Surgery

Samuel David Gross (1805–1884), Emil Theodor Kocher (1841–1917)

In 1886, the American surgeon Samuel Gross wrote of the difficulties of trying to remove a thyroid gland that had swelled tremendously in the neck due to a condition known as goiter: "No sensible man will . . . attempt to extirpate a goitrous thyroid gland. Should a surgeon be so adventurous or foolhardy . . . every stroke of his knife will be followed by a torrent of blood, and lucky will it be for him if his victim lives long enough to enable him to finish his horrid butchery."

Goiter is caused by a lack of dietary iodine, required by the thyroid gland to synthesize hormones needed for metabolism and growth. The era of modern successful thyroid surgery began with Swiss surgeon Emil Kocher, who performed thousands of surgeries starting in 1872. Kocher won the Nobel Prize for his work on the physiology, pathology, and surgery of the thyroid gland. Unfortunately, although people can live without a thyroid for years, the lack of thyroid hormones eventually leads to mental and physical deterioration, causing Kocher to lament, "I have doomed people with goiter . . . to a vegetative existence [turning many into] cretins, saved for a life not worth living."

The neck's thyroid gland has two lobes, resembling the wings of a butterfly. The two principle hormones secreted by the gland are triiodothyronine and thyroxine. Hyperthyroidism involves a thyroid that produces too much of these hormones (causing weight loss, racing heartbeat, and weakness), and hypothyroidism involves too little (causing fatigue and other symptoms). Fortunately, hyperthyroidism can be treated in several ways, including with radioactive iodine, which accumulates in the thyroid gland and can destroy all or part of the gland. As a result of this treatment, the individual may exhibit hypothyroidism, which can be treated by daily pills containing synthetic thyroxine. If thyroid hormone levels are low, the brain's hypothalamus secretes thyrotropin-releasing hormone (TRH) that causes the pituitary gland to release thyroid-stimulating hormone (TSH), which in turn triggers the thyroid's hormone production. If thyroid hormone levels are high, TRH and TSH production is suppressed.

SEE ALSO *Halstedian Surgery (1904)*, Human Growth Hormone (1921), and Autoimmune Diseases (1956).

Thyroid gland (red) with its left and right lobes together with the pyramidal lobe (central part with upward projection). Behind the thyroid are schematic representations of the trachea (windpipe) and thyroid cartilage.

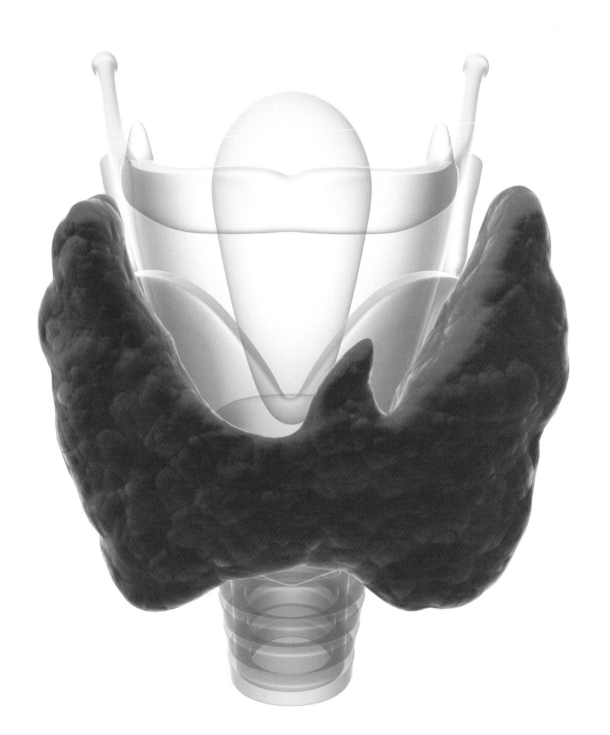

Cause of Leprosy

Gerhard Henrik Armauer Hansen (1841–1912)

In 1948, British physician Ernest Muir wrote, "Leprosy is dreaded most of all diseases, not because it kills, but because it leaves alive. . . . Mask face, unclosing eyes, slavering mouth, claw-hands, limping feet . . . and eyes drawing on toward blindness—such is the picture conjured in the mind." Some considered it the curse of God, visited on sinners. Others thought it was an inherited condition. Because the disease causes nerve damage and associated loss of sensation, afflicted individuals may frequently injure their hands or feet, leading to their eventual loss. Through history, these disfigured "lepers" were often ostracized by society and placed in leper colonies.

The disease may have originated on the Indian subcontinent—a 4,000-year-old skeleton from India showed erosion patterns suggestive of leprosy. By 1200, approximately 19,000 leprosy **hospitals** existed in Europe. In 1873, Norwegian physician G. H. Armauer Hansen finally discovered that the cause of the leprosy was the bacterium *Mycobacterium leprae*—the first bacterium to be identified as causing disease in humans. In unstained sections of tissue from infected individuals, the bacteria resemble small rods.

Hansen's study of the bacteria was hampered, not only because he could not seem to infect test animals, like rabbits, but because the bacteria do not grow in artificial culture media in the laboratory, since they lack many genes that are required for survival independent of a host. Desperate to better understand leprosy, Hansen attempted to inoculate the eye of a woman with leprosy bacteria, without permission. In 1880, she sued him in court, and he was removed from his post as resident physician of Bergen's leprosy hospital. Fortunately, scientists eventually discovered that the bacteria can be grown in mouse foot pads and in nine-banded armadillos.

Most adults are actually immune to the disease, which can take several years to develop after initial exposure and appears to be communicable through mucus of the nose and throat. Today, leprosy is treatable by administering a collection of three drugs: dapsone, rifampicin, and clofazimine.

SEE ALSO Panum's "Measles on the Faroe Islands" (1846), Cause of Bubonic Plague (1894), Cause of Rocky Mountain Spotted Fever (1906), Imprisonment of Typhoid Mary (1907), and Thalidomide Disaster (1962).

Today, leprosy is treatable by administering a collection of drugs. Shown here is prevention-campaign graffiti on a public wall in Ladakh, India.

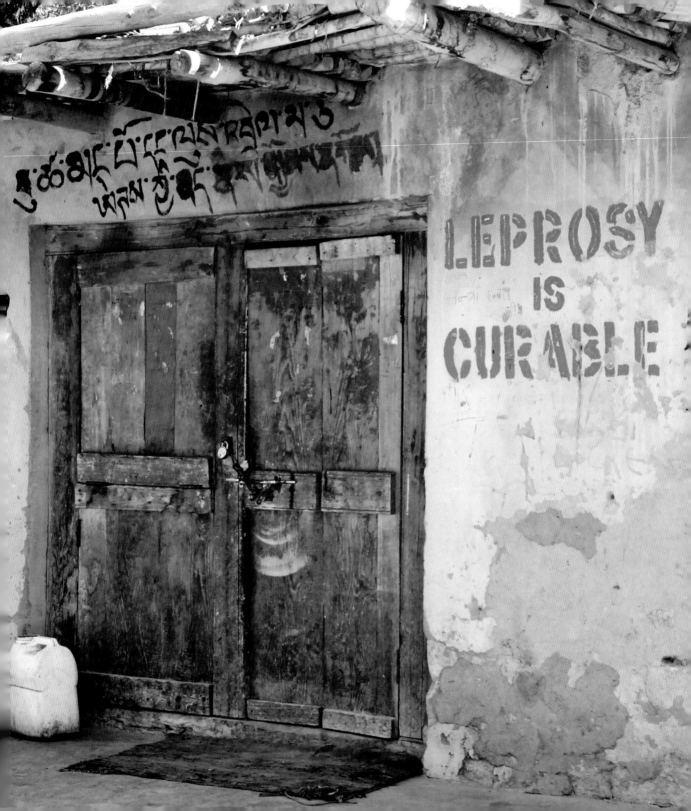

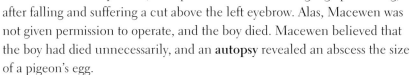

Modern Brain Surgery

William Macewen (1848–1924), **Rickman John Godlee** (1849–1925), **Victor Alexander Haden Horsley** (1857–1916)

The actor Michael J. Fox, who suffers from Parkinson's disease, asked a neurosurgeon, "Why do you think it is that brain surgery, above all else—even rocket science—gets singled out as the most challenging of human feats, the one demanding the utmost of human intelligence?" The neurosurgeon paused and replied, "No margin for error."

Crude forms of brain surgery are among the oldest medical procedures, and holes have been made in the skulls of living people since prehistoric times (see entry "**Trepanation**"). Even the Greek physician Hippocrates described brain injuries he felt could be treated by trepanation. However, it was not until the 1800s that the world saw the first *modern* and successful neurological operations.

Consider the case of Scottish surgeon William Macewen who, in 1876, diagnosed a brain abscess (inflamed and swollen tissue) in the left frontal brain area in a boy who suffered from convulsions and aphasia (an impairment related to language processing)

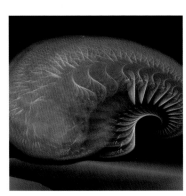

after falling and suffering a cut above the left eyebrow. Alas, Macewen was not given permission to operate, and the boy died. Macewen believed that the boy had died unnecessarily, and an **autopsy** revealed an abscess the size of a pigeon's egg.

In 1879, Macewen began to successfully perform brain operations to treat patients suffering from brain abscesses. This work occurred before the invention of **X-rays**, and Macewen relied on patient symptoms and recent research into the function of various brain regions (see entry "**Cerebral Localization**") to help him predict the appropriate location at which to open the skull. For example, he might observe pupil reflexes, location of pain, and the nature and location of convulsive behavior. Macewen's work would not have been possible without the previous breakthroughs in **anesthesia** and **antiseptics**.

In 1884, English surgeon Rickman John Godlee became the first to remove a brain tumor (an abnormal growth of tissue). In 1887, English surgeon Victor Horsley performed the first successful surgery to remove a tumor of the spinal cord.

SEE ALSO Trepanation (6500 B.C.), Cerebrospinal Fluid (1764), General Anesthesia (1842), Cerebral Localization (1861), Antiseptics (1865), and Levodopa for Parkinson's Disease (1957).

LEFT: *Futuristic depiction of a human brain (c. 2050), with cybernetic, fractal heat-dissipation units, by Slovenian artist Teja Krašek.* RIGHT: *A horizontal section through the head of an adult man, from the Visible Human Project. A cadaver was frozen, sliced into thin sections, and photographed. This section shows the cerebral cortex and underlying white matter.*

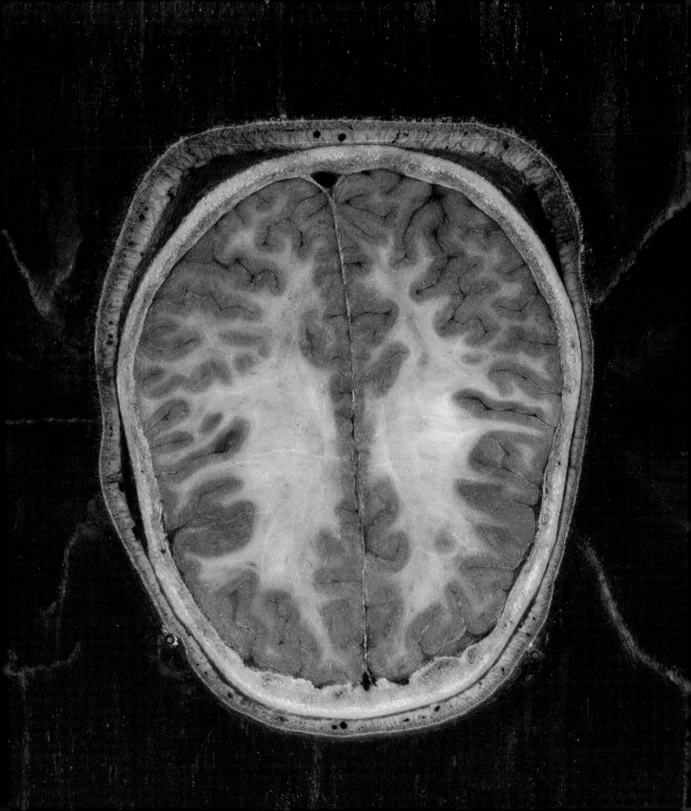

Sphygmomanometer

Stephen Hales (1677–1761), Samuel Siegfried Karl Ritter von Basch (1837–1905), Scipione Riva-Rocci (1863–1937), Nikolai Sergeyevich Korotkov (or Korotkoff) (1874–1920)

Blood pressure measurement provides an example of the physician's dependence on technology for the care of patients. Today, arterial blood pressure is often measured using a sphygmomanometer, a device that traditionally employed a column of mercury to measure pressure. The systolic pressure reflects the pressure when the ventricles of the heart contract—for example, a normal adult pressure of 120 millimeters of mercury. The diastolic pressure is a minimum pressure in the arteries, which occurs when the ventricles are being filled with blood. In adults, a diastolic pressure of 80 millimeters of mercury falls within the normal range.

The evolution of sphygmomanometers has a fascinating history filled with ingenious inventors. For example, in 1733, English physiologist Stephen Hales provided the first well-documented measurements of blood pressure in an animal when he described connecting a long glass tube to a horse's neck artery and noted that the blood rose nine feet, six inches (2.9 m) into the tube. In 1881, Austrian physician Samuel von Basch used a rubber bulb filled with water to apply pressure to the artery until the pulse disappeared. The rubber bulb was attached to a mercury device that was used to measure the systolic pressure while the artery was compressed. In 1896, Italian physician Scipione Riva-Rocci made use of an inflatable cuff worn around the arm in order to produce a uniform pressure on the artery. Finally, in 1905, Russian physician Nikolai Korotkov used a stethoscope to listen to the sounds from the artery as pressure from the cuff was released, thus leading to the measuring of the diastolic pressure. After 1910, U.S. physicians regularly reported systolic and diastolic blood pressures in their clinical reports on patients.

Today the sphygmomanometer allows doctors to diagnose low and high blood pressure, the latter of which is a risk factor for strokes, heart attacks, and kidney failure. Mercury sphygmomanometers are still used today, along with electronic and aneroid devices that do not require the use of liquids.

SEE ALSO Pulse Watch (1707), Stethoscope (1816), Spirometry (1846), Ophthalmoscope (1850), and Medical Thermometer (1866).

An aneroid sphygmomanometer, used by doctors to diagnose low and high blood pressure.

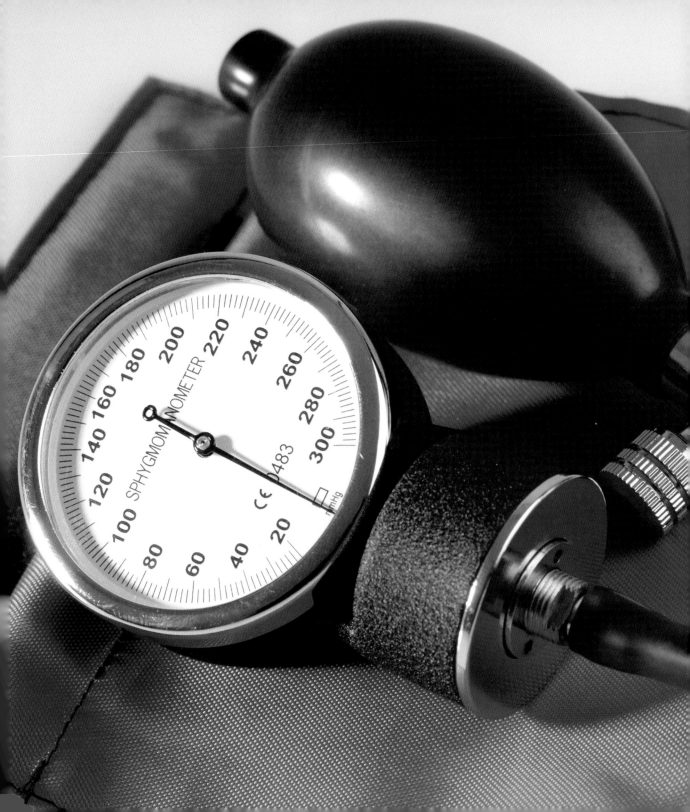

Cesarean Section

Max Sänger (1853–1903)

Medical historian Jane Sewell writes that in the United States today, "Women may be afraid of the pain of childbirth, but they do not expect it to kill them [or their babies]. Such could not be said of many women as late as the nineteenth century. . . . The cesarean section [once was an] operation that virtually always resulted in a dead woman and dead fetus and now almost always results in a living mother and baby."

A cesarean section (CS) today usually involves a horizontal incision made through the pregnant woman's abdomen and uterus to deliver a baby—often performed when either the mother's or child's life is at risk. The name may be derived from a legend about an ancestor of Roman emperor Julius Caesar, who was delivered by this kind of surgery. For most of history, an emergency CS was not intended to save the mother's life, because surgical techniques were not sufficiently advanced. Surgeons did not have the skills to repair a uterine incision without causing infection and in a way that would properly hold together the uterine muscle, with its contractions following delivery. The first recorded case of a woman surviving a CS comes from 1500, when Jakob Nufer, a Swiss castrator of pigs, allegedly performed the surgery on his wife. In 1794, Dr. Jesse Bennett performed the first successful CS in the United States when he operated on his wife.

Finally, in 1882, German obstetrician Max Sänger, the father of the modern CS, developed a special arrangement of **sutures** made of silver wires that produced minimal tissue reaction and had low rates of infection. His surgery to close the uterus revolutionized the practice of CS and saved the lives of countless women.

Today, the CS is often recommended for pregnancy complications, including severe preeclampsia (which includes high blood pressure during pregnancy), multiple births, diabetes, HIV infection of the mother, placenta previa (placenta partially covering the cervix), and a very narrow birth canal.

SEE ALSO Sutures (3000 B.C.), Abortion (70), Obstetrical Forceps (1580), Hunter's *Gravid Uterus* (1774), Hysterectomy (1813), Salpingectomy (1883), Modern Midwifery (1925), Self-Surgery (1961), and First Test-Tube Baby (1978).

Schematic representation of a fetus in the womb in a normal head-down presentation. Other presentations are more difficult to deliver or may not be deliverable by natural means.

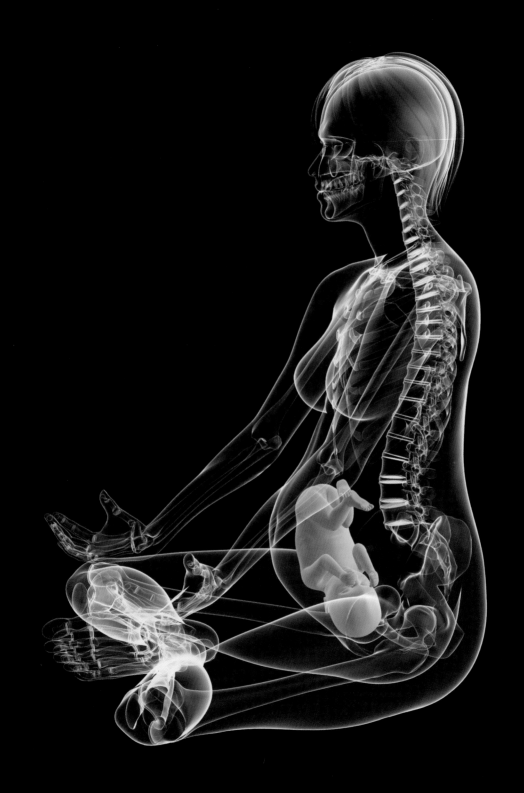

Koch's Tuberculosis Lecture

Heinrich Hermann Robert Koch (1843–1910), **Selman Abraham Waksman** (1888–1973)

In 1882, the German physician Robert Koch gave a landmark lecture announcing his discovery of the bacterial cause of tuberculosis. According to the folks at *Nobelprize.org*, this lecture is often considered "the most important in medical history" because it "was so innovative, inspirational, and thorough that it set the stage for the scientific procedures of the twentieth century." Not only did Koch demonstrate the presence of the bacterium *Mycobacterium tuberculosis* using an innovative microscopy staining procedure, he also proved that the bacterium caused the disease.

Surrounded by microscopes and animal-tissue specimens, Koch began his talk by describing the horrifying history of the disease: "If the importance of a disease for mankind is measured by the number of fatalities it causes, then tuberculosis must be considered much more important than those most feared infectious diseases, plague, cholera, and the like. One in seven of all human beings dies from tuberculosis." The Nobel Laureate Paul Ehrlich, who attended the talk, later remarked, "I hold that evening to be the most important experience of my scientific life."

Tuberculosis can be spread through the air by coughing. It usually affects the lungs and is associated with symptoms such as coughing up blood, but it can also affect other parts of the body, such as the bones and intestines. Today, infected people can often harbor bacteria without exhibiting symptoms—and, incredibly, about one-third of all people on Earth are infected. Unfortunately, the inactive bacteria may become active in people with weakened immune symptoms, such as people with AIDS (acquired immunodeficiency syndrome).

In 1944, American microbiologist Selman Waksman and colleagues finally discovered the antibiotic streptomycin, which cured patients with tuberculosis. However, the bacteria soon became resistant to this drug, and today patients are sometimes treated with as many as four different antibacterial drugs for many months to combat the disease.

From 1700 to 1900 alone, tuberculosis killed around one billion people. The disease was once called consumption because the bodies of the afflicted appeared to be "consumed" from within.

SEE ALSO Panum's "Measles on the Faroe Islands" (1846), Broad Street Pump Handle (1854), Searches for the Soul (1907), Tobacco Smoking and Cancer (1951), and Reverse Transcriptase and AIDS (1970).

Transmission electron micrograph of Mycobacterium tuberculosis *bacteria, which cause tuberculosis.*

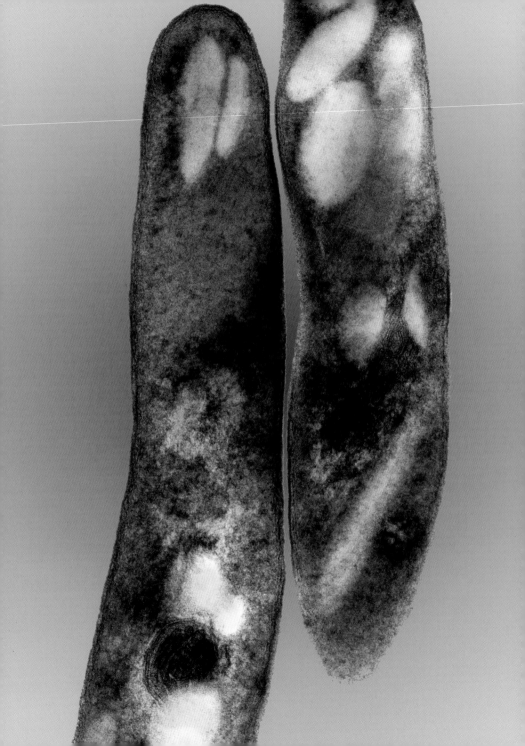

Phagocytosis Theory

Ilya Ilyich Mechnikov (1845–1916)

Within our bodies is an immune system of enormous complexity that helps protect us from a variety of diseases. As a result of his studies of starfish larvae, the Russian biologist Ilya Mechnikov was the first to discover how one component of this system worked. In particular, in 1882, he observed certain cells move toward a thorn he had placed in the body of a larva. He theorized that such cells, soon to be called phagocytes (from the Greek *phagein*, meaning "to devour"), functioned like single-celled creatures that engulf and destroy smaller particles as part of their normal digestive process. He later studied tiny daphnia crustaceans and discovered that their mobile phagocytes destroyed fungal spores in the body of the creatures. He also observed that phagocytes of mammals engulf and destroy anthrax bacteria. Mechnikov proposed that phagocytes were a major defense mechanism against invading organisms, such as bacteria, and that such a process probably evolved from the simple digestive processes of single-celled creatures like amoebas. The function of *eating to feed* had expanded to include *eating to defend*. He likened the behavior of phagocytes in the body to an army fighting infection.

Many scientists of Mechnikov's time resisted his idea of a phagocytic defense mechanism, in part because prevailing theories suggested that these kinds of cells actually served to *spread* pathogens in the body rather than destroy them. However, he eventually won the 1908 Nobel Prize for his monumental discovery. Today we know that the phagocytes studied by Mechnikov were probably monocytes and neutrophils, just two kinds of leukocytes (white blood cells) that are part of the immune system and produced in bone marrow. During an infection, chemical signals attract phagocytes to the areas of invasion. Phagocytes also play a role in ridding the body of dead or dying cells every day of our lives. The number of leukocytes in the blood often is an indicator of specific diseases, such as those involving infections.

SEE ALSO Lymphatic System (1652), Structure of Antibodies (1959), and Thymus (1961).

Scanning electron micrograph of a neutrophil (a phagocyte, colored yellow) engulfing rod-shaped anthrax bacteria (orange). Neutrophils are the most abundant white blood cells and the first line of defense against invading microbes. (Courtesy of Volker Brinkmann.)

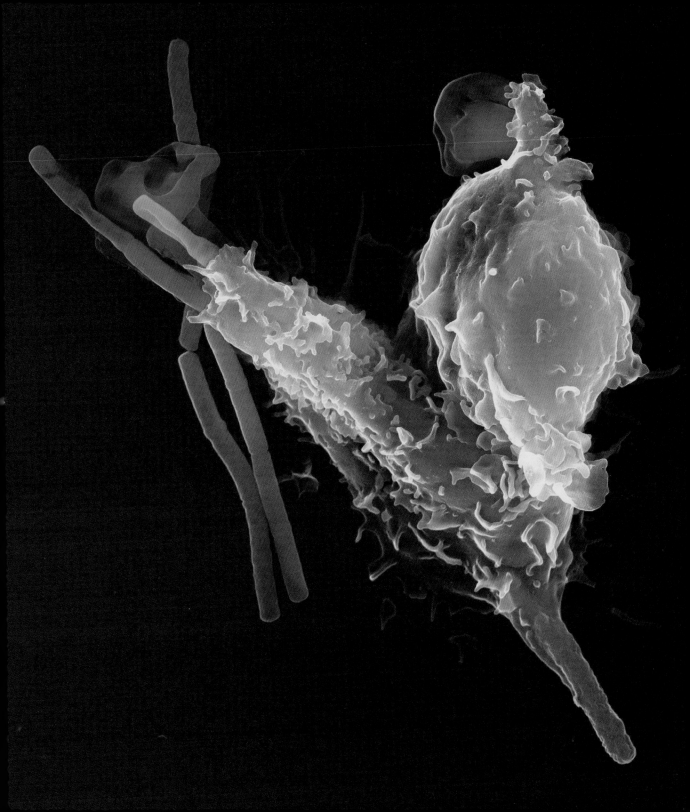

Health Insurance

Otto Eduard Leopold von Bismarck (1815–1898)

Health insurance helps protect individuals from incurring high medical expenses and may be supplied by governments or private insurance companies. In 1883, Prussian-German statesman Otto von Bismarck implemented one of the earliest forms of national health insurance programs, and it provided health care for a large segment of industrial workers. National health plans were later established in England (1911), Sweden (1914), and France (1930).

Health insurance in the United States is relatively new, partly because, prior to 1920, most people were treated in their homes at low cost, and the state of medical technology could do little for many patients. Even surgery was performed in private homes until the 1920s. The first individual insurance plans in the United States began during the Civil War (1861–1865) but only provided coverage against accidents related to travel by steamboat or rail. As early as 1847, Massachusetts Health Insurance of Boston offered relatively comprehensive group policies. In 1929, teachers in Dallas, Texas, formed the first modern group health insurance plan by contracting with Baylor **Hospital** for medical services for a fixed monthly fee. This was as a precursor to Blue Cross hospital insurance in the United States. Hospitalization plans benefited from risk pooling—spreading the risk across a population of mostly healthy consumers. In 1939, the California Medical Association started Blue Shield, designed to pay physician fees.

During World War II, the U.S. government prohibited employers from raising wages, so they began to compete for employees by offering improved health-care insurance benefits. Created in 1965, Medicare is a public program for the elderly and certain disabled individuals. Medicaid covers certain very-low-income children and their families.

In the United States, government control of health care has often been passionately debated. In 1935, Morris Fishbein, editor of the *Journal of the American Medical Association*, said that publically funded medical service would "communize" America, and that Americans would "become a nation of automatons, moving, breathing, living, suffering and dying at the will of politicians and political masters."

SEE ALSO Acupuncture *Compendium* (1601), Hospitals (1784), American Medical Association (1847), and Hospice (1967).

Trains could be quite dangerous in the late 1800s, and the first individual insurance plans in the United States provided coverage against accidents related to travel by steamboat or rail. Shown here is a Granville-Paris Express wreck in October 1895.

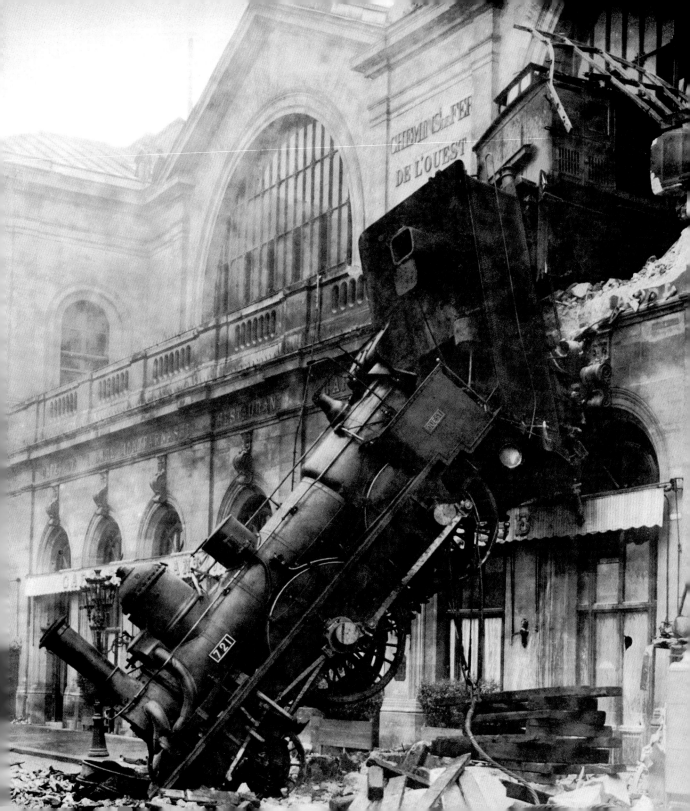

Salpingectomy

Robert Lawson Tait (1845–1899)

Surgeon Harold Ellis writes, "Until 1883, a ruptured ectopic pregnancy was a death sentence." Although some pioneering surgeons did successfully remove ovarian cysts from suffering women as far back as 1809, "for some inexplicable reason, the surgeon would stand helplessly by the bedside and watch a young woman . . . exsanguinate from her ruptured tube."

Normally, an egg becomes fertilized in the fallopian tube, which leads from a woman's ovaries to the uterus. Once it enters the uterus, the fertilized egg, or zygote, implants in the uterine wall, and the embryo develops within the uterus. Sometimes, however, in an ectopic pregnancy (EP), the zygote implants outside the uterus—for example, in the wall of the narrow fallopian tube. If the fallopian tube ruptures or is about to rupture, surgical removal of the tube may be necessary to protect the life of the woman.

In 1883, Scottish surgeon Lawson Tait performed the first surgical removal of a tube in a surgery referred to as salpingectomy—a procedure that has since saved countless lives. He writes of his first salpingectomy: "The right fallopian tube was ruptured and from it a placenta was protruding. I tied the tube and removed it. I searched for, but could not find, the fetus, and I suppose it got lost among the folds of intestine and there was absorbed. The patient made a very protracted convalescence, but she is now perfectly well."

A salpingectomy may also be performed for tubal **cancer** or dangerous infections. Today, a salpingectomy can sometimes be avoided if the EP is discovered early in the pregnancy, at which point the drug methotrexate is given to terminate the growth of the developing embryo. In some cases, if the EP has not irreparably damaged the fallopian tube, the physician can instead perform a salpingostomy, making a small incision in the tube to remove the misplaced embryo. Minimally invasive **laparoscopic surgery** may be performed on the fallopian tubes.

SEE ALSO Abortion (70), Hunter's *Gravid Uterus* (1774), Hysterectomy (1813), Cesarean Section (1882), "The Rabbit Died" (1928), IUD (1929), First Test-Tube Baby (1978), and Laparoscopic Surgery (1981).

Photo of an opened oviduct with an ectopic pregnancy and a 10-millimeter embryo about five weeks old. The portion of the oviduct above the uterus is referred to as the fallopian tube. (Courtesy of Ed Uthman, M.D.)

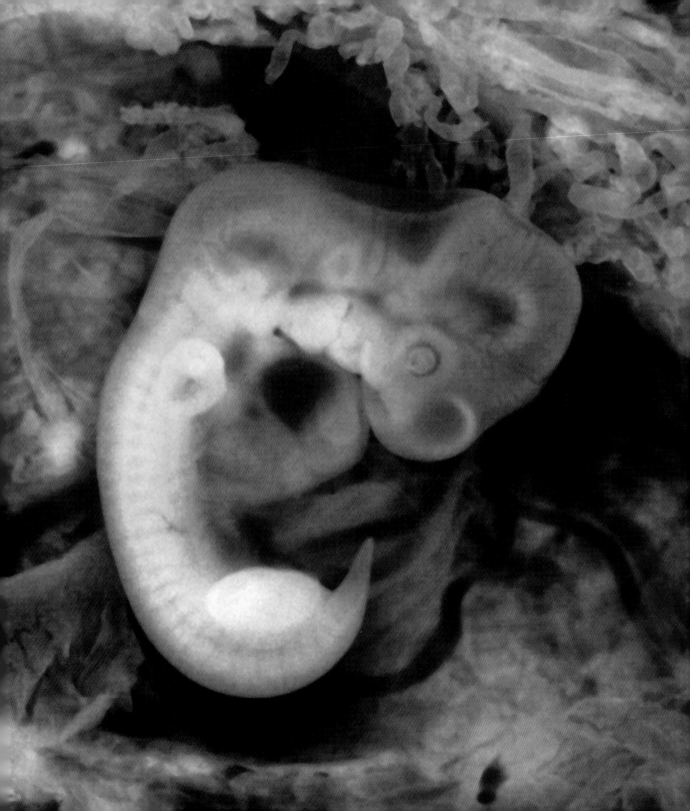

Cocaine as Local Anesthetic

Friedrich Gaedcke (1828–1890), **Albert Friedrich Emil Niemann** (1834–1861), **Thomas Hardy** (1840–1928), **William Stewart Halsted** (1852–1922), **Sigmund Freud** (1856–1939), **Karl Koller** (1857–1944)

In 1882, British novelist Thomas Hardy portrayed what it was like to undergo eye cataract surgery by recalling the words of an old man: "It was like a red-hot needle in yer eye whilst he was doing it. But he wasn't long about it. Oh no. If he had been long I couldn't ha' beared it. He wasn't a minute more than three-quarters of an hour at the outside." Imagine the sheer torment of a needle in your eye for 45 minutes with no local anesthetic to numb the pain!

In the 1880s, Austrian neurologist Sigmund Freud was researching cocaine as a possible treatment for morphine addiction when he suggested to a young Austrian eye doctor, Karl Koller, that cocaine might be used to numb particular areas of the body. In a famous experiment in 1884, Koller applied a solution of cocaine to his own eye and then pricked his eye with a pin. He felt no pain, and thus heralded a new kind of painless surgery involving local anesthetics—drugs that can block pain perception by inhibiting nerve-signal propagation in specific body regions while the patient is fully conscious. Soon after hearing of Koller's discovery, American surgeon William Halsted followed up by injecting cocaine into nerves to create specific nerve-block anesthesia. (Unfortunately, Halsted soon became a cocaine addict.) Of course, **general anesthesia** was possible in the form of ether or various gases that induce a state of unconsciousness, but this had drawbacks, including vomiting and the inability to interact with the patient during the procedure.

For centuries, South American indigenous peoples chewed the leaves of coca plants for their cocaine-induced stimulant effect. The natives also used saliva from chewing the leaves to relieve painful wounds. However, it was not until 1855 that German chemist Friedrich Gaedcke actually isolated the cocaine chemical compound. German chemist Albert Niemann improved the process in 1859 and called the compound cocaine. Today, cocaine has largely been replaced by safer and less addictive synthetic local anesthetics, including benzocaine, lidocaine, and many others.

SEE ALSO Snow Anesthesia (1812), General Anesthesia (1842), Aspirin (1899), Psychoanalysis (1899), Halstedian Surgery (1904), Patent Medicines (1906), Neurotransmitters (1914), and Medical Self-Experimentation (1929).

Erythroxylum coca is a plant native to South America. Coca contains alkaloids, which include cocaine.

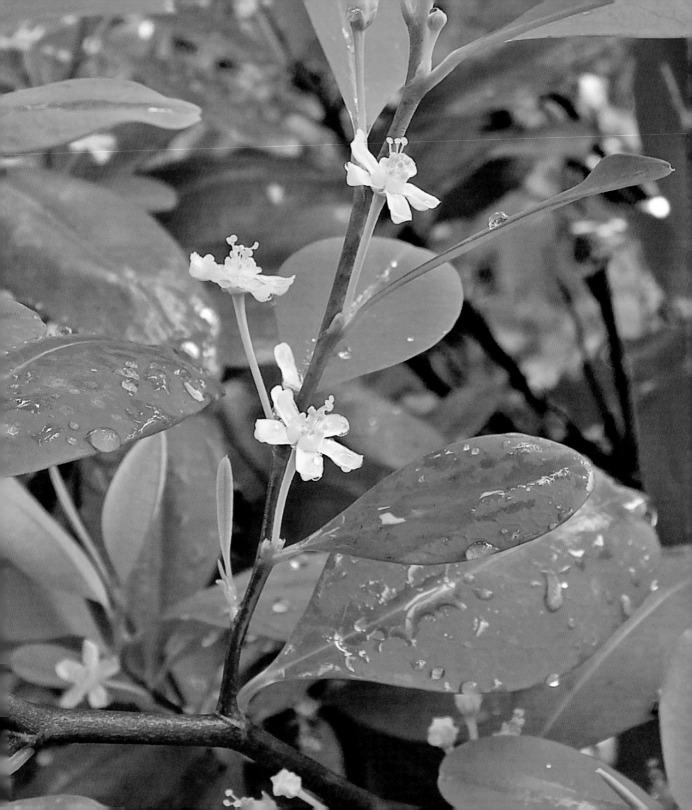

Antitoxins

Shibasaburo Kitasato (1853–1931), **Paul Ehrlich** (1854–1915), **Emil Adolf von Behring** (1854–1917), **Erich Arthur Emanuel Wernicke** (1859–1928)

Historian Derek Linton writes, "In 1901, Emil von Behring received the first Nobel Prize in medicine for serum therapy against diphtheria, a disease that killed thousands of infants annually. Diphtheria serum was the first major cure of the bacteriological era and its development generated novel procedures for testing . . . drugs." Von Behring's serum therapy required the turning of sheep and horses into antitoxin factories.

Some bacteria wreak their havoc on the body by producing harmful toxins. For example, the bacterium *Corynebacterium diphtheriae* causes diphtheria by producing a protein that is broken into two fragments that spread through the bloodstream and affect the heart, kidneys, and nerves. The bacterium *Clostridium tetani* produces a protein neurotoxin called tetanospasmin, causing spasms in the muscles of the jaw and other parts of the body. Tetanus usually comes from an infected wound and was a major killer on the battlefields of World War I.

Around 1890, German scientists von Behring and Erich Wernicke developed the first effective antiserum against diphtheria toxin. At about the same time, von Behring also developed an antiserum against tetanus toxin with Japanese bacteriologist Shibasaburo Kitasato. The researchers immunized animals with sterilized broth cultures of tetanus or diphtheria bacteria that contained the toxins and found that the animals' sera (part of the blood separated from blood cells and clotting factors) could be injected into diseased animals and cure them by rendering the toxins harmless. This transfer of antibodies made by one animal into another animal (via serum) provides a short-term immunization referred to as passive immunity. Antibodies in the antiserum bind to the harmful agents, allowing the recipient to mount a more intense immune response.

The German scientist Paul Ehrlich helped von Behring refine the techniques so that horses and sheep could be injected with a safe amount of toxin, and then their blood was conveniently used to produce lifesaving antisera with appropriate amounts of antitoxin. Unlike vaccines, antisera can cure people that already have the disease.

SEE ALSO Mithridatium and Theriac (100 B.C.), Biological Weapons (1346), Polio Vaccine (1955), and Structure of Antibodies (1959).

Clostridium tetani with its characteristic "drumstick" shape. C. tetani *can be found as spores in soil. It produces a toxin that causes tetanus, which can lead to powerful muscular spasms and death.*

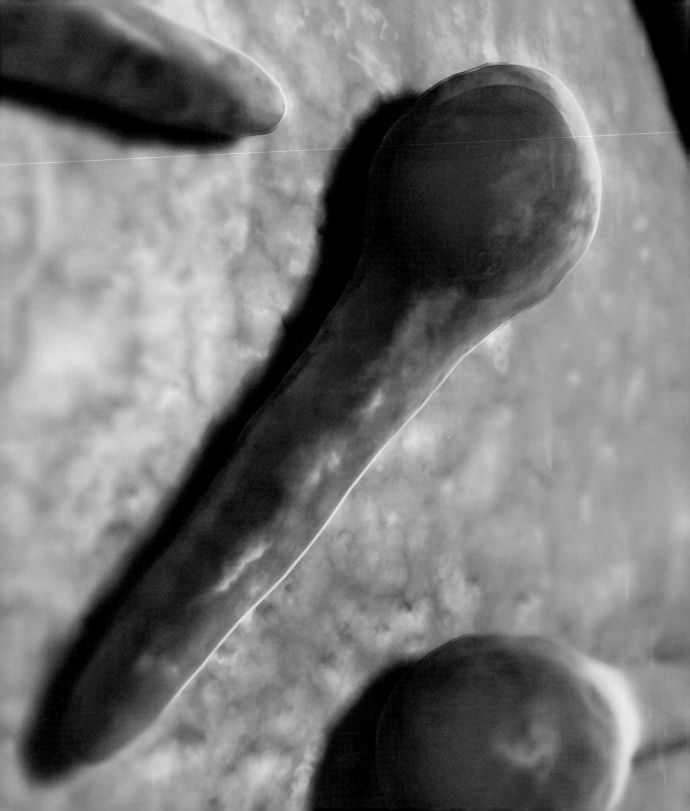

Latex Surgical Gloves

Joseph Lister (1827–1912), William Stewart Halsted (1852–1922)

Before the rise of **antiseptic** techniques and an understanding of the need for cleanliness when treating patients, surgeons used their bare hands and sometimes wore only protective aprons that resembled the aprons of a butcher. Many physicians were proud of the accumulation of blood, gore, and pus on their aprons and wore them as a badge of honor. Around 1865, British surgeon Joseph Lister dramatically reduced postoperative infections through the use of carbolic acid, now called phenol, for sterilizing wounds and surgical instruments.

In 1890, American surgeon William Halsted was the first to use sterilized medical gloves, prompted by the needs of his surgical assistant, Caroline Hampton, who had developed severe skin irritation on her hands as a result of repeated washing with carbolic acid and other harsh substances. Halsted contacted the Goodrich Rubber Company, requesting samples of rubber gloves that could be sterilized after use, and he gave them to Hampton. Her skin recovered, and not long afterward, Halsted married her!

Today, medical gloves are routinely used to prevent the spread of infections between patients and their caregivers. Such gloves are made from latex, vinyl, and other materials. Lycopodium powder and talc are two ingredients that were once used to make the gloves easier to apply and remove. However, both of these ingredients were later shown to be harmful if they contaminated surgical wounds, and cornstarch became most commonly used starting around the 1970s. Today, many gloves are powder-free and created through a process that makes the glove material less sticky. Latex provides very fine control and tactile sensitivity, but is sometimes avoided due to latex **allergies** among caregivers and patients.

Physicians before Halsted did try various materials for gloves, ranging from gloves made from sheep intestines (1758) to thick rubber gloves (in the 1840s), but these were rather clumsy and unsuitable for the delicate needs of surgery. Around 1844, Goodyear developed vulcanization (chemical modification) methods that enabled the creation of lighter, stretchier forms of rubber.

SEE ALSO Condom (1564), Semmelweis's Hand Washing (1847), Antiseptics (1865), Halstedian Surgery (1904), Allergies (1906), and Band-Aid Bandage (1920).

Medical gloves are routinely used to prevent the spread of infections between patients and their caregivers.

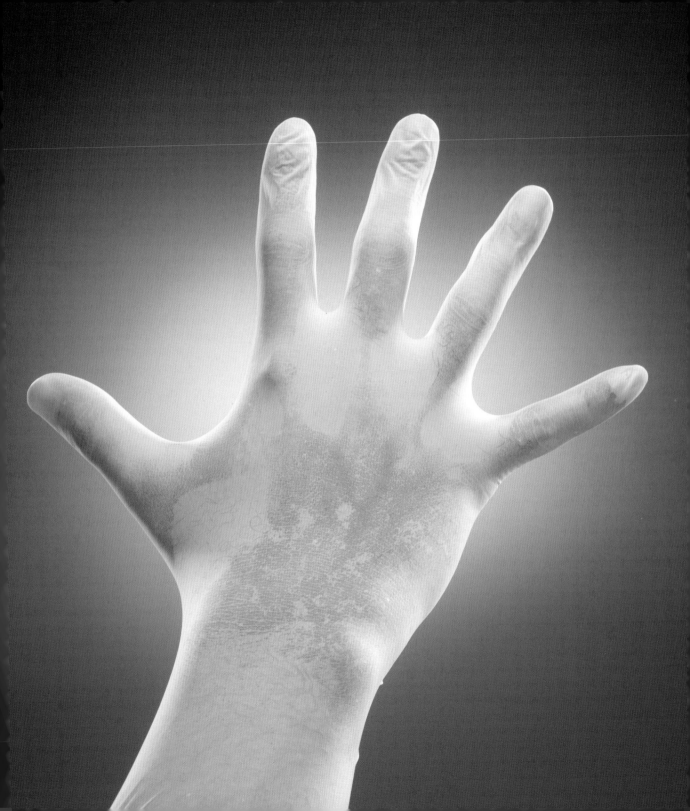

Neuron Doctrine

Heinrich Wilhelm Gottfried von Waldeyer-Hartz (1836–1921), Camillo Golgi (1843–1926), Santiago Ramón y Cajal (1852–1934)

According to neurobiologist Gordon Shepherd, the Neuron Doctrine is "one of the great ideas of modern thought [comparable to] quantum theory and relativity in physics [and] the periodic table and the chemical bond in chemistry." Having its birth in microscopy studies in the late 1800s, the Neuron Doctrine posits that distinct cells called neurons serve as the functional signal units of the nervous system and that neurons connect to one another in several precise ways. The doctrine was formally stated in 1891 by German anatomist Wilhelm von Waldeyer-Hartz, based on the observations of Spanish neuroscientist Santiago Cajal, Italian pathologist Camillo Golgi, and other scientists. Cajal improved upon the special silver stains of Golgi that allowed them to better microscopically visualize the incredible detail of cell branching processes.

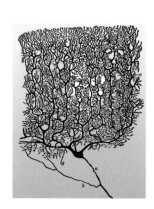

Although modern scientists have found exceptions to the original doctrine, most neurons contain dendrites, a soma (cell body), and an axon (which can be as long as three feet, or one meter!). In many cases, signals may propagate from one neuron to another by **neurotransmitter** chemicals that leave the axon of one neuron, travel through a tiny junction space called a chemical synapse, and then enter the dendrite of an adjacent neuron. If the net excitation caused by signals impinging on a neuron is sufficiently large, the neuron generates a brief electrical pulse called an action potential that travels along the axon. Electrical synapses, called gap junctions, also exist and create a direct connection between neurons.

Sensory neurons carry signals from sensory receptor cells in the body to the brain. Motor neurons transmit signals from the brain to muscles. Glial cells provide structural and metabolic support to the neurons. While neurons in adults tend not to reproduce, new connections between neurons can form throughout life. Each of the roughly 100 billion neurons can have more than 1,000 synaptic connections.

Multiple sclerosis results from insufficient myelin (chemical insulation) around axons. Parkinson's disease is associated with a lack of the neurotransmitter dopamine, normally produced by certain neurons in the midbrain.

SEE ALSO Cranial Nerves Classified (1664), Cerebellum Function (1809), Bell-Magendie Law (1811), Alzheimer's Disease (1906), Neurotransmitters (1914), Human Electroencephalogram (1924), and Levodopa for Parkinson's Disease (1957).

LEFT: *Cajal's complex drawing of a Purkinje neuron in a cat's cerebellar cortex.* RIGHT: *Neuron with multiple dendrites, a cell body, and one long axon. The capsulelike bulges on the axon are myelin-sheath cells.*

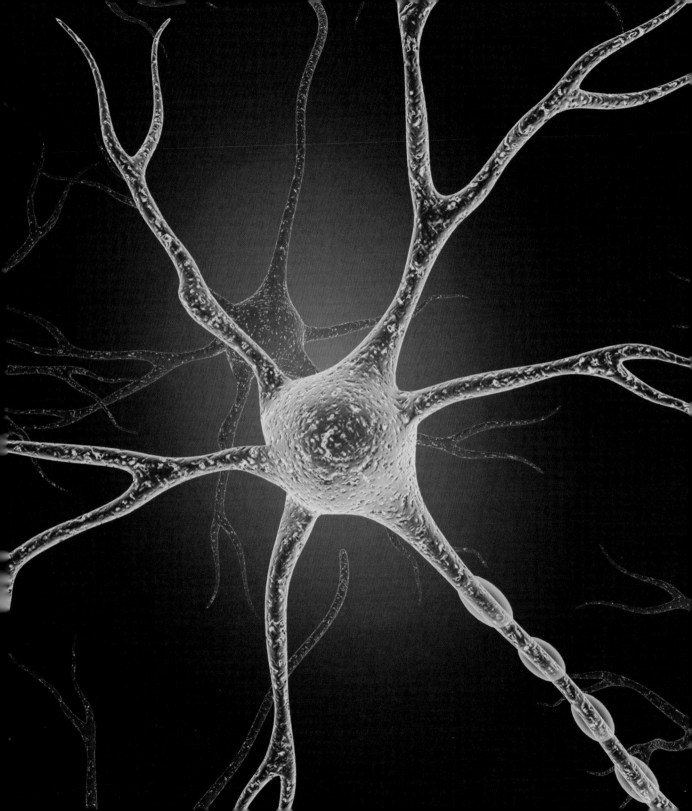

Discovery of Viruses

Martinus Willem Beijerinck (1851–1931), Dimitri Iosifovich Ivanovsky (1864–1920)

Science journalist Robert Adler writes, "Rabies, smallpox, **yellow fever**, dengue fever, poliomyelitis, influenza, AIDS . . . The list [of diseases caused by viruses] reads like a catalog of human misery. . . . The scientists who deciphered the secrets of viruses were literally groping in the dark, trying to understand something they could not see . . . and, for many years, could not even imagine."

Viruses exist in a strange realm between the living and nonliving. They do not possess all of the required molecular machinery to reproduce themselves on their own, but once they infect animals, plants, fungi, or bacteria, they can hijack their hosts in order to generate numerous viral copies. Some viruses may coax their host cells into uncontrolled multiplication, leading to **cancer**. Today, we know that most viruses are too small to be seen by an ordinary light microscope, given that an average virus is about one one-hundredth the size of the average bacterium. The virions (virus particles) consist of genetic material in the form of **DNA** or RNA and an outer protein coating. Some viruses also have an envelope of lipids (small organic molecules) when the virus is outside a host cell.

In 1892, Russian biologist Dimitri Ivanovsky took one of the early steps toward understanding viruses when he attempted to understand the cause of tobacco mosaic disease, which destroys tobacco leaves. He filtered an extract of crushed diseased leaves by using a fine porcelain filter designed to trap all bacteria. To his surprise, the fluid that had flowed through the filter was still infectious. However, Ivanovsky never understood the true viral cause, believing that toxins or bacterial spores might be the causative agent. In 1898, Dutch microbiologist Martinus Beijerinck performed a similar experiment and believed that this new kind of infectious agent was liquid in nature, referring to it as "soluble living germs." Later researchers were able to grow viruses in media containing guinea pig cornea tissue, minced hen kidneys, and fertilized chicken eggs. It was not until the 1930s that viruses could finally be seen via the electron microscope.

SEE ALSO Biological Weapons (1346), Causes of Cancer (1761), Common Cold (1914), Pap Smear Test (1928), Stanley's Crystal Invaders (1935), HeLa Cells (1951), Radioimmunoassay (1959), Reverse Transcriptase and AIDS (1970), and Oncogenes (1976).

Most animal viruses are symmetrical (e.g., icosahedral) and nearly spherical in shape, as depicted in this artistic representation. Viruses are generally much smaller than bacteria.

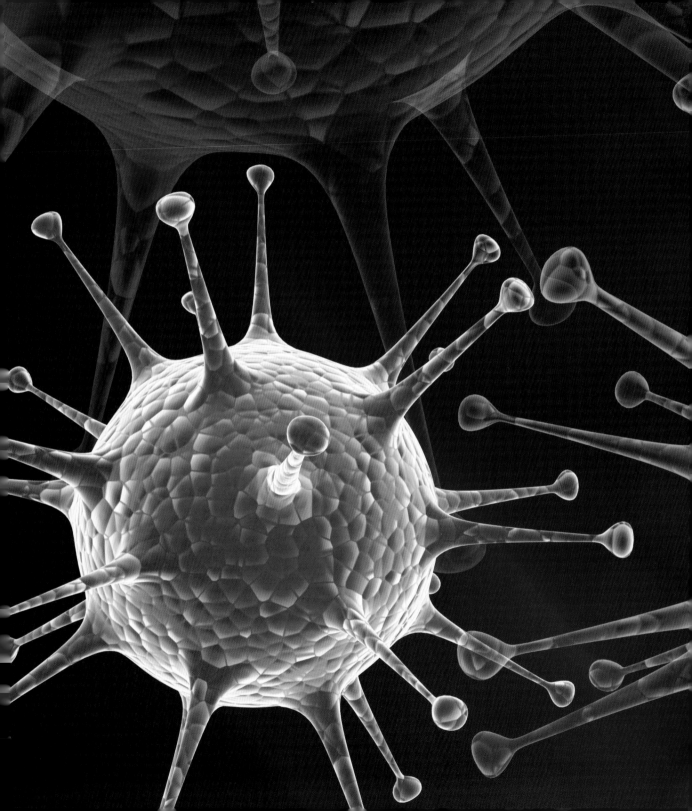

Osteopathy

Andrew Taylor Still (1828–1917)

Osteopathy is a field of healthcare that emphasizes the role of the musculoskeletal system in the prevention and treatment of health problems. After Civil War army surgeon Andrew Taylor Still lost most of his children to infectious diseases, he founded the first school of osteopathy in Kirksville, Missouri, in 1892. According to Still's philosophy, most diseases were caused by mechanical interference of nerves and blood flow, and they were curable by manipulation of "deranged, displaced bones, nerves, muscles—removing all obstructions—thereby setting the machinery of life moving." In his autobiography, Still claimed that he could "shake a child and stop scarlet fever, croup, diphtheria, and cure whooping cough in three days by a wring of its neck." Although statements such as these may seem far-fetched by today's standards, his methods had success relative to conventional medicine simply because he killed fewer patients than many physicians. Surgery and drugs of his time were often harmful, so many people questioned the effectiveness of common methods involving **bloodletting**, rectal feedings, and agents that contained toxic quantities of arsenic and mercury. Still wrote that, during the Civil War, in those parts "of Missouri and Kansas where the doctors were shut out, the children did not die."

Today, in the United States, an American-trained D.O. (Doctor of Osteopathic Medicine) is educated in a manner similar to a traditional medical doctor and is essentially the legal equivalent of an M.D. (In the European and Commonwealth nations, an osteopath is not a physician.) A majority of osteopaths enter family practice. In addition to conventional medical approaches and the use of drugs, a modern D.O. in the United States also emphasizes diet, posture, and therapeutic manipulation. However, strong debates take place today with respect to exaggerated claims of the benefits of cranial osteopathy to relieve pain or treat other ailments. Cranial osteopathy involves the manipulation of skull bones and is used by a minority of practitioners.

SEE ALSO Phrenology (1796), D.D. Palmer and Chiropractic (1895), and Flexner Report and Medical Education (1910).

Andrew Taylor Still, one of the founders of osteopathic medicine, c. 1914.

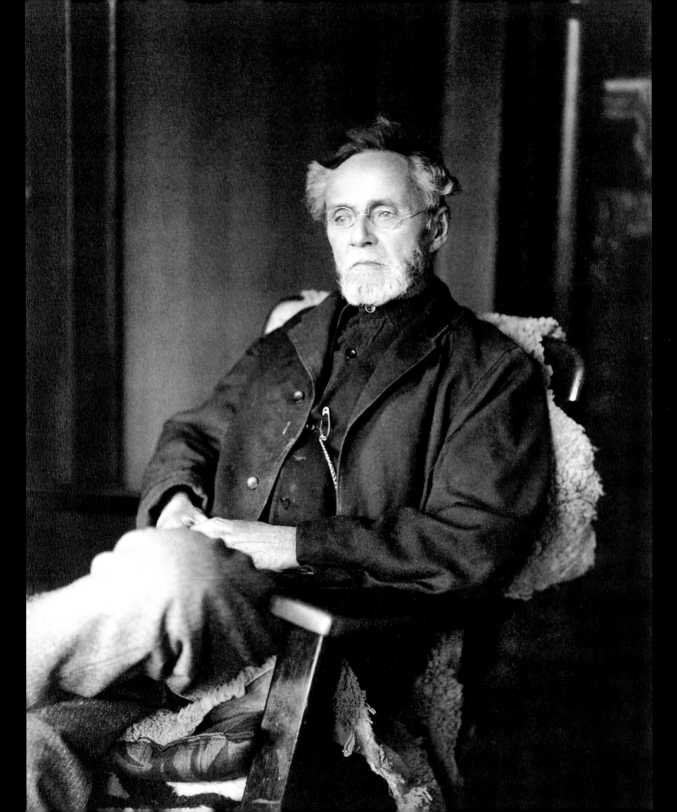

Discovery of Adrenaline

George Oliver (1841–1915), **Edward Albert Sharpey-Schafer** (born Schäfer; 1850–1935), **Jokichi Takamine** (1854–1922)

The discovery of adrenaline is notable, in part, because it was the first glandular hormone to be isolated and produced in the laboratory. Hormones are chemical "messengers" released by a cell in one part of the body that affect cells elsewhere.

Starting in 1893, English physician George Oliver and English physiologist Edward Sharpey-Schafer performed the first systematic studies of the effects of adrenaline. Oliver had been experimenting on his son by giving him extracts of adrenal glands (which are located atop the kidneys), and Oliver observed a change in the diameter of his son's blood vessels. Next, Oliver urged Sharpey-Schafer to inject the extract into a dog. To their amazement, the mercury blood-pressure device showed a very dramatic change in the dog's blood pressure. They soon showed that the gland's active substance, known today as either adrenaline or epinephrine, had a profound effect on the constriction of arterioles (small-diameter blood vessels), resulting in increased blood pressure. Anatomist Stephen Carmichael writes, "Their publication in 1894, resulting from their subsequent experiments, is heralded as the first demonstration of a hormonal effect. Many historians regard this study of the adrenal medulla [the organ's core] as a milestone in endocrinology."

Japanese chemist and samurai Jokichi Takamine is usually credited as the first person to isolate and, to a large extent, purify adrenaline around 1901. Although his assistant had actually obtained the first crystalline product, Takamine filed the patent involving the blood pressure–raising principle, which made him rich. Adrenaline eventually found uses in hemorrhage control, cardiology, obstetrics, and the treatment of allergies.

Adrenaline is vital for normal bodily functions. It is secreted in larger quantities during times of stress, when it increases heart rate as well as the volume of blood pumped from heart ventricles with each beat, resulting in an increase of blood flow to muscles. It triggers smooth-muscle relaxation in the airways and causes peripheral arteries and veins (those far from the heart) to constrict. However, it causes vasodilation (vessel widening) in the muscles, liver, and heart.

SEE ALSO Thyroid Surgery (1872), Allergies (1906), Human Growth Hormone (1921), Cortisone (1948), Pineal Body (1958), and Beta-Blockers (1964).

Adrenaline is produced by the adrenal glands (dull orange organs shown atop the kidneys) from the amino acids phenylalanine and tyrosine.

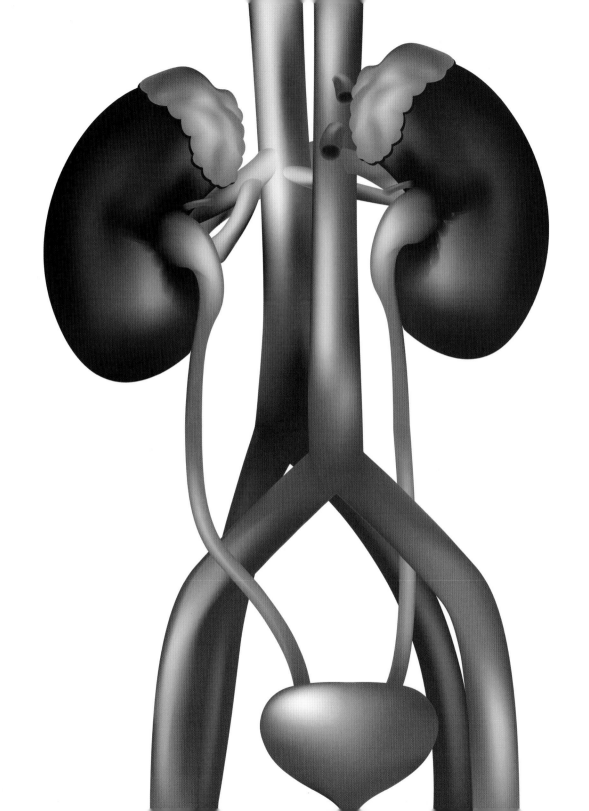

Cause of Bubonic Plague

Shibasaburo Kitasato (1853–1931), Alexandre Emile Jean Yersin (1863–1943)

Journalist Edward Marriott writes, "Plague. The very word carries an unholy resonance. No other disease can claim its apocalyptic power: it can lie dormant for centuries, only to resurface with nation-killing force." Not until 1894, when bubonic plague was rampant in Hong Kong, did a frenetic and unfriendly race between Hong Kong's two top scientists—French-Swiss physician Alexandre Yersin and Japanese physician Shibasaburo Kitasato—finally elucidate the bacterial origin of bubonic plague. Yersin explicitly linked the plague with the rod-shaped bacterium, now called *Yersinia pestis.*

Historian Norman F. Cantor writes, "The Black Death of 1348–49 was the greatest biomedical disaster in European and possibly world history." Arab historian Ibn Khaldun noted that "civilization both East and West was visited by a destructive plague that devastated nations and caused populations to vanish. It swallowed up many of the good things of civilization and wiped them out in the entire inhabited world."

During the fourteenth-century bubonic plague—often called the Black Death—roughly 75 million people worldwide perished, including more than one-third of Europe's population. Plagues visited Europe numerous times, with varying mortality rates, until the 1700s. Although scientists still debate whether all of the plagues were in fact the same disease, the cause is usually attributed to *Yersinia pestis* or its variants, which are carried by rodents and fleas. People who are infected by the plague display buboes, or swellings of lymph nodes, and they die within a few days. Europeans quickly developed theories as to the cause of the disease, ranging from astrological forces or God's wrath to the poisoning of wells by Jews. As a result, tens of thousands of Jews were exterminated.

Authors Lloyd and Dorothy Moote write, "Building on the foundational work of Koch and Pasteur and the achievements of Yersin and Kitasato, twentieth-century microbe hunters would go on to develop the long-sought wonder drugs [antibiotics] that could cure plague. The end of an ancient scourge of humankind was at last clearly in sight."

SEE ALSO Persecution of Jewish Physicians (1161), Biological Weapons (1346), Panum's "Measles on the Faroe Islands" (1846), Germ Theory of Disease (1862), and Cause of Leprosy (1873).

Rat fleas in the hair of a rat. Bubonic plague is an infection of the lymphatic system, usually resulting from the bite of a rat flea that harbors Y. pestis *bacilli in its gut.*

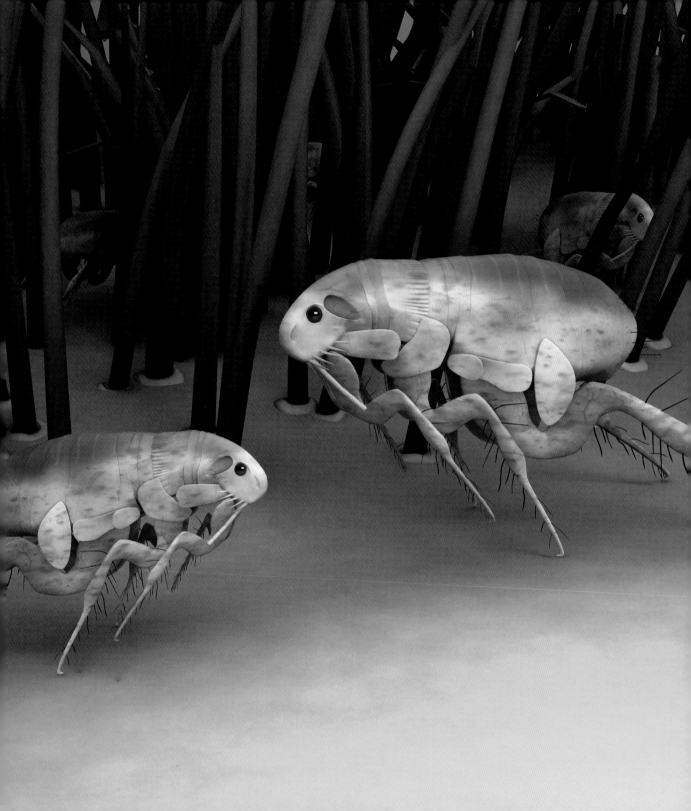

D.D. Palmer and Chiropractic

Daniel David "D.D." Palmer (1845–1913), **Bartlett Joshua "B.J." Palmer** (1882–1961)

"Americans have a love affair with chiropractors," writes physician Edward Schneider. "We are more likely to see a chiropractor than any other alternative-care provider." For this reason, this health-care discipline deserves a place in this book. The practice of chiropractic began in 1895, when Daniel "D.D." Palmer claimed to have improved a man's hearing by manipulating the man's back. Palmer, a former beekeeper and grocer, wrote that he received the idea of chiropractic from the spirit of a diseased physician.

Although Louis Pasteur's **germ theory of disease**, proposed in the 1860s, was well known, Palmer still lived in a time where odd treatments and **patent medicines** were popular and sold with colorful names and exaggerated claims. Palmer wrote in 1909, "Chiropractors have found in every disease that is supposed to be contagious, *a cause in the spine*. In the spinal column we *will* find a subluxation that corresponds to every type of disease. If we had one hundred cases of small-pox, I can prove to you where, in one, you will find a subluxation and you will find the same conditions in the other ninety-nine. I adjust one and return his functions to normal. . . . There is no contagious disease. . . . There is no infection." Palmer's son B.J. was also a pioneer of chiropractic treatment.

Chiropractic today usually involves the treatment of musculoskeletal pain and other diseases by manipulation of the spine and other joints. Traditional chiropractors have often made reference to vertebral subluxation, a kind of spinal joint dysfunction, as interfering with the functioning of the body and its organs. Palmer initially hypothesized that subluxations caused pinched nerves but later suggested that they cause nerves to be too slack or tense, thus affecting the health of organs in which they interact. Diseases were caused by the disrupted flow of "innate intelligence." Many modern chiropractors are receptive to mainstream medicine when appropriate. Debate continues as to the degree to which the **placebo effect** plays a role in chiropractic treatment for pain relief.

SEE ALSO Alternative Medicine (1796), Germ Theory of Disease (1862), Osteopathy (1892), Patent Medicines (1906), and Placebo Effect (1955).

Chiropractic today usually involves the treatment of musculoskeletal pain and other diseases by manipulation of the spine and other joints. Back pain (also known as dorsalgia) may originate from the nerves, muscles, joints or other structures near the spine.

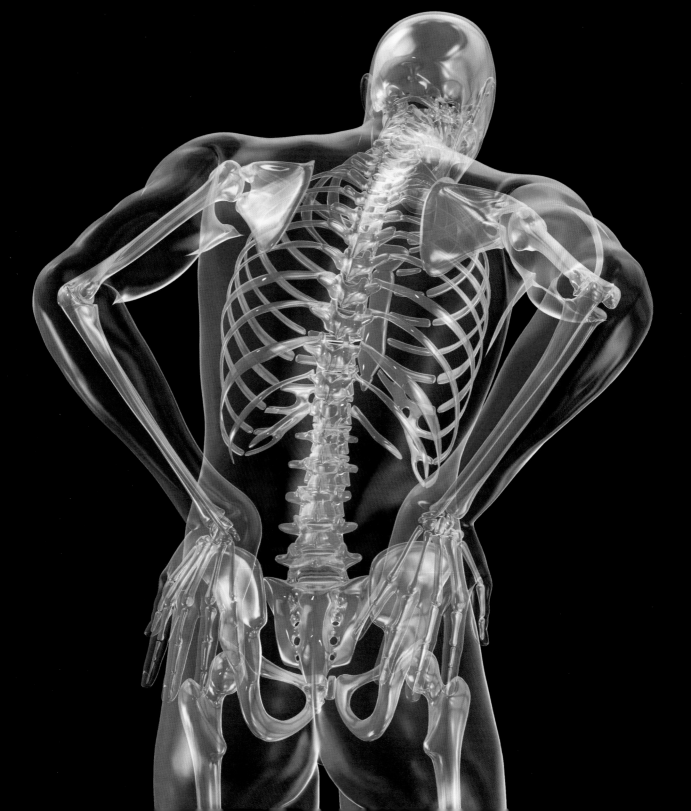

X-rays

Wilhelm Conrad Röntgen (1845–1923), Hermann Joseph Muller (1890–1967)

Upon seeing her husband's X-ray image of her hand, Wilhelm Röntgen's wife "shrieked in terror and thought that the rays were evil harbingers of death," writes author Kendall Haven. "Within a month, Wilhelm Röntgen's X-rays were the talk of the world. Skeptics called them death rays that would destroy the human race. Eager dreamers called them miracle rays that could make the blind see again and could beam . . . diagrams straight into a student's brains." However, for physicians, X-rays marked a turning point in the treatment of the sick and wounded.

On November 8, 1895, the German physicist Röntgen was experimenting with a cathode-ray tube when he found that a discarded fluorescent screen lit up more than a meter (three feet) away when he switched on the tube, even though the tube was covered with a heavy cardboard. He realized that the tube emitted some form of invisible rays, and he soon found that they could penetrate various materials, such as wood, glass, and rubber. When he placed his hand in the path of the invisible rays, he saw a shadowy image of his bones. It was later shown that X-rays are electromagnetic waves, like light, but of a higher energy and a shorter wavelength.

In 1914, X-ray stations were used on the battlefields of World War I to help diagnose wounded soldiers. Aside from skeletal structures, X-rays today can be used to visualize arteries and veins in angiography, which involves the injection of an opaque contrast agent into the blood vessels. **Radiation therapy** may employ X-rays to destroy some forms of **cancer**. X-rays may also be used to identify lung and breast diseases and intestinal obstructions. Computed tomography (CT) uses computer processing to combine many X-ray images in order to generate cross-sectional views and three-dimensional visualizations.

In 1926, American biologist Hermann Muller clearly and quantitatively demonstrated that X-rays can create mutations in cells, thus calling attention to the potential dangers of overexposure to X-rays.

SEE ALSO Radiation Therapy (1903), Mammography (1949), Medical Ultrasound (1957), CAT Scans (1967), and Magnetic Resonance Imaging (MRI) (1977).

X-ray of the side view of a human head, showing screws used to reconstruct the jawbones.

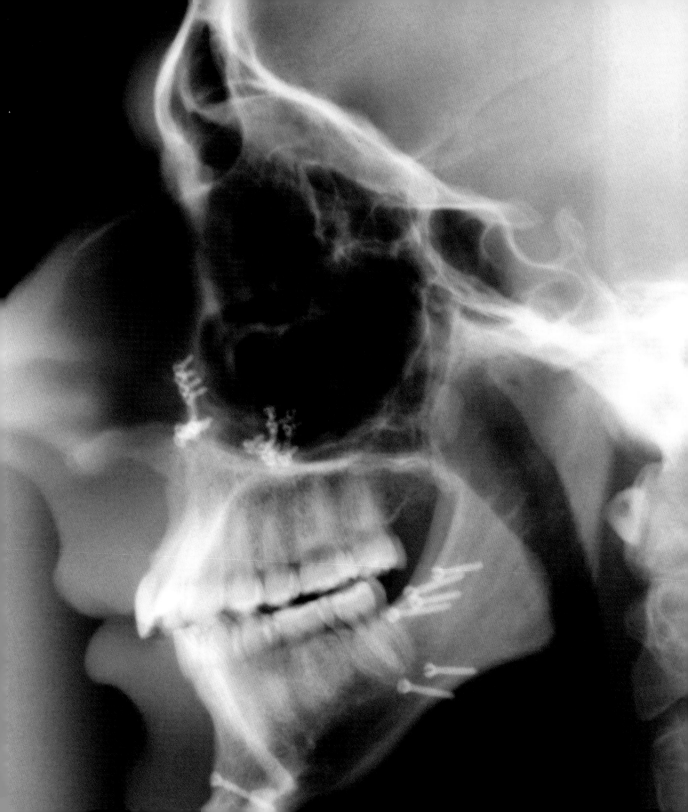

Cause of Malaria

Charles Louis Alphonse Laveran (1845–1922), Sir Ronald Ross (1857–1932)

According to physicians Charles Poser and G. W. Bruyn, malaria has defeated conquering armies, devastated papal conclaves, affected the fate of besieged cities, and likely contributed to the decline of Greek civilization and the Roman Empire. Historians studying the response of physicians to this disease observe an evolution in medical thinking, beginning in superstition and, around 1900, ending in hard science.

Malaria is notable, not only because it kills more than a million people each year in places like sub-Saharan Africa, but also because it is probably the first disease for which a complex unicellular organism (a protist) was definitively identified as its cause. People are infected when the malaria parasite in the salivary glands of a female *Anopheles* mosquito enters the bloodstream when a person is bitten. After spending time in the liver, the parasite multiplies within red blood cells, causing fevers, coma, and, in severe cases, death. In modern times, malaria has been treated with combinations of drugs that often contain derivatives of artemisinin (which is found in Chinese medicinal herbs) or quinine (which originally came from tree bark).

Five species of the parasite (genus *Plasmodium*) can cause the disease, with *Plasmodium falciparum* being the most dangerous. The body's immune system has difficulty killing the parasite because it is somewhat protected when it resides within the liver and blood cells. Young children are particularly vulnerable, but the spread of malaria can be slowed by using mosquito nets treated with insecticides and by draining standing water, in which mosquitoes lay eggs.

In 1880, French army physician Charles Laveran discovered malaria parasites in the blood of a patient. In 1897, while working in India, the British physician Ronald Ross finally proved that malaria is transmitted by mosquitoes after observing the parasites in mosquito salivary glands.

Interestingly, individuals with only one gene for the **sickle-cell anemia** blood disease have substantial protection against malaria. Science historian Charles Rosenberg writes, "No disease illustrates the complex interdependencies that shape disease incidence and experience better than malaria."

SEE ALSO Sewage Systems (600 B.C.), Mendel's Genetics (1865), Cause of Sleeping Sickness (1902), Cause of Rocky Mountain Spotted Fever (1906), Ehrlich's Magic Bullets (1910), Cause of Yellow Fever (1937), and Cause of Sickle-Cell Anemia (1949).

Female Anopheles albimanus *mosquito feeding on a human host and becoming engorged with blood.*

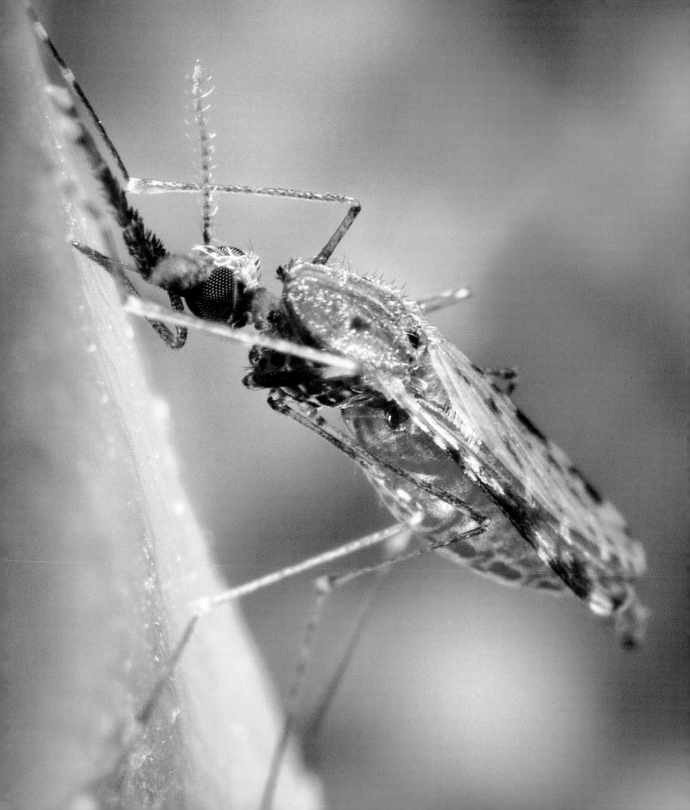

Aspirin

Hippocrates of Cos (460 B.C.–377 B.C.), **Charles Frédéric Gerhardt** (1816–1856), **Heinrich Dreser** (1860–1924), **Arthur Eichengrün** (1867–1949), **Felix Hoffmann** (1868–1946), **Sir John Robert Vane** (1927–2004)

Historian Edward Shorter writes, "Since its introduction in 1899, aspirin (acetylsalicylic acid) has been the most popular drug of all time. In the United States alone, some 10,000 to 20,000 tons of aspirin are used annually." Aspirin relieves pain, reduces fever, and decreases blood clotting—therefore making aspirin potentially useful for reducing the incidence of strokes and heart attacks. Aspirin was the first-discovered member of the class of drugs called nonsteroidal anti-inflammatory drugs (NSAIDs).

Over the millennia, Africans, Chinese, ancient Sumerians, and others have used medicines derived from plants and trees. The ancient Egyptians knew of the pain-relieving effects of potions made of willow leaves, and the ancient Greek physician Hippocrates also recommended the juices of willow bark and leaves for pain. Scientists later discovered that the active ingredient in these potions was the chemical salicin, which the body converts to salicylic acid. These chemicals were rather harsh on users' digestive systems, which, in 1897, motivated researchers at the Bayer company in Germany to modify the compound to form acetylsalicylic acid (ASA), a pain reliever that is less harsh on the stomach. These researchers included Felix Hoffmann, Heinrich Dreser, and Arthur Eichengrün, with some debate as to who should be given the most credit. (Note that in 1853, the French chemist Charles Gerhardt had prepared ASA, but used an approach that was not cost-effective.)

Finally, in 1899, Bayer marketed and manufactured ASA on a large scale and called it aspirin. In 1971, British pharmacologist John Vane and colleagues showed that aspirin worked by inhibiting prostaglandins and thromboxanes in the body. Prostaglandins play a role in causing inflammation and regulating pain. Thromboxanes are responsible for aggregation of platelets during blood-clot formation. Today, we know that aspirin inactivates the cyclooxygenase enzyme, which is required for prostaglandin and thromboxane synthesis.

The invention of aspirin has stimulated further research in the quest for new anti-inflammatory painkillers and is a good example of the role of pharmacognosy, which involves the study of medicines derived from natural sources.

SEE ALSO Hippocratic Oath (400 B.C.), Dioscorides's *De Materia Medica* (70), Digitalis (1785), Cocaine as Local Anesthetic (1884), and Heparin (1916).

White willow, from Otto Wilhelm Thomé's Flora von Deutschland, Österreich und der Schweiz *(1885). In 1765, the Reverend Edmund Stone from England observed that a tincture of willow bark reduced fever. The active extract of the bark is salicin.*

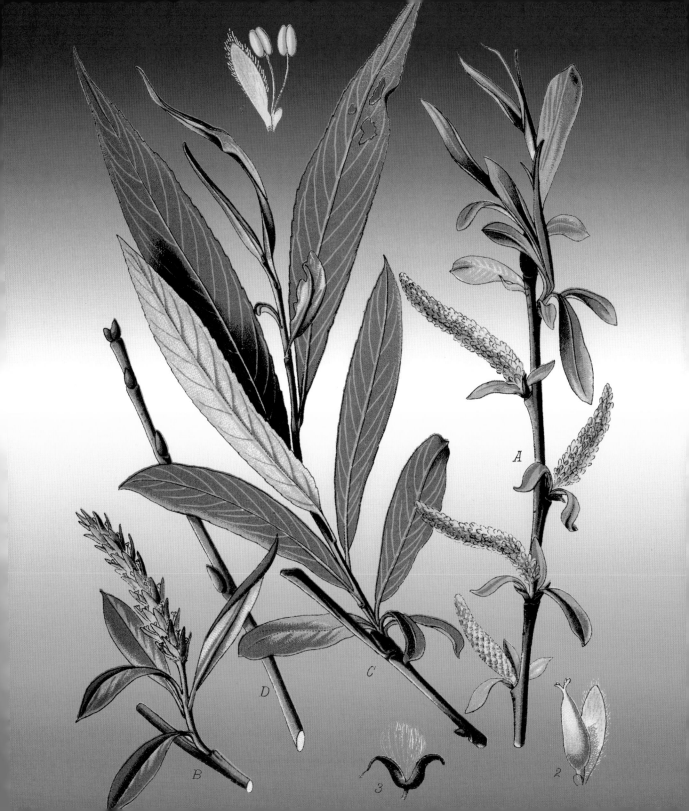

Defibrillator

Peter Christian Abildgaard (1740–1801), **Jean-Louis Prévost** (1838–1927), **Frederic Batelli** (1867–1941), **Claude Schaeffer Beck** (1894–1971)

In 1775, Danish veterinarian Peter Abildgaard published a scientific paper discussing the electrical resuscitation of a chicken: "With a shock to the head, the animal was rendered lifeless, and arose with a second shock to the chest; however, after the experiment was repeated rather often, the hen was completely stunned, walked with some difficulty, and did not eat for a day and night; then later it was very well and even laid an egg." At the time, scientists had little understanding of the heart physiology involved in chicken resurrection.

The normal heart has its own internal electrical system that controls the heart rate and rhythm. The electrical signal begins in a group of cells called the sinoatrial node at the top of the heart and spreads to the bottom to coordinate timing of the heart pumping. First, the heart's two upper chambers (atria) contract, and then the bottom chambers (ventricles) contract to pump blood to the body.

Defibrillation refers to the treatment of cardiac arrhythmias (abnormal electrical activity in the heart) that include ventricular fibrillation (VF, or ineffective quivering of the ventricle muscles) and ventricular tachycardia (VT, or abnormally rapid ventricular heart rhythms). Defibrillator devices can deliver a sudden electric current to the heart and help reestablish a natural rhythm.

In 1899, Swiss physiologists Jean-Louis Prévost and Frederic Batelli discovered that they could induce VF in dogs with small electric shocks and then reverse the condition with larger charges. The first use of a defibrillator on a human occurred in 1947, when American cardiac surgeon Claude Beck placed internal paddles on either side of the heart of a 14-year-old boy experiencing VF and delivered a charge to the heart, causing it to return to a normal rhythm.

Today, automated external defibrillators (AEDs) can actually analyze the heart rhythm and then, if warranted, deliver a therapeutic charge. Implantable cardioverter-defibrillators (ICDs) are small, battery-powered devices placed under the skin. The ICDs detect arrhythmias and then deliver the appropriate electrical impulses for treatment.

SEE ALSO Digitalis (1785), Stethoscope (1816), Electrocardiograph (1903), Cardiopulmonary Resuscitation (1956), Artificial Pacemaker for Heart (1958), and Near-Death Experiences (1975).

Manual external defibrillator. Medical personnel may determine what charge (in joules) to apply and then will deliver the shock through paddles placed on the chest.

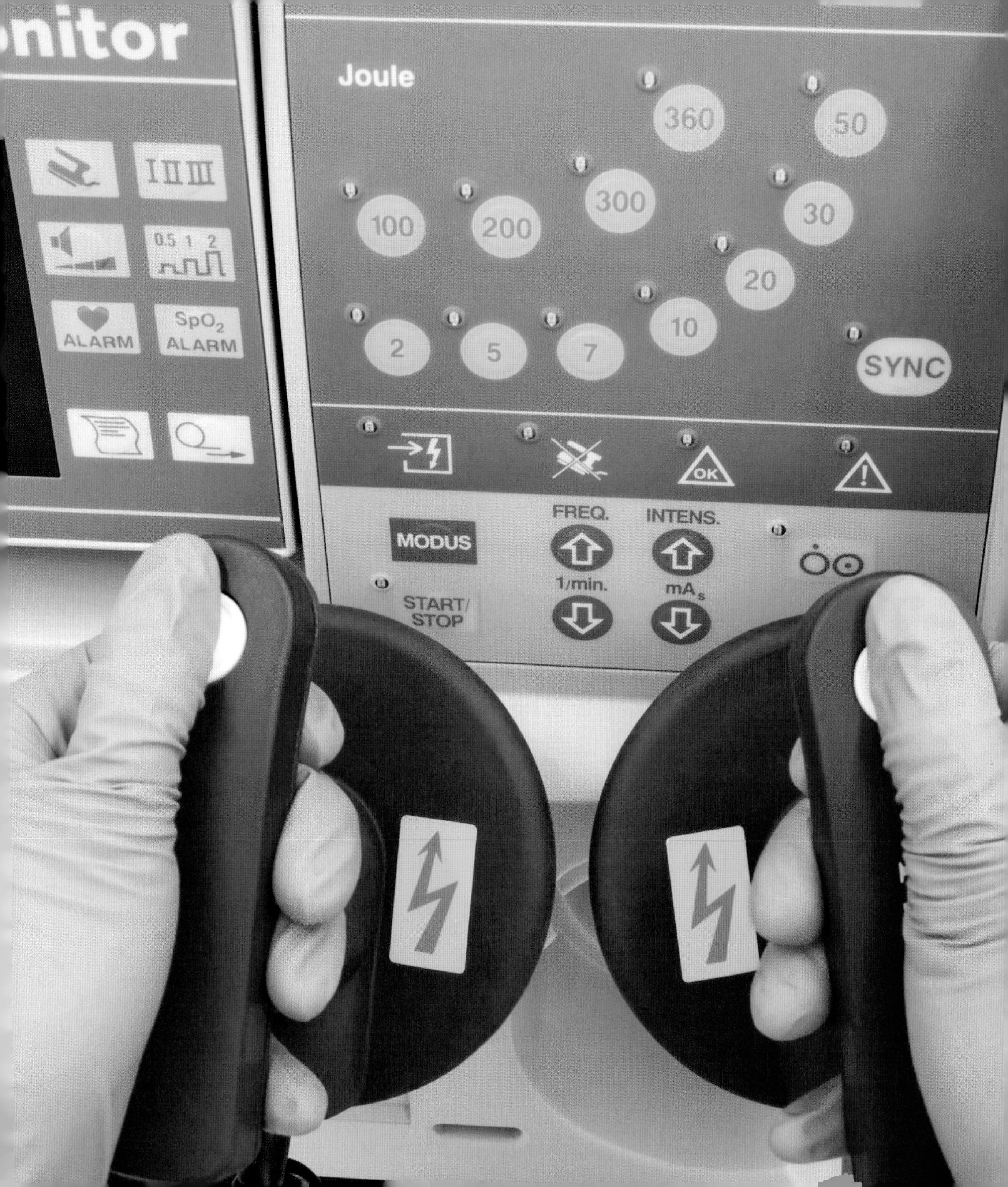
nitor
Joule
360
50
300
30
100
200
20
10
2
5
7
SYNC
0.5 1 2
SpO2
ALARM
ALARM
OK
MODUS
FREQ.
INTENS.
1/min.
mAs
START/
STOP

Hearing Aids

Giambattista della Porta (1535–1615), **Thomas W. Graydon** (1850–1900), **Miller Reese Hutchison** (1876–1944)

The evolution of hearing aids—devices used to amplify sounds to help hearing-impaired individuals—starts in ancient times, when people used hollow animal horns placed by the ear. In his 1558 book *Natural Magick*, Italian scholar Giambattista della Porta describes wooden hearing aids in the shape of animal ears. Starting in the 1600s, various funnel-like "ear trumpets" were used for directing sound into the ear. In 1880, physician Thomas Graydon invented the Dentaphone, a bone-conduction hearing aid with a vibrating diaphragm that transmitted sound to the user's teeth. Vibrations were then transmitted to the inner ear via bone conduction. In 1899, American inventor Miller Hutchison created one of the first electric hearing devices: the battery-powered Akoulalion. This table model used a carbon microphone and had several earphones.

The earliest "useful" electrical hearing aids in the 1900s employed vacuum tubes for sound amplification but were large and unwieldy. Starting in the 1950s, the

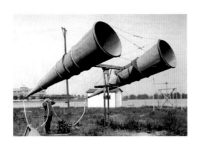

transistor allowed hearing aids to become smaller and more sophisticated in their ability to process and transmit sounds. Some hearing aids were even built into eyeglass frames. Today, many styles of hearing aids exist, including behind-the-ear aids in which a case (with amplification system) sits behind the flap of the ear with a tube coming down toward the ear canal. Other hearing aids may reside entirely in the ear canal. Bone-anchored hearing aids vibrate the skull and inner ear.

In general, hearing aids have a means for sound capture (a microphone) and for processing to provide amplification and clarity. Today's hearing aids are quite sophisticated and may feature electronic noise reduction circuits to reduce undesirable background noise, programmability, and selectable modes so that users may alter signal-processing characteristics. Certain frequency ranges may be emphasized. Hearing aids may use both omnidirectional and directional microphones, the latter of which are useful when communicating with a particular person. Telecoils allow electronic audio sources to be connected to hearing aids.

SEE ALSO Eyeglasses (1284), Exploring the Labyrinth (1772), Stethoscope (1816), and Cochlear Implants (1977).

Small "ear trumpet" hearing aids of the 1600s eventually evolved into these amazing devices. LEFT: *A huge two-horn system at Bolling Field, Washington, D.C. (1921).* RIGHT: *Photograph of Swedish soldiers operating an acoustic locator in 1940. Such devices were used to locate aircraft before radar became common.*

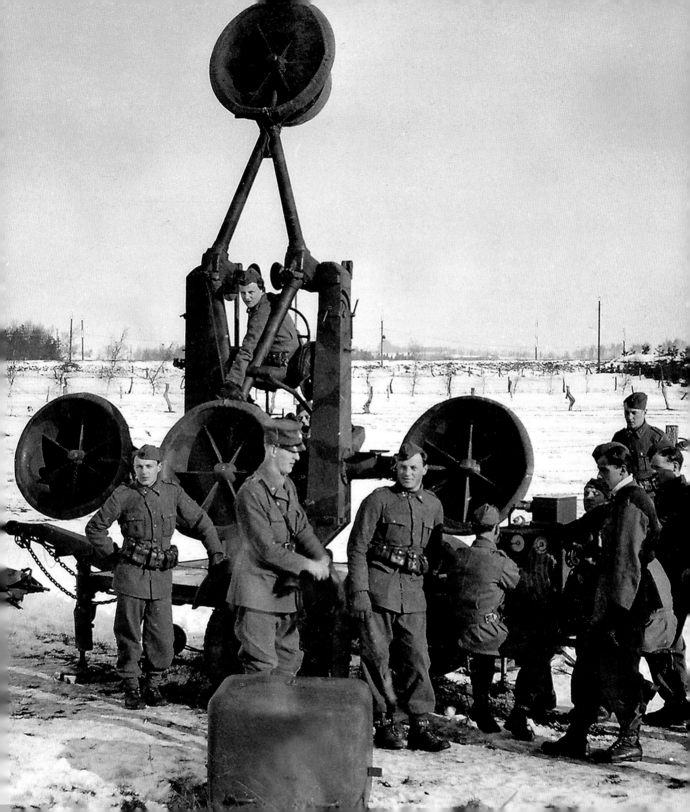

Psychoanalysis

Sigmund Freud (1856–1939)

According to author Catherine Reef, the Austrian physician Sigmund Freud "explored the human mind more thoroughly than anyone who had come before him. He pioneered a new method for diagnosing and treating mental illness, a method he called psychoanalysis. He simply talked to his patients, and, more important, he listened." Freud emphasized the importance of unconscious mental processes in shaping human behavior and emotions, and he encouraged his patients to "freely associate" and speak about images from fantasies and dreams. He encouraged patients to act as though they were travelers "sitting next to the window of a railway carriage and describing to someone outside the carriage the changing views" seen outside. When waiting for his patients' words to reveal hidden messages, Freud often felt like an archeologist unearthing precious relics in ancient cities. His goal was to interpret unconscious conflicts that caused harmful symptoms, thereby giving the patients insight and resolutions to their problems, which might include abnormal fears or obsessions. *The Interpretation of Dreams*, published in 1899, was his greatest work.

In general, Freud often suggested that patients' repressed sexual fantasies and early childhood experiences played an important role in later dysfunctional behavior. His most famous psychoanalytic model divided the mind into three separate parts: the id (concerned with basic drives such as sexual satisfaction), the superego (concerned with socially acquired controls and moral codes), and the ego (the conscious mind that motivates our decisions through the tension between the id and superego).

Although it is still difficult to discern what fraction of his often controversial ideas will ultimately be considered correct or even useful, his ideas on psychology "have completely revolutionized our conception of the human mind," according to author Michael Hart. Rather than condemn or ridicule those with behavioral anomalies, Freud sought understanding. Psychiatrist Anthony Storr writes, "Freud's technique of listening to distressed people over long periods rather than giving them orders or advice has formed the foundation of most modern forms of psychotherapy, with benefits to both patients and practitioners."

SEE ALSO *De Praestigiis Daemonum* (1563), Phrenology (1796), Truth Serum (1922), Jung's Analytical Psychology (1933), Electroconvulsive Therapy (1938), Transorbital Lobotomy (1946), Antipsychotics (1950), and Cognitive Behavioral Therapy (1963).

Freud's psychoanalytic couch, on which his patients reclined. Freud would sit out of sight in the green chair, listening to their free associations. (Freud Museum, London.)

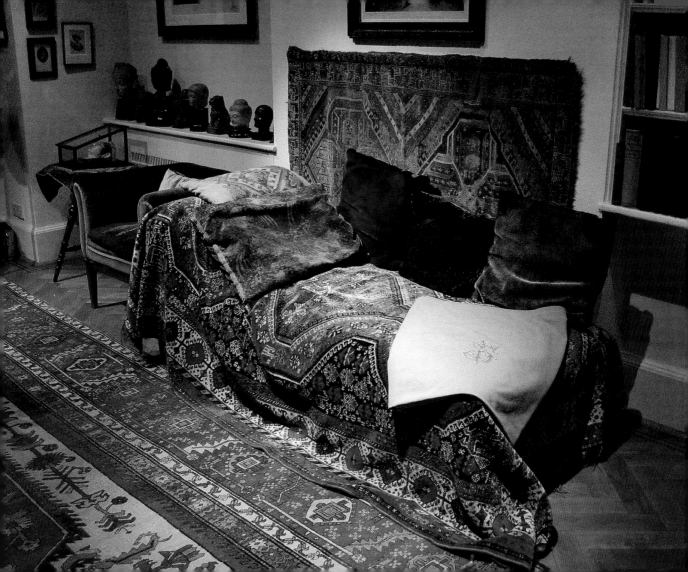

Caduceus

For most Americans, the caduceus—an ancient symbol featuring two snakes winding about a winged staff—symbolizes medicine, medical care, and medical personnel. Although the association of the caduceus with alchemy and wisdom can be traced back to the Renaissance, it is likely that its current symbolic use is based on confusion with the similar-looking Rod of Asclepius. Asclepius was the Greek god of medicine and healing, and his rod shows a *single* serpent winding about a staff that contains no wings. In mythology, Asclepius was such a great healer that he could bring people back from the dead. This power displeased Zeus, who struck Asclepius with a lightning bolt. Nevertheless, for centuries, sick people visited temples built in honor of Asclepius and hoped to be cured—perhaps not unlike people who visit certain Christian shrines today.

The caduceus has traditionally represented Hermes, the great messenger of the Greek gods and a guide to the underworld. The caduceus as a symbol for medicine became popular after the U.S. Army Medical Corps adopted the symbol in 1902 and added it to uniforms, perhaps mistaking it for the Rod of Asclepius. Today, some U.S. health-care professionals and associations use the caduceus, and others use the Rod of Asclepius.

The use of serpents in the context of healing has had a long history, perhaps in part because the ancients observed snakes shedding their old skins in a periodic process of renewal. In the Bible, God tells Moses to create a bronze serpent (later called Nehushtan), mounted on a pole. If any of Moses's followers were bitten by a dangerous snake, they could then look at the bronze serpent and be cured. The earliest known symbol of two snakes spiraling around a vertical rod appears in representations of Ningishzida, a Mesopotamian deity of the underworld. The symbol for Ningishzida predates the caduceus, Rod of Asclepius, and Nehushtan by many centuries.

SEE ALSO Barber Pole (1210), Stethoscope (1816), American Medical Association (1847), and Red Cross (1863).

Several examples of the caduceus, an ancient symbol featuring two snakes winding about a winged staff.

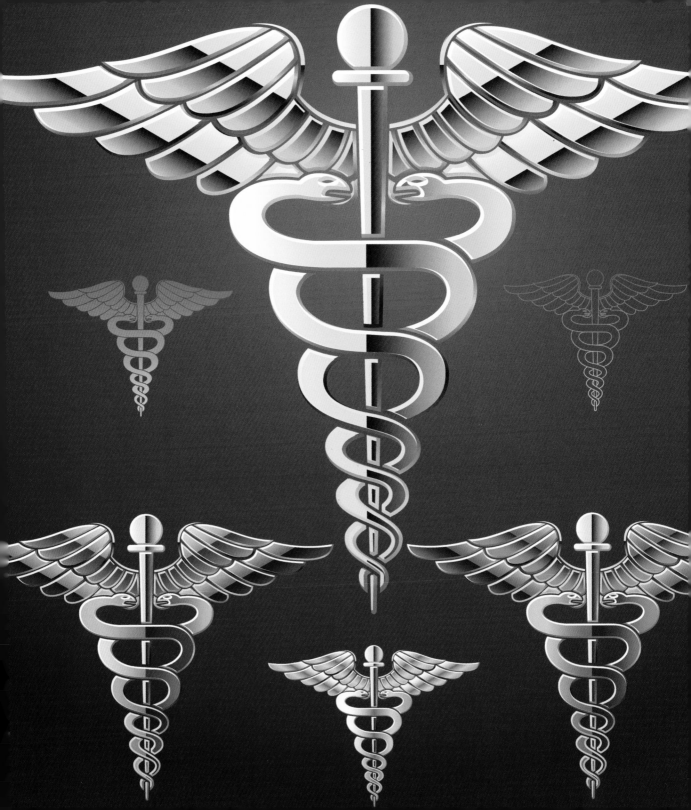

Chromosomal Theory of Inheritance

Theodor Heinrich Boveri (1862–1915), Walter Stanborough Sutton (1877–1916)

Chromosomes are threadlike structures, each made of a long coiled **DNA** molecule wrapped around a protein scaffold. Chromosomes are visible under a microscope during cell division. Human body cells contain 23 pairs of chromosomes—one member of the pair contributed by the mother and one by the father. **Sperm** and egg each contain 23 unpaired chromosomes. When the egg is fertilized, the number of chromosomes is restored to 46.

Around 1865, Austrian priest Gregor Mendel observed that organisms inherit traits via discrete units that we now refer to as genes (see **Mendel's genetics**), but it was not until 1902 that German biologist Theodor Boveri and American geneticist and physician Walter Sutton independently identified chromosomes as the carrier of this genetic information.

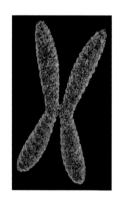

While studying sea urchins, Boveri concluded that sperm and egg each had a half set of chromosomes. However, if sperm and egg united to create sea urchin embryos with abnormal numbers of chromosomes, the embryos developed abnormally. Boveri concluded that different chromosomes affected different aspects of the creatures' development. Sutton's studies of grasshoppers demonstrated that matched pairs of chromosomes separate during the generation of sex cells. Not only did Boveri and Sutton suggest that the chromosomes carry parental genetic information, they also showed that chromosomes were independent entities that persisted even when they were not visible, during various stages of a cell's life, which was counter to one prevailing belief that the chromosomes simply "dissolved" during the course of cell division and reformed in the daughter cells. Their work provided a foundation for the new field of cytogenetics, the combination of cytology (the study of cells) and genetics (the science of heredity).

Today we know that during the creation of sperm and egg, matching chromosomes of parents can exchange small parts in a "crossover" process, so that new chromosomes are not inherited solely from either parent. Incorrect numbers of chromosomes can lead to genetic disorders. People with Down syndrome have 47 chromosomes.

SEE ALSO Discovery of Sperm (1678), Cell Division (1855), Mendel's Genetics (1865), Inborn Errors of Metabolism (1902), Genes and Sex Determination (1905), Amniocentesis (1952), DNA Structure (1953), Epigenetics (1983), Telomerase (1984), and Human Genome Project (2003).

LEFT: *Artist's representation of a chromosome.* RIGHT: *Within each chromosome, strands of DNA are coiled around proteins to form a nucleosome (shown here). Nucleosomes, in turn, are folded into even more complex structures within the chromosome, thus providing additional regulatory control of gene expression.*

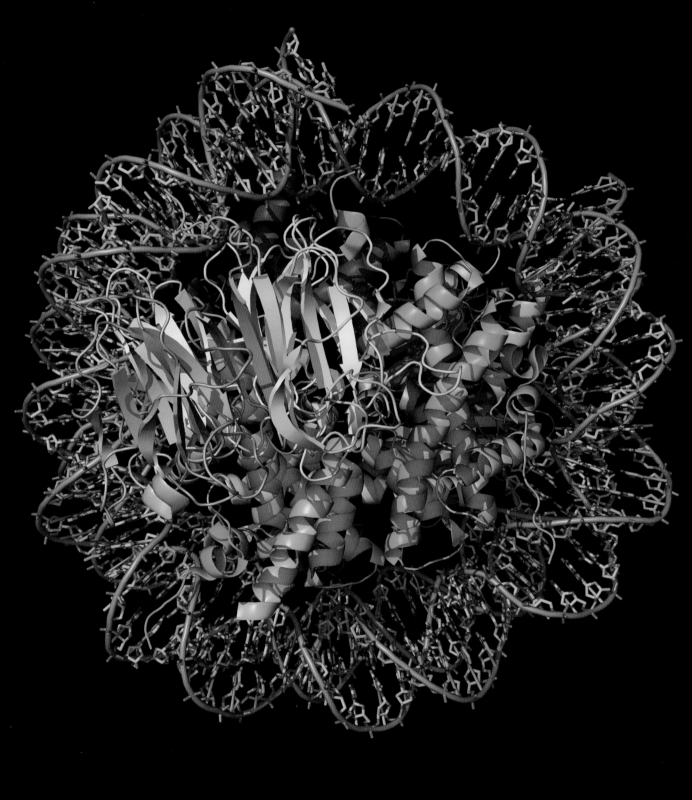

Inborn Errors of Metabolism

Archibald Edward Garrod (1857–1936)

Imagine the fear of parents who suddenly discover that their infant is producing black urine. The disease, alkaptonuria, was researched in 1902 by English physician Archibald Edward Garrod, who came to believe that this and certain other diseases were caused not by some infectious agent but rather by inherited inborn errors of metabolism (IEM), in which certain chemical pathways in the body were disrupted. Today, we know that these genetic diseases are usually caused by recessive genes, which means that an infant will exhibit the disease if it receives a defective gene from both the father and mother. In most cases, these defective genes lead to an underproduction of or a flaw in an enzyme, which controls chemical reaction rates.

Think of the cells in the body as functioning as a complex set of roadways in which the chemicals in a multistep sequence of reactions are represented as cars. If a traffic light remains red (a defective enzyme), then cars will pile up (representing an overabundance of certain chemicals that can harm the body).

Today, we know of several hundred IEM, a few of which are listed here. Alkaptonuria results from a defective enzyme involved in the degradation of tyrosine, an amino acid. A toxic tyrosine by-product accumulates and may damage cartilage and heart valves. Phenylketonuria (PKU) is caused by a deficiency in a liver enzyme needed to metabolize the amino acid phenylalanine. If detected early, PKU can be controlled by restricting foods rich in phenylalanine (e.g., meat and milk). If untreated, PKU can cause severe mental retardation. Thalassemias are a group of metabolic disorders that affect hemoglobin synthesis. Tay-Sachs disease, which occurs more frequently in Jews of eastern European descent, involves the deficiency of an enzyme required for metabolism of a certain class of fats. Mental ability deteriorates, with eventual death by about the age of four. Possible treatments for IEM continue to be explored, including bone marrow and organ transplants, as well as gene transfers.

SEE ALSO Urinalysis (4000 B.C.), Mendel's Genetics (1865), Chromosomal Theory of Inheritance (1902), Cause of Sickle-Cell Anemia (1949), and Gene Therapy (1990).

Many inborn errors of metabolism are inherited in an "autosomal recessive" pattern, depicted here. At top, both the father and mother carry one copy of the defective gene (orange). One out of four of their children inherits both defective genes (right) and exhibits the disease.

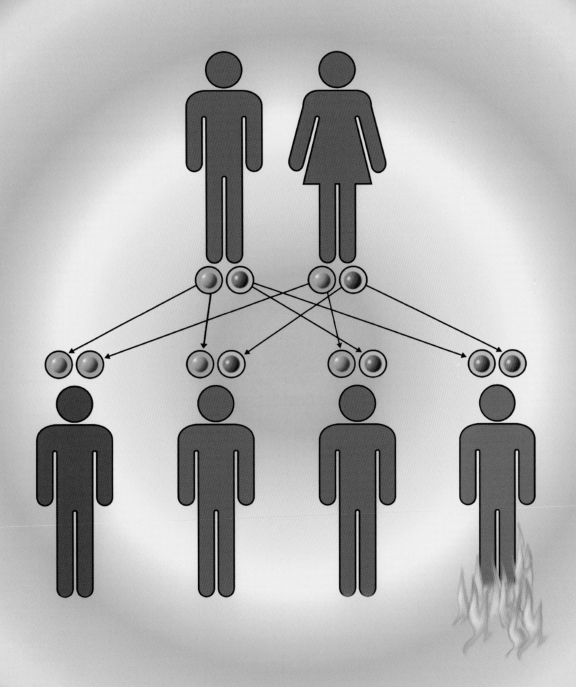

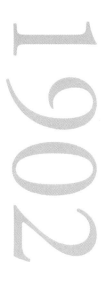

Cause of Sleeping Sickness

Paul Ehrlich (1854–1915), **David Bruce** (1855–1931), **Kiyoshi Shiga** (1871–1957)

Journalist Melody Peterson describes sleeping sickness as "a disease far more lethal and terrifying than its name implies. . . . The jewel-eyed yellowish brown flies . . . inject deadly parasites into their human victims. As the parasites multiply, their human hosts appear to go mad. The victims grow agitated and confused, slur their speech, and stumble."

Sleeping sickness, also known as African trypanosomiasis, is caused by a flagellate (a protozoan with a propulsive tail) that lives in the blood of the host and is transmitted by the bite of a tsetse fly. The disease is endemic in parts of Africa. In the first stage of the disease, a person experiences fever and joint pain. The parasites invade the bloodstream and **lymphatic system** and cause swelling of lymph nodes. In the later stages, when the parasite invades the brain, victims' sleep patterns become erratic, after which they lose bladder control, become difficult to wake, and finally die.

Two forms of the parasite affect humans: *Trypanosoma brucei gambiense* (TBG) and *Trypanosoma brucei rhodesiense* (TBR). TBG is widespread in central and western parts of Africa and is a slower-developing, more chronic form of the disease. TBR is more common in eastern and southern Africa and is more likely to infect several kinds of mammals. TBR is the more aggressive parasite, causing all stages of the sleeping sickness to develop rapidly, usually killing an individual within a year if the victim is not quickly treated.

In 1901, sleeping sickness erupted and killed more than 250,000 people in Uganda. In 1902, the Scottish microbiologist David Bruce was among the first to conclusively identify the causative agent (the flagellate) and vector (the fly). A few years later, German scientist Paul Ehrlich and Japanese physician Kiyoshi Shiga developed atoxyl, an arsenic-containing treatment that sometimes helped but could cause blindness in recipients. Today, treatments include pentamidine, suramin, melarsoprol, and/or eflornithine, depending on the disease stage and parasite form.

SEE ALSO Lymphatic System (1652), *Micrographia* (1665), Cause of Malaria (1897), Cause of Rocky Mountain Spotted Fever (1906), Ehrlich's Magic Bullets (1910), and Cause of Yellow Fever (1937).

The sleeping sickness parasite, Trypanosoma brucei gambiense, *shown in a colorized blood smear photomicrograph.*

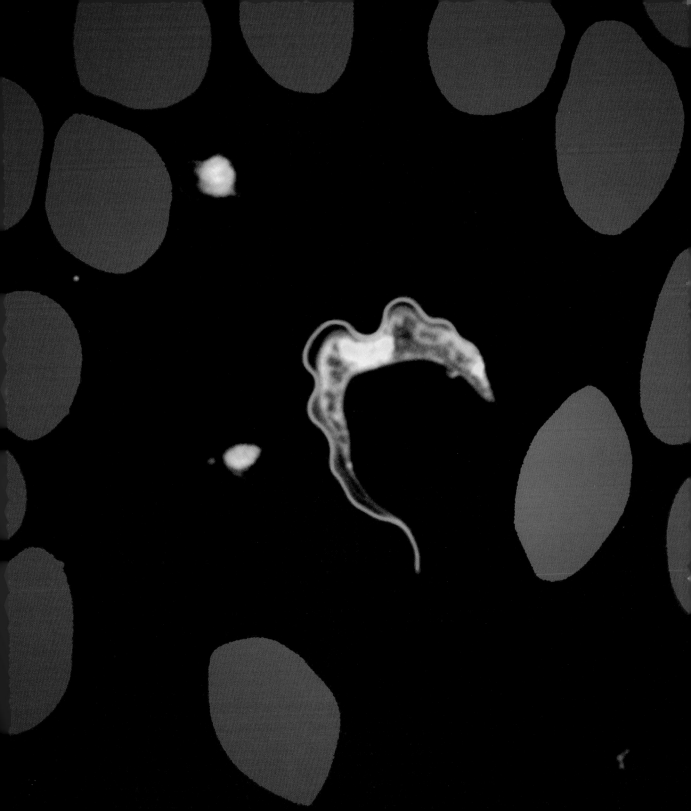

Vascular Suturing

Alexis Carrel (1873–1944), Charles Augustus Lindbergh (1902–1974)

The surgeon Julius Comroe Jr. once wrote, "Between 1901 and 1910, [French surgeon] Alexis Carrel, using experimental animals, performed every feat and developed every technique known to vascular surgery today." Carrel's groundbreaking work performing surgical grafts and reconnecting arteries and veins led to his Nobel Prize in 1912.

Before the methods of Carrel, the suturing (surgically joining) of blood vessels often injured the interior lining of the vessels, leading to fatal blood clots. Surgeons avoided vascular surgery, and many people who might have been saved by the procedure died. Carrel was so determined to make such surgery possible that he took sewing lessons from expert local embroideresses who used the finest needles and threads. Amazingly, Carrel soon developed a new method of suturing blood vessels—published in 1902 and still in use today—that involved turning back the ends of cut vessels like cuffs in order to minimize certain kinds of damage. He also coated his thin needles and **sutures** with Vaseline to further minimize damage to the delicate vessels. Prior to this time, the treatments for wounded vessels often involved ligation (tying) (see entry "**Paré's 'Rational Surgery'**") and possible amputation of involved limbs.

In 1908, Carrel performed what some have called the first modern **blood transfusion**, in which he sutured a father's artery to a vein in the leg of his sick baby. Because the blood types were compatible, the father served as a blood pump and supply for the baby, who suffered from intestinal bleeding. Carrel was also able to transplant a kidney from one dog to another, but problems of immune rejection prevented him from performing such transplants on humans. In the 1930s, together with aviator Charles Lindbergh, he developed a perfusion pump that allowed organs to survive outside the body during surgery. Lindburgh once stated, "Carrel's mind flashed with the speed of light in space between the logical world of science and the mystical world of God." Carrel's pioneering methods eventually led the way to successful organ transplants, modern heart surgery and bypass operations, and **tissue grafts**.

SEE ALSO Sutures (3000 B.C.), Paré's "Rational Surgery" (1545), Tissue Grafting (1597), Ligation of the Abdominal Aorta (1817), Blood Transfusion (1829), and Nanomedicine (1959).

Artistic depiction of a neatly cut artery, illustrating the three main layers of the wall, starting from the inside: the tunica intima, tunica media, and tunica adventitia. Disclike red blood cells are seen pouring from the opening.

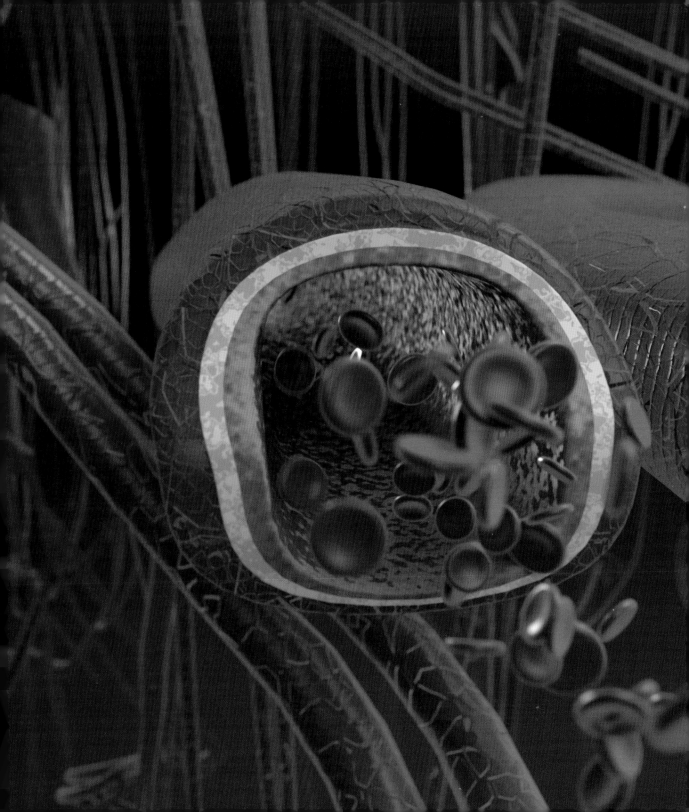

Electrocardiograph

Augustus Desiré Waller (1856–1922), **Willem Einthoven** (1860–1927)

The electrocardiograph (ECG or EKG, from the German *Elektrokardiogramm*) is an indispensable device for monitoring the electrical activity of the heart, using electrodes placed on the skin. By observing the resultant traces through time, physicians can often diagnose abnormal heart rhythms, which may be caused by heart damage, hormone and electrolyte imbalances, and other factors.

In 1887, the English physiologist Augustus D. Waller was the first to record the heart's electrical activity from a person's skin, using a device containing a column of mercury in a thin glass tube known as the Lippmann Electrometer. The movement of the mercury underwent slight changes in concert with the electrical activity of the heart. However, the device was impractical, partly because of the friction and inertia of the moving mercury and the device's sensitivity to external vibrations. Dutch physician and physiologist Willem Einthoven was aware of Waller's work and, in 1901, started to develop new ultrasensitive string galvanometers to monitor the heart. These devices employed a thin electrical-sensing needle suspended between the poles of a magnet. Because the heart's electrical activity is so weak, Einthoven created his lightweight needle using a superfine filament of silver-coated quartz.

Although Einthoven was among the first to promote the electrocardiograph for clinical use, his earliest version weighed 600 pounds (272 kg), occupied two rooms, and required five operators! The patient sat with both arms and left leg immersed in pails of salt solutions, which acted as electrodes to conduct the current from the skin surface to the filament. In 1903, Einthoven described various waves on the electrocardiogram (the recorded electrical trace) that are still relevant today. For example, the P wave characterizes the activity of the heart's atria, while the QRS wave complex and the T wave characterize the action of the heart's ventricles. Einthoven won the Nobel Prize in 1924 for his work.

Today, electrocardiographs are portable, and other approaches used to study the heart include the echocardiogram, which employs sound waves to create an image of the heart in action.

SEE ALSO Pulse Watch (1707), Stethoscope (1816), Defibrillator (1899), Human Electroencephalogram (1924), and Artificial Pacemaker for Heart (1958).

A patient's cardiogram displayed on an operating room machine. The top trace represents heart electrical activity, and the bottom trace represents the arterial pressure values acquired with an artery catheter.

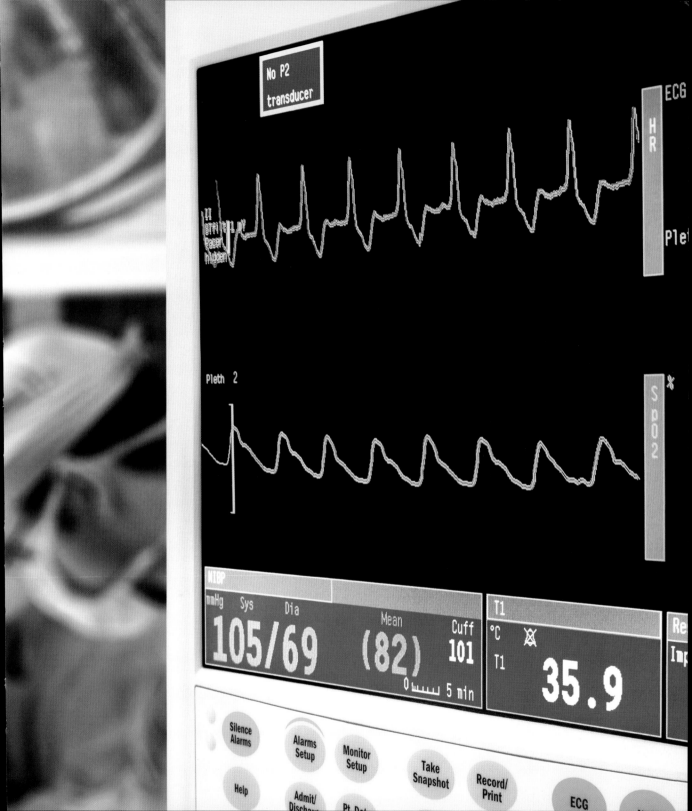

Radiation Therapy

Wilhelm Conrad Röntgen (1845–1923), **Antoine Henri Becquerel** (1852–1908), **Pierre Curie** (1859–1906), **Marie Skłodowska Curie** (1867–1934), **Georg Clemens Perthes** (1869–1927), **Claudius Regaud** (1870–1940), **Henri Coutard** (1876–1950)

Radiation therapy (or radiotherapy) makes use of ionizing radiation to destroy **cancer** cells by damaging the **DNA** (genetic material) within such cells. The term *ionizing radiation* refers to electromagnetic waves (e.g., **X-rays**) or beams of subatomic particles (e.g., protons) that have sufficient energy to remove electrons from atoms or molecules. Radiation can harm both normal and cancer cells, but rapidly growing cancer cells are often more sensitive to such radiation. Note that radiotherapy may damage DNA directly or create charged particles or free-radical molecules that subsequently damage the DNA.

Radiation may be delivered from a machine or, with brachytherapy, it may be delivered by radioactive material placed in the body near cancer cells. Systemic radiation therapy involves swallowable or injectable substances, such as radioactive iodine or substances attached to antibodies that travel to the cancer cells.

There are several milestones in the history of discoveries related to radiation. For example, French scientist Henri Becquerel discovered uranium radioactivity in 1896, and German physicist Wilhelm Conrad Röntgen accidentally discovered X-rays about a year before while experimenting with electrical discharge tubes. In 1898, physicists Marie and Pierre Curie discovered two new radioactive elements, polonium and radium. At his Nobel lecture in 1903, Becquerel suggested that radium might be used to cure cancer. The same year, the German surgeon Georg Perthes advanced the use of X-ray therapy in the treatment of breast cancer and skin cancer.

During the 1920s and 1930s, French researchers Claudius Regaud and Henri Coutard discovered that by administering *fractionated* doses of radiation (e.g., smaller doses each day rather than a large single dose), they could destroy tumors with less damage to nearby healthy tissue. Also, by giving many doses, the cancer cells are likely to be exposed at different stages of the cell-division cycle, making them more vulnerable.

Today, computers play an invaluable role in helping visualize tumor location, aligning the patient during treatment, and calculating radiation dosages.

SEE ALSO Causes of Cancer (1761), X-rays (1895), Cancer Chemotherapy (1946), and DNA Structure (1953).

A 1957 photograph of the first patient treated with linear-accelerator radiation therapy for retinoblastoma, a cancer of the retina, the light-sensing tissue of the eye. One eye was treated successfully.

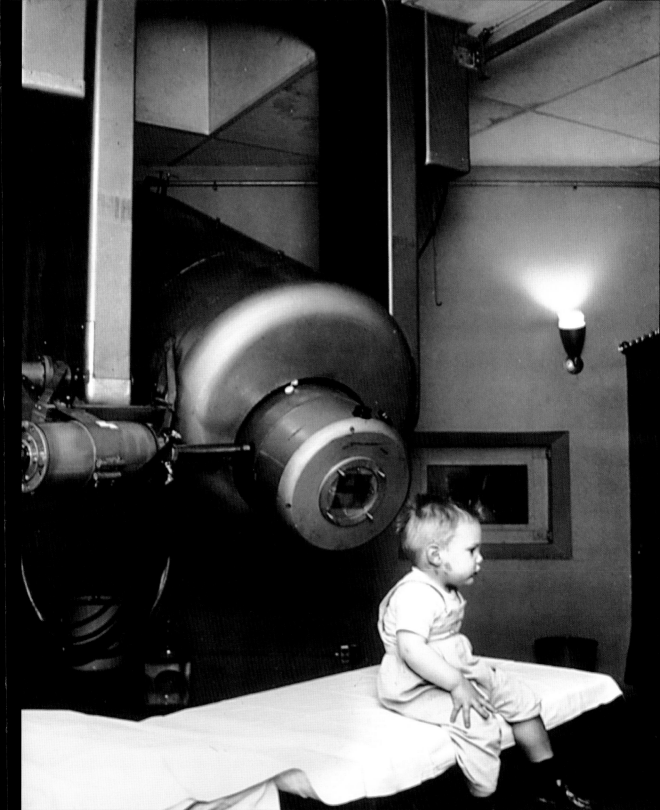

Halstedian Surgery

William Stewart Halsted (1852–1922)

In 1889, Johns Hopkins Hospital opened in Baltimore and developed a system of training surgeons that led to our modern programs in which a student enters a university-sponsored program that is associated with a **hospital**, where the students gradually develop skills and assume clinical responsibilities. American surgeon William Halsted, the first chief of the Department of Surgery at Johns Hopkins Hospital, started the first formal surgical residency training program in the United States. Halsted insisted that residents not only train to be surgeons but also be teachers of surgery. His residents often became respected surgeons at other schools and promoted his ideas.

Halsted is also famous for "Halstedian surgical techniques," a slow, methodical approach in which a surgeon respects human tissues, handling them with utmost gentleness to minimize damage and blood loss. In an age when catgut was still used for **sutures**, he emphasized the use of fine silk to minimize tissue damage and infection. He introduced rubber gloves and scrubs in the operating room. His famous operations on thyroids, intestines, and hernias were successfully designed to restore proper form and function.

In 1913, surgeon Harvey Cushing commented on Halsted's approach: "Observers no longer expected to be thrilled in an operating room; the spectacular public performances of the past, no longer condoned, are replaced by quiet, rather tedious procedures. . . . The patient on the table, like the passenger in a car, runs greater risks if he has a loquacious driver . . . who exceeds the speed limit."

When Halsted trained in medical school, many surgeons operated in street clothes and with bare hands. Surgeons of the past, who bragged about 30-second amputations, were now replaced by careful Halstedian dissectors who also closed tissue layers one at a time. In 1904, in an address titled "Training of the Surgeon," Halsted said, "We need a system, and we will surely have it, which will produce not only surgeons, but surgeons of the highest type, who will stimulate the finest youths of their country to study surgery."

SEE ALSO Sutures (3000 B.C.), Hospitals (1784), Thyroid Surgery (1872), Cocaine as Local Anesthetic (1884), Latex Surgical Gloves (1890), Vascular Suturing (1902), Flexner Report and Medical Education (1910), Laser (1960), and Robotic Surgery (2000).

Portrait of William Stewart Halsted, Yale College class of 1874. (Photograph courtesy of Yale University.)

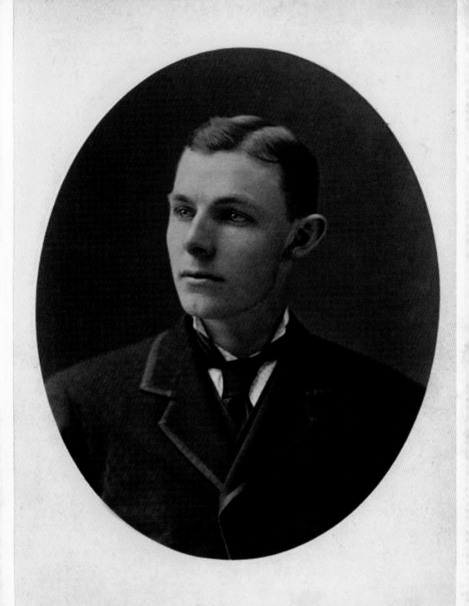

William Stewart Halsted
W. Halsted 1852-1922

Corneal Transplant

Eduard Konrad Zirm (1863–1944)

The July 1946 issue of *LIFE* magazine proclaimed, "Hundreds of people in the U.S. who once were blind are able to see today with the help of dead people's eyes. . . . To be blind for minor reasons [of damage to the cornea] when the rest of the eye is good has always seemed particularly unbearable."

The cornea is the clear dome-shaped surface in front of the iris and pupil of the eye, and blindness can occur if it becomes damaged. The cornea is responsible for a majority of the "focusing power" of the eye. Today, keratoplasties, also known as corneal transplants, can restore vision and have become the most common and among the most successful forms of solid-tissue transplants. During the transplant, the damaged cornea is sometimes removed with a trephine (an instrument resembling a circular cookie cutter), and the cornea of a recently deceased person is attached in its place.

In 1905, Austrian ophthalmologist Eduard Zirm performed the first successful human corneal transplant—probably making it the first successful person-to-person transplant ever performed—on Alois Glogar, a laborer blinded in an accident while working with lime. The corneas came from an 11-year-old boy who was blinded by deep injuries to his eyes. Because Zirm did not have modern fine material to sew the cornea to the eye, he used strips of conjunctiva—a layer in the white of the eye—to help hold down the cornea while healing took place.

The tissue rejection that would normally occur in transplants is decreased (but not absent) for corneas due to partial immune privilege, which results from several factors, including cornea anatomy and the presence of naturally occurring immunosuppressive compounds in the watery substance between the lens and the cornea. Around 90 percent of corneal grafts are successful a year after the operation. Today, **lasers** are often used in place of cutting blades, and research continues in the quest to use artificial materials and stem cells for corneal replacement.

SEE ALSO Eye Surgery (600 B.C.), Eyeglasses (1284), Tissue Grafting (1597), Kidney Transplant (1954), Autoimmune Diseases (1956), Structure of Antibodies (1959), and Growing New Organs (2006).

The cornea is the clear, dome-shaped surface in front of the iris and pupil of the eye, shown here with a light reflecting off its surface.

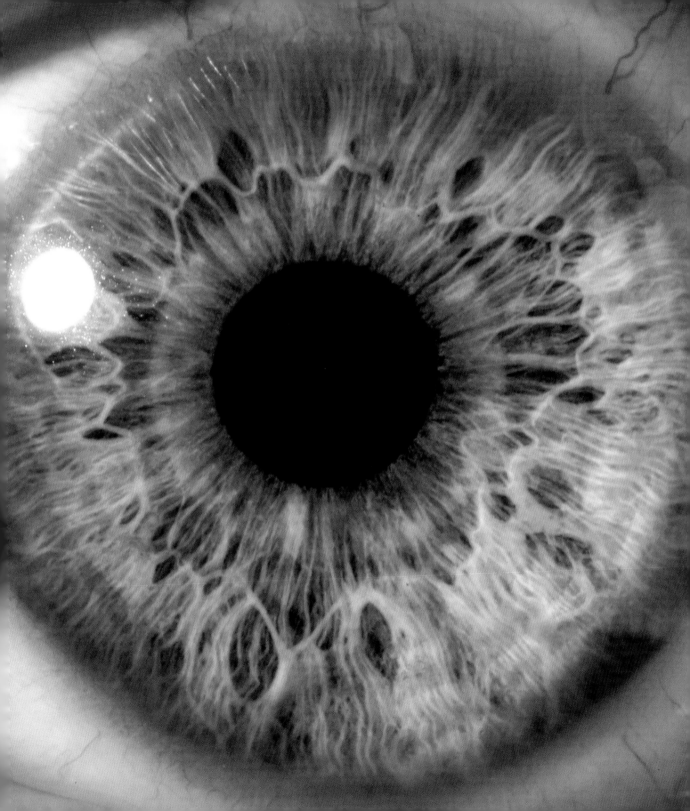

Genes and Sex Determination

Edmund Beecher Wilson (1856–1939), **Nettie Maria Stevens** (1861–1912)

For centuries, physicians wondered about how the gender of infants was determined in the womb. In 355 B.C., Aristotle erroneously suggested that hot semen generated males and cold semen made females. Today, we know that sex differentiation depends on genes located on our chromosomes. Usually, a woman has two X chromosomes (symbolically written as XX), and a male has one X and one much smaller Y chromosome (XY). A son receives his Y chromosome from his father. This XY sex-determination system was first described by American geneticists Nettie Stevens and Edmund Wilson in 1905.

Interestingly, women with Turner's syndrome exist with only one X and no Y chromosome, which suggests that the genes on the Y are not required for survival, but rather are needed to trigger maleness in the developing embryo. Males with one Y chromosome and two X chromosomes (XXY, or Klinefelter syndrome) frequently have reduced facial hair and small testes. XXX females exist and have normal intelligence, but females with even more X chromosomes are mentally handicapped. XYY males are taller than average. Generally speaking, a single copy of Y contains the male-determining gene and, even in the presence of several Xs, produces an individual who looks male. However, XY individuals with androgen insensitivity syndrome resemble women whose vaginas end blindly, with no uterus present.

Around 1990, a team of scientists discovered the SRY gene on the Y chromosome that plays an important role in the chain of events that leads an embryo to maleness. XX men do exist—they lack the Y chromosome but have a copy of the SRY region on one of their other chromosomes. Also, XY women can exist who have a mutation that disables the SRY gene.

Developing human embryos have the potential to be either male or female and have a bipotential gonad that can become either testes or ovaries, depending on which genes are subsequently activated. The testes secrete testosterone, the hormone responsible for male traits.

SEE ALSO Discovery of Sperm (1678), Mendel's Genetics (1865), and Chromosomal Theory of Inheritance (1902).

Genetics and sex. At left are the chromosomes of a male (XY, top) and female (XX, bottom). At the center and right are representations of the DNA molecule that contributes to the genetic code and structure of each chromosome.

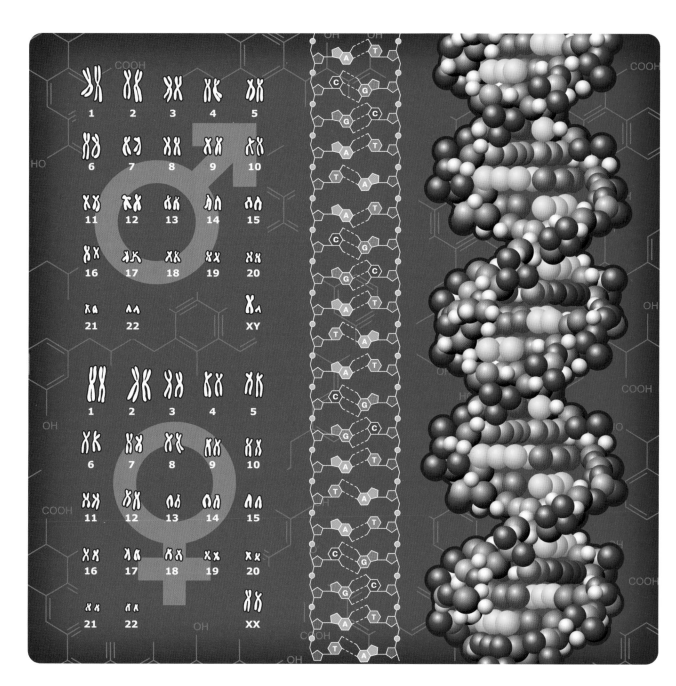

"Analytic" Vitamin Discovery

Christiaan Eijkman (1858–1930), **Sir Frederick Gowland Hopkins** (1861–1947), **Gerrit Grijns** (1865–1944)

Author Kendall Haven writes, "We label foods by their vitamin content. We spend billions of dollars every year buying vitamin supplements. The discovery of vitamins revolutionized nutritional science . . . and the study of how the human body functions."

Generally speaking, vitamins are chemicals required by organisms in small amounts in the diet. Some vitamins, such as vitamin D, are not absolutely required in human diets because we can synthesize vitamin D if exposed to sufficient sunlight. Vitamins help regulate metabolism and growth and perform other functions, and some vitamins bind to enzymes (proteins that speed chemical reaction rates). Inadequate vitamin intake leads to diseases (see entry "*A Treatise on Scurvy*").

This history of vitamin discovery is long and involves numerous researchers. Biochemist Gerald F. Combs Jr. writes, "The analytical phase of vitamin discovery, indeed modern nutrition research itself, was entered with the finding of an animal model for beriberi in the 1890s." Beriberi is a disease that is caused by a deficiency of vitamin B_1, leading to fatigue, irregular heart rate, and eventual death. In 1897, Dutch physician Christiaan Eijkman discovered that when more expensive polished (white) rice was fed to chickens, they developed beriberi symptoms. When returned to a diet of brown rice with hulls, the chickens became healthy again.

In 1906, Eijkman and Dutch physician Gerrit Grijns published a now-classic paper in which they wrote, "There is present in rice polishings a substance different from protein . . . that is indispensable to health and the lack of which causes nutritional polyneuritis." Their discussion of an anti-beriberi substance (later referred to as vitamin B_1) is one of the earlier recognitions of the vitamin concept. Around the same time, British biochemist Frederick Hopkins showed that rats needed to have diets with special "accessory food items," later shown to be vitamins.

The 13 vitamins for humans are classified as either fat-soluble (A, D, E, and K) or water-soluble—B_1 (thiamine), B_2 (riboflavin), B_3 (niacin), B_5 (pantothenic acid), B_6, B_7 (biotin), B_9 (folic acid), B_{12}, and C.

SEE ALSO *A Treatise on Scurvy* (1753), American Medical Association (1847), Banishing Rickets (1922), and Liver Therapy (1926).

Microcrystals of ascorbic acid (vitamin C) in polarized light.

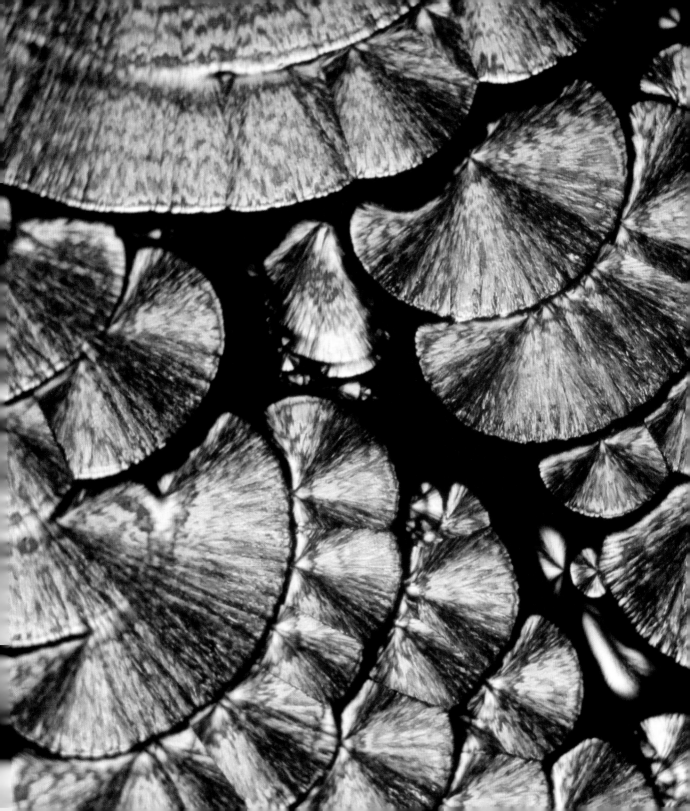

Allergies

Abu Bakr Muhammad ibn Zakariya al-Razi (865–925), **Charles Richet** (1850–1935), **Paul Portier** (1866–1962), **Clemens Peter Freiherr von Pirquet** (1874–1929), **Béla Schick** (1877–1967)

Allergic diseases have been known since antiquity. Around 900 A.D., Persian physician al-Razi, also known as Rhazes, described seasonal rhinitis (nasal inflammation) triggered by the scent of roses. In 1902, French physiologists Charles Richet and Paul Portier discussed anaphylaxis (an acute allergic reaction that can lead to multiple-organ failure and death) when observing that dogs died when exposed a second time to toxins from sea anemones. In 1906, Austrian pediatrician Clemens von Pirquet considered the anemone experiments along with his own studies of "serum sickness" carried out with Hungarian pediatrician Béla Schick. In particular, they noticed that children immunized against common infectious diseases had quicker, more severe reactions upon a second exposure to the vaccine. Pirquet coined the term *allergy* for what appeared to be the abnormal response of an overactive or supersensitized immune system.

Consider the modern explanation in which a person encounters a possible allergen, such as flower pollen or bee venom, for the first time. In certain individuals, various white blood cells may begin to overreact. In particular, a T_H2 lymphocyte responds by producing interleukin-4 (a protein-signaling molecule), which may stimulate B cells to overproduce IgE antibodies that bind to mast cells and basophils. At this point, the IgE-coated cells are sensitized to the particular allergen and "remember" it. If the person is exposed to the allergen again, the activated mast cells and basophils release histamine and other inflammatory chemicals into surrounding tissues, causing itchiness, rashes, hives, and possible anaphylaxis—which can sometimes be treated with antihistamines, steroids, or injections of epinephrine.

The likelihood of having allergies is greater in developed nations and is inherited from parents. According to one theory, the relative sterility of modern urban environments means that the immune system is not sufficiently exposed to pathogens to keep it "busy." Allergies are also less common in children from larger families, with a presumably greater exposure to microbes and parasites, the latter of which have sometimes been shown to be able to beneficially suppress the immune system.

SEE ALSO Zoo Within Us (1683), Latex Surgical Gloves (1890), Discovery of Adrenaline (1893), Antihistamines (1937), Cortisone (1948), Autoimmune Diseases (1956), and Structure of Antibodies (1959).

Colorized electron microscope image of pollen from a variety of common plants such as the sunflower, morning glory, hollyhock, lily, primrose, and castor bean (Dartmouth Electron Microscope Facility).

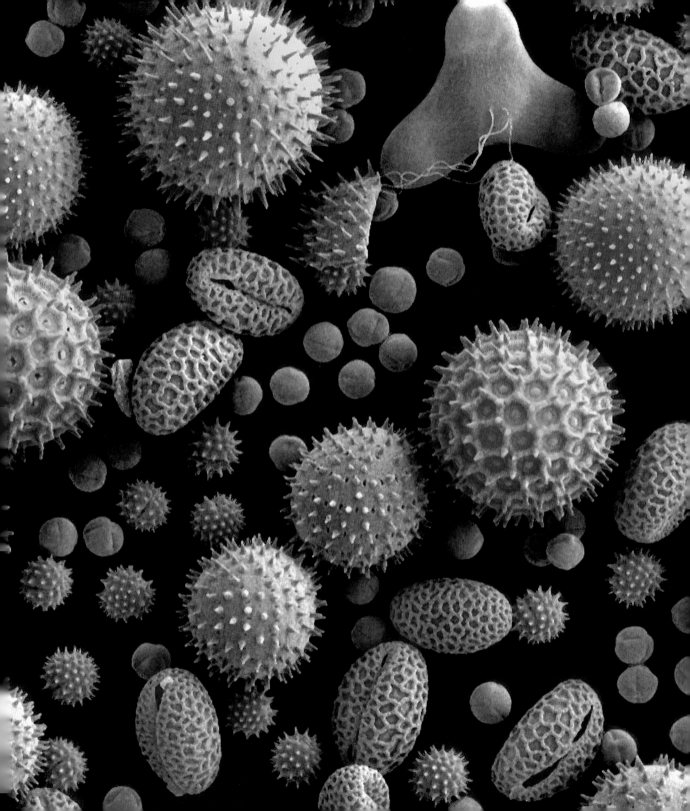

Alzheimer's Disease

Aloysius "Alois" Alzheimer (1864–1915)

In 1994, former U.S. President Ronald Reagan wrote, "I have recently been told that I am one of the millions of Americans who will be afflicted with Alzheimer's disease. . . . I now begin the journey that will lead me to the sunset of my life." A year later, diners in a restaurant applauded him, but he did not know why they were clapping and that he had once been president.

Alzheimer's disease (AD) is a form of dementia, a general term that refers to the abnormal loss of memory and other intellectual abilities. AD destroys brain cells and interferes with the ability to acquire new memories. As the disease progresses, long-term memories are lost and language abilities disappear. The mean life expectancy after initial diagnosis is about seven years.

Brain plaques and tangles are two abnormal features of AD. The plaques accumulate *between* nerve cells and contain protein fragments called beta-amyloid (BA). Tangles form *within* dying cells and consist of tangled fibers of a microtubule-associated protein called tau. Studies continue regarding the role of plaques and tangles in AD and how they may block signals between nerve cells and cause cell death.

In 1906, German psychiatrist and neuropathologist Alois Alzheimer presented the case of Mrs. Auguste Deter, who initially had memory problems at age 51 and soon exhibited delusions and more severe mental problems before dying. An **autopsy** revealed dramatic shrinkage of Deter's cerebral cortex (outer layer of the brain that plays a role in memory, thought, and language), along with BA plaques and neurofibrillary tangles.

Today, AD is usually diagnosed from the patient's behavior. Advanced medical imaging methods such as **CAT**, **MRI**, and **PET** can be used to exclude other possible causes of dementia. **Cerebrospinal fluid** may be analyzed for the presence of BA or tau proteins in order to help diagnose the disease even before symptoms are obvious. Most people with AD develop the disease after age 65, and one form of a gene called APOE is correlated with a higher chance of developing AD.

SEE ALSO Cerebrospinal Fluid (1764), Mendel's Genetics (1865), Neuron Doctrine (1891), Prosopagnosia (1947), Nerve Growth Factor (1948), Antipsychotics (1950), Levodopa for Parkinson's Disease (1957), CAT Scans (1967), Positron Emission Tomography (PET) (1973), Magnetic Resonance Imaging (MRI) (1977), and Prions (1982).

A cross section of a healthy brain (top) and of the brain of someone afflicted with Alzheimer's disease (bottom), showing a dramatic shrinkage of the cerebral cortex.

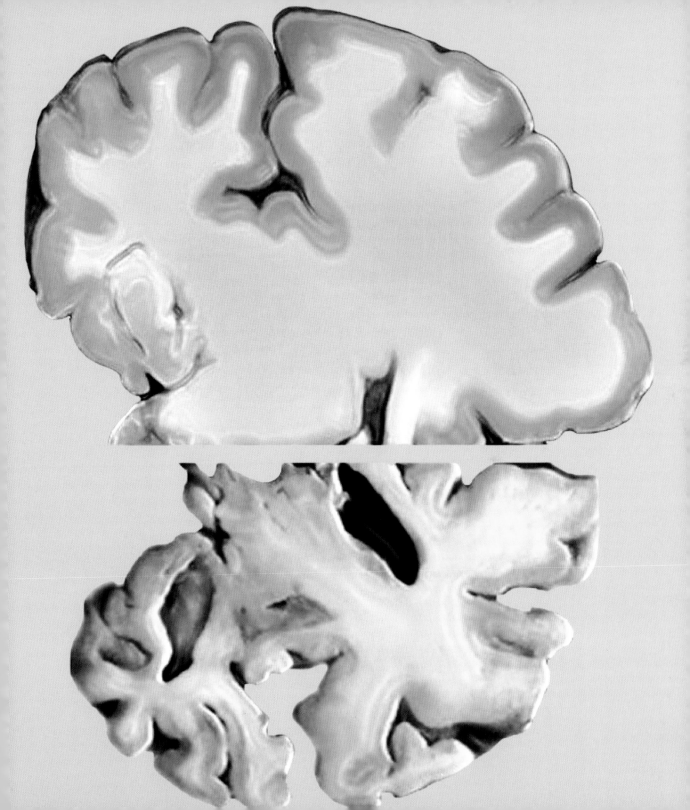

Meat Inspection Act of 1906

Theodore "Teddy" Roosevelt (1858–1919), Charles Patrick Neill (1865–1942), Upton Beall Sinclair Jr. (1878–1968)

American author Upton Sinclair's 1906 novel *The Jungle* was based on his undercover work of 1904 in the meatpacking plants of Chicago stockyards. In *The Jungle*, he wrote of the unsanitary conditions in which workers did not bother to remove poisoned rats before meat was ground into sausage. Workers washed their hands "in the water that was to be ladled into the sausage." Every spring, other workers cleaned out waste barrels full of old meat and "dirt and rust and old nails and stale water—and cartload after cartload of it would be taken up and dumped into the hoppers with fresh meat, and sent out to the public's breakfast." Other men fell into open vats on the floor and were left there "till all but the bones of them had gone out to the world as Durham's Pure Leaf Lard!"

Sinclair also wrote, "Men welcomed tuberculosis in the cattle they were feeding, because it made them fatten more quickly," and that old moldy sausage "would be dosed with borax and glycerine, and dumped into the hoppers, and made over again for home consumption." Meat was reused after it sat on the floor in dirt and sawdust and was spat upon by workers.

President Theodore Roosevelt believed that Sinclair's descriptions were exaggerated and sent Labor Commissioner Charles P. Neill to inspect the meatpacking facilities. Neill confirmed that the factory conditions were "revolting." Public pressure finally led to the passage of the Meat Inspection Act of 1906, which mandated that the U.S. Department of Agriculture inspect meat processing plants that conducted business across state lines. Inspectors were to examine the sanitary conditions of slaughterhouses as well as livestock (e.g., cattle, sheep, and pigs) before and after slaughter. These and subsequent national reforms became part of a war on food-borne illnesses that resulted from tapeworms, bacteria (e.g., *Salmonella* and *Campylobacter*), and other contaminants. Modern beef production can involve slaughter plants that process 400 cattle in an hour, a speed that can sometimes lead to accidental fecal contamination through rushed butchering.

SEE ALSO Sewage Systems (600 B.C.), *The Sanitary Condition of the Labouring Population of Great Britain* (1842), Semmelweis's Hand Washing (1847), Broad Street Pump Handle (1854), Chlorination of Water (1910), and Prions (1982).

Meat workers split hog backbones and prepare them for final inspection. These hogs are ready for the cooler at Swift & Co., Chicago, 1906.

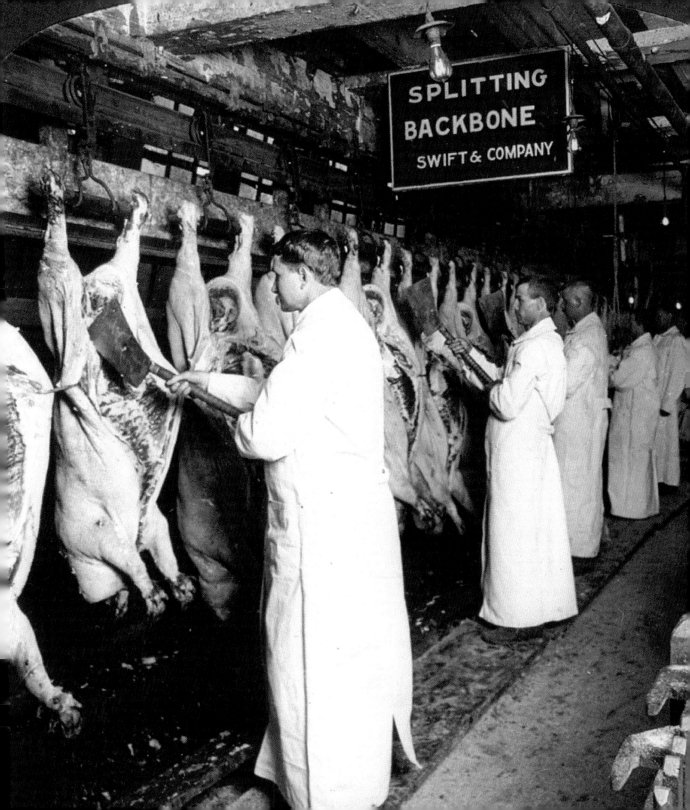

Patent Medicines

Ebenezer Sibly (1751–1800), **Lydia Estes Pinkham** (1819–1883), **Samuel Hopkins Adams** (1871–1958)

Throughout the 1800s of America, "patent medicines" were all the rage. These pills and tonics had colorful names, eye-catching packaging, and secret ingredients. Although some of these medicines did provide pain relief due to their high alcoholic content and use of **cocaine**, most were ineffective for treating other ailments, beyond functioning as powerful **placebos** for hopeful people seeking cures. Despite the name, these products were usually not patented—a process that would require revealing the ingredients to competitors and to the public—but their names were often trademarked. During the height of their popularity, when doctors and real cures were scarce, many people self-medicated. Around 1900, more advertising money was spent to promote patent medicines than for any other products. Fantastic advertising stunts included traveling circus–like shows and multipage advertisements in newspapers and almanacs for products said to treat diabetes, female complaints, baldness, asthma, kidney diseases, **cancer**, and more. Claimed ingredients ranged from snake oil to sulfuric acid, mercury, licorice, and unspecified swamp roots. In the late 1700s in England, Ebenezer Sibly actually promoted his Solar Tincture to "restore life in the event of sudden death."

In 1905, American instigative journalist Samuel H. Adams published a series of articles in *Collier's Weekly* titled "The Great American Fraud," in which he exposed the bogus claims and possible dangers associated with patent medicines. His articles stirred Congress to pass the Pure Food and Drug Act in 1906. Among other things, this act required that ingredients be labeled in drugs that included alcohol, cocaine, heroin, morphine, and cannabis. Adams also discussed Kopp's Baby Friend, made of morphine and sweetened water to calm babies, along with competitor Dr. Windlow's Soothing Syrup that "makes 'em lay dead 'til morning."

In 1879, when Lydia Pinkham's picture was added to the label of her Vegetable Compound for "female complaints," sales soared, and she became one of the most recognized women in America. In 1886, Coca-Cola contained cocaine and was sold as a patent medicine for curing diseases.

SEE ALSO Mithridatium and Theriac (100 B.C.) and Placebo Effect (1955).

Advertisement (c. 1890) for Hamlin's Wizard Oil, an American patent medicine, which was claimed to be useful for everything from diphtheria and sore throat to cancer and diarrhea. Ingredients included alcohol, camphor, ammonia, chloroform, sassafras, cloves, and turpentine.

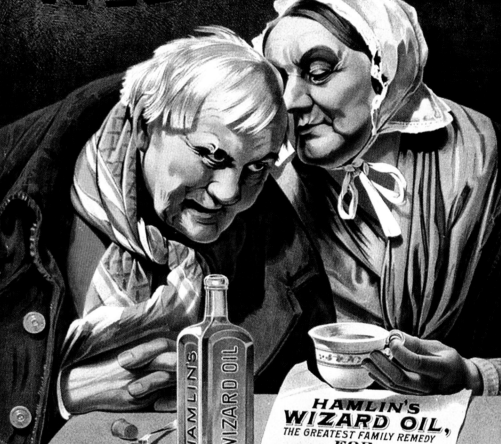

Cause of Rocky Mountain Spotted Fever

Howard Taylor Ricketts (1871–1910)

According to the September 7, 1942, issue of *LIFE* magazine, "For years before the scientists came, people had sickened mysteriously in the valley, burned with sudden fever, flamed with red-purple rash, and died. The farmers said it was from drinking melted snow water." But the medical detectives found that Rocky Mountain spotted fever (RMSF) was transmitted by a hard-skinned bloodthirsty tick.

In 1906, American pathologist Howard Ricketts traveled to the frontier of western Montana in a dangerous quest to determine the source of the life-threatening disease that broke out there every spring. He performed much of his research in tents set up on the grounds of a hospital in Bitterroot Valley. Using guinea pigs, he proved that the cause of the disease was the bacterium now called *Rickettsia rickettsii* in his honor. Ricketts also showed that the RMSF bacterium was transmitted through the bites of ticks. By 1938, a laboratory in the Bitteroot Valley was producing a vaccine for RMSF, but it was not very effective and practical; today, antibiotics such as doxycycline, tetracycline, and chloramphenicol are used for treatments.

RMSF is currently the most lethal rickettsial illness in the United States. Initial symptoms may include fever, headache, and muscle pain, followed by a rash that starts at the wrists and ankles and moves toward the trunk. The bacterium infects the cells that line blood vessels throughout the body and, thus, can affect many organs, causing paralysis as well as gangrene (death of tissues). Although original research was focused on the Rocky Mountain region of the United States, the disease is actually distributed throughout the continental United States and also penetrates Canada and Central and South America. The two most important vectors (transmitters) of RMSF are the American dog tick (*Dermacentor variabilis*) and the Rocky Mountain wood tick (*Dermacentor andersoni*).

Note that, today, Lyme disease is the most common tick-borne disease in the Northern Hemisphere, caused by bacteria of the genus *Borrelia* and transmitted by ticks of the genus *Ixodes*.

SEE ALSO Discovery of *Sarcoptes Scabiei* (1687), Cause of Malaria (1897), Cause of Sleeping Sickness (1902), and Cause of Yellow Fever (1937).

American dog ticks (Dermacentor variabilis), *a vector of Rocky Mountain Spotted Fever.*

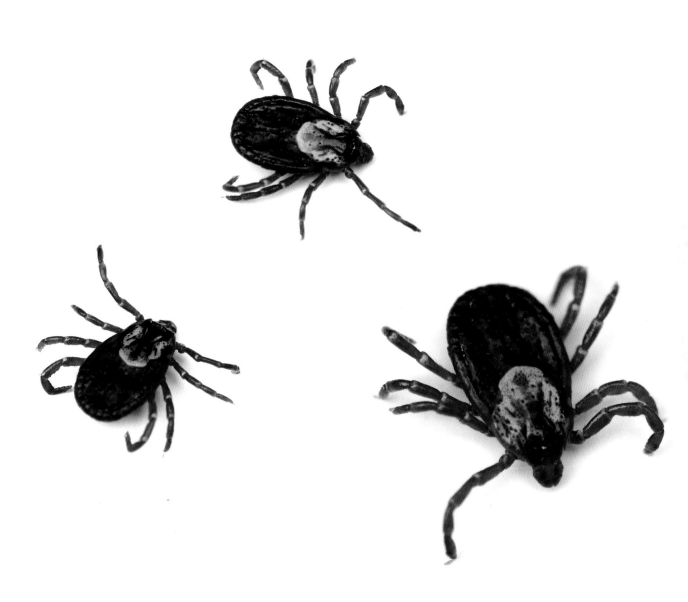

Imprisonment of Typhoid Mary

Mary Mallon (1869–1938), George A. Soper (1870–1948)

The 1907 imprisonment of Typhoid Mary marks an important medical milestone, not only because Mary was the first famous, seemingly healthy person known to have caused an "epidemic" in the United States, but because her case raises profound questions about the role of society in imposing lifetime confinement for disease carriers.

Typhoid fever is a worldwide disease transmitted by consuming food or water contaminated with feces that contain the bacterium *Salmonella typhi*. Symptoms of the disease may include high fever, diarrhea or constipation, intestinal perforation, and, in severe cases, death. Chlorinated drinking water in the United States has decreased the incidence, and today the disease can be treated with various antibacterial drugs. Some individuals may be infected with the bacterium and be contagious without exhibiting symptoms. The most famous of these "carriers" was Mary Mallon, more commonly known as Typhoid Mary.

Born in Ireland, Mary came to the United States as a teenager and eventually cooked in the homes of the New York City elites. In 1906, sanitation engineer George Soper discovered that typhoid outbreaks frequently occurred in homes in which Mary cooked. Soper asked Mary for specimens of her feces, and she responded by chasing him away with a carving fork! Finally, doctors confirmed that Mary was a typhoid carrier, and in 1907 she was confined to a small cottage on North Brother Island in the East River, near the Bronx. She was released in 1910 after being told never to work again preparing food—advice she did not heed, causing more typhoid outbreaks. When news of Mary spread, one newspaper cartoonist drew her breaking egg-size skulls into a frying pan. Historians attribute more than 50 cases of typhoid (and at least three deaths) to Mary, but those she infected probably infected more people. She was sent back to the island, where she spent the rest of her life. Her case caused much debate and helped established the role of epidemiology (the study of factors affecting the health of populations) in shaping public policy.

SEE ALSO Zoo Within Us (1683), *The Sanitary Condition of the Labouring Population of Great Britain* (1842), Semmelweis's Hand Washing (1847), Broad Street Pump Handle (1854), Meat Inspection Act of 1906 (1906), Chlorination of Water (1910), and Sterilization of Carrie Buck (1927).

A historical poster warning about the dangers of improper food handling and suggesting how Typhoid Mary spread disease.

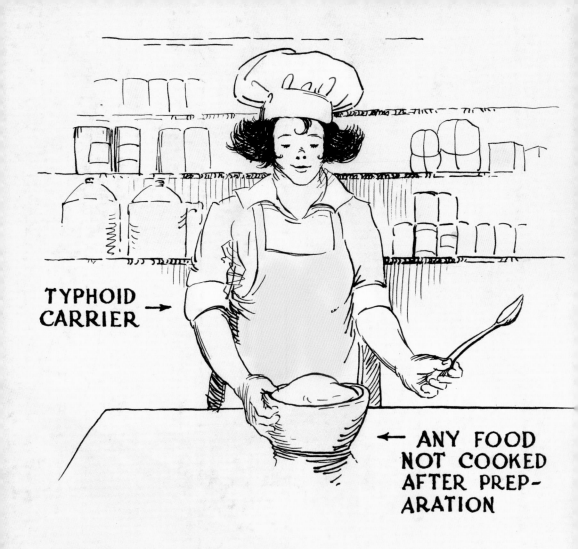

TYPHOID CARRIER →

← ANY FOOD NOT COOKED AFTER PREP-ARATION

IN THIS MANNER THE FAMOUS "TYPHOID MARY" INFECTED FAMILY AFTER FAMILY

Searches for the Soul

Herophilus of Chalcedon (335 B.C.–280 B.C.), **René Descartes** (1596–1650), **Duncan MacDougall** (1866–1920)

Various futurists have suggested that as we learn more about the structure of the brain, technologists may one day be able to simulate a mind or upload it to a computer. These speculations assume a materialist view, in which the mind arises from brain activity. On the other hand, French philosopher René Descartes, in the mid-1600s, supposed that the mind, or "soul," exists separately from the brain, but is connected to the brain via an organ like the **pineal body**, which acts as a portal between brain and mind. The ancient Greek physician Herophilus dissected heads and decided that the soul was located in the fluid-filled cavity of the brain. In particular, he believed that the seat of the soul was the *calamus scriptorius*, a cavity in the floor of the fourth cerebral ventricle.

In 1907, American physician Duncan MacDougall placed dying tuberculosis patients on a scale. He reasoned that at the moment of death, the scale should indicate a drop in weight as the soul disembarked. As a result of his experiments, MacDougall measured the soul to be 21 grams (0.7 ounce). Alas, MacDougall and other researchers were never able to duplicate this finding. These various views concerning the separation of soul and matter represent a philosophy of mind-body dualism.

A more materialist view of the mind and body may be supported by experiments that suggest our thoughts, memory, and personality can be altered by damage to regions of the brain, and that brain imaging studies can map both feelings and thoughts. As just one curious example, injury to the brain's right frontal lobe can lead to a sudden, passionate interest in fine restaurants and gourmet foods—a condition called gourmand syndrome. Of course, the dualist Descartes might have argued that damage to the brain alters behavior because the mind operates through the brain. If we excise the car's steering wheel, the car behaves differently, but this does not mean that there is no separate driver.

SEE ALSO Cranial Nerves Classified (1664), Cerebrospinal Fluid (1764), Koch's Tuberculosis Lecture (1882), Jung's Analytical Psychology (1933), Prosopagnosia (1947), Pineal Body (1958), Cryonics (1962), Near-Death Experiences (1975), and Human Cloning (2008).

Artist's concept of searching for the soul within the brain. Herophilus believed that the seat of the soul was the calamus scriptorius, *a narrow, lower end of the floor of one of the brain's cerebral ventricles.*

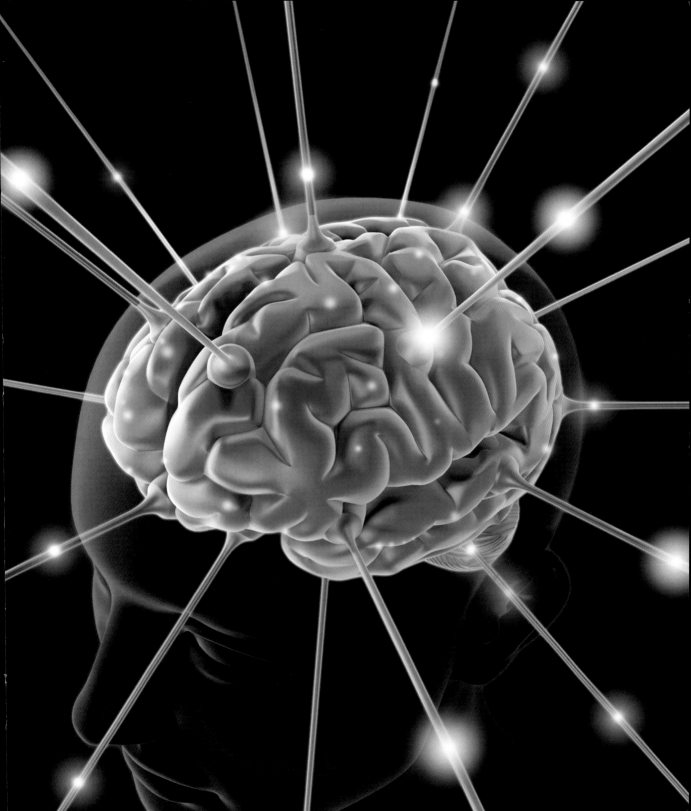

Chlorination of Water

Carl Rogers Darnall (1867–1941), William J. L. Lyster (1869–1947)

In 1997, *LIFE* magazine declared, "The filtration of drinking water plus the use of chlorine is probably the most significant public health advancement of the millennium." Adding chlorine, a chemical element, to water is usually an effective treatment against bacteria, viruses, and amoebas, and has played a large role in the dramatic increase in life expectancy in developed countries during the 1900s. For example, in the United States, waterborne bacterial diseases such as typhoid and cholera became rare after drinking water was chlorinated. Because chlorine remains in the water supply after initial treatment, it continues to fight contamination from possible pipe leaks.

Chlorination was known to be an effective disinfectant in the 1800s, but water chlorination systems for public water supplies were not in continuous use until the early 1900s. Around 1903, the community in Middelkerke, Belgium, used chlorine gas for disinfection of drinking water, and in 1908 a water utility in Jersey City, New Jersey, used sodium hypochlorite for water chlorination. In 1910, Brigadier General Carl Rogers Darnall, a U.S. Army chemist and surgeon, used compressed liquefied chlorine gas to purify water for troops on the battlefield. The basic ideas in his invention of a mechanical liquid-chlorine purifier are now used throughout the developed world. Army scientist Major William Lyster subsequently invented the Lyster cloth bag, containing sodium hypochlorite and used to conveniently treat water by troops in the field.

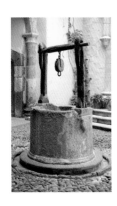

The chlorine applied during water disinfection can react with organic compounds in the water to produce trihalomethanes and haloacetic acids, which have the potential to cause **cancer**. However, the risk of these compounds is low when compared with the risk of waterborne diseases. Alternatives to chlorination include disinfection with ozone, chloramine, and ultraviolet light.

According to spokespeople for the Darnall Army Medical Center, "It is safe to say that more lives have been saved and more sickness prevented by Darnall's contribution to sanitary water than by any other single achievement in medicine."

SEE ALSO Sewage Systems (600 B.C.), *The Sanitary Condition of the Labouring Population of Great Britain* (1842), Broad Street Pump Handle (1854), Germ Theory of Disease (1862), Imprisonment of Typhoid Mary (1907), and Fluoridated Toothpaste (1914).

LEFT: *Water well in a medieval village in Spain.* RIGHT: *A water well at the Great Mosque of Kairouan, Tunisia (postcard from 1900, overlaid on patterns from the door of the prayer hall). In modern times, wells are sometimes periodically cleaned with a chlorine solution to reduce bacterial levels.*

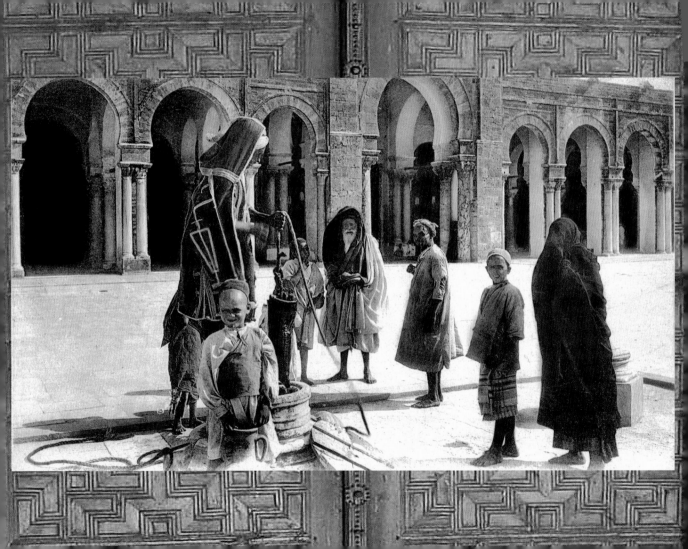

Ehrlich's Magic Bullets

Paul Ehrlich (1854–1915), Sahachiro Hata (1873–1938)

In 1900, very few drugs existed to combat the causes of infectious diseases. One famous example is quinine, used as early as 1630 by Europeans for treatment of **malaria**, which is caused by a protozoan parasite carried by mosquitoes. Mercury was used as early as 1495 to treat syphilis, a sexually transmitted bacterial disease. However, mercury treatments could be quite toxic to humans. The quest for chemical agents that exhibited selective toxicity against the infectious causes of disease, while sparing the human patient, began in earnest with the pioneering work of German scientist Paul Ehrlich, one of the famous founders of modern chemotherapy. Of course, Ehrlich's very systematic search for such useful chemicals could not have been implemented before the **germ theory of disease** was established in the late 1800s and before microorganisms could be identified.

Ehrlich was particularly interested in arsenic compounds that might be used to selectively destroy *Treponema pallidum*, the bacterium that causes syphilis. On a daily basis, Ehrlich directed his army of researchers to test numerous arsenic compounds. In 1909, Japanese bacteriologist Sahachiro Hata, an expert on testing syphilitic rabbits, was working in Ehrlich's laboratory. When he tested arsenic compound number 606, he found it to be effective against syphilis. In 1910, Ehrlich announced the discovery of 606 to the world. Salvarsan, the trade name for 606, was the first practical success of Ehrlich's quest for chemotherapeutic agents, which he called magic bullets. This name refers to the fact that Ehrlich believed that such drugs functioned as selective weapons that could target specific chemical receptors present on the parasite and not harm the cells of the host.

According to science writer John Simmons, "While Louis Pasteur and Robert Koch developed the germ theory of disease, Paul Ehrlich is responsible for the generalization that illness is essentially chemical." Interestingly, some church officials were opposed to Salvarsan on the grounds that venereal diseases were God's punishment for immorality. In the 1940s, **penicillin** came to be used for treating syphilis.

SEE ALSO Germ Theory of Disease (1862), Cause of Malaria (1897), Penicillin (1928), Sulfa Drugs (1935), Cancer Chemotherapy (1946), and Reverse Transcriptase and AIDS (1970).

Syphilis is a sexually transmitted disease caused by the spirochete bacteria Treponema pallidum, *shown here. Spirochetes have long, helically coiled cells.*

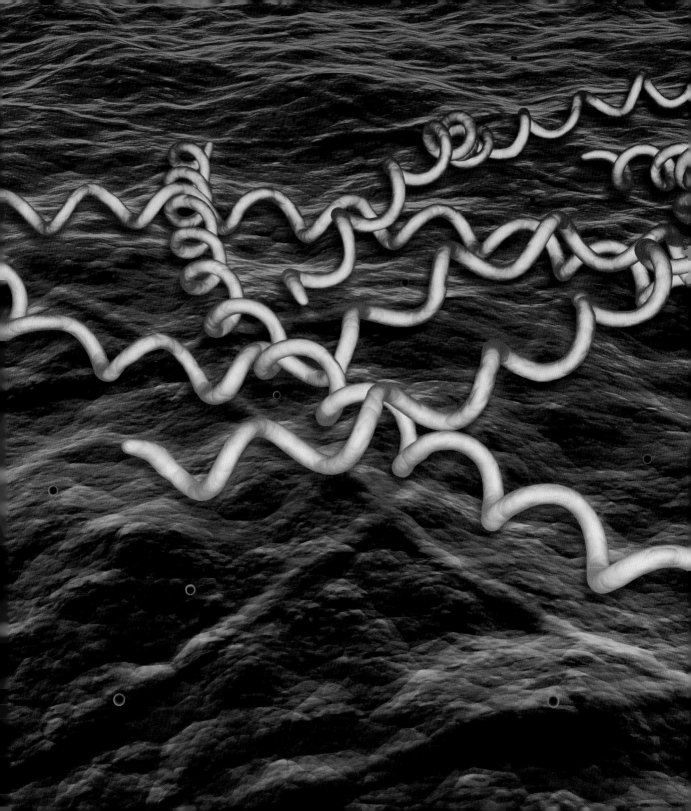

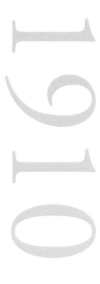

Flexner Report and Medical Education

Abraham Flexner (1866–1959)

In 1900, medical school education in much of the United States was relatively informal. Admissions standards were lax, and in many cases, only a high-school education was required. Many physicians were poorly trained. A pivotal moment in the history of medicine occurred with the 1910 publication of *Medical Education in the United States and Canada*, a study by American educator Abraham Flexner. Much of today's medical education in the United States has its roots in the recommendation of this report.

To provide research for his report, Flexner visited all 155 medical schools in the United States and Canada. Although some schools he visited, such as Johns Hopkins University School of Medicine and Wake Forest University School of Medicine, received high praise, especially disconcerting were the existing "proprietary" schools— small trade schools that were unaffiliated with a college or university and run by a few doctors to make a profit. In these schools, dissection was not required, and many instructors were local doctors who were often unaware of state-of-the-art practices.

Flexner recommended that the medical schools require a high-school education and at least two years of college or university study devoted to basic science. According to his report, a mere 16 of the 155 medical schools had such requirements. He also suggested that medical education should be four years in duration—the first two years devoted to basic science and the last two years devoted to hands-on clinical training. Flexner wrote, "An education in medicine involves both learning and learning how; the student cannot effectively know, unless he knows how." Many schools closed, and by 1935 only 66 medical schools operated in the United States. One possible downside of the Flexner report was the forced closure of rural and smaller proprietary schools that had admitted African Americans, women, and lower-class students. After instituting the Flexner recommendations, medical education was usually only within reach of the upper-class white males. The Medical College Admission Test (MCAT) was developed in 1928 to serve as a standardized test for medical school admissions.

SEE ALSO Hospitals (1784), Women Medical Students (1812), American Medical Association (1847), Osteopathy (1892), and Halstedian Surgery (1904).

Pictured here is the John Morgan Hall at the University of Pennsylvania School of Medicine, founded in 1765. This was the first school of medicine in the American colonies.

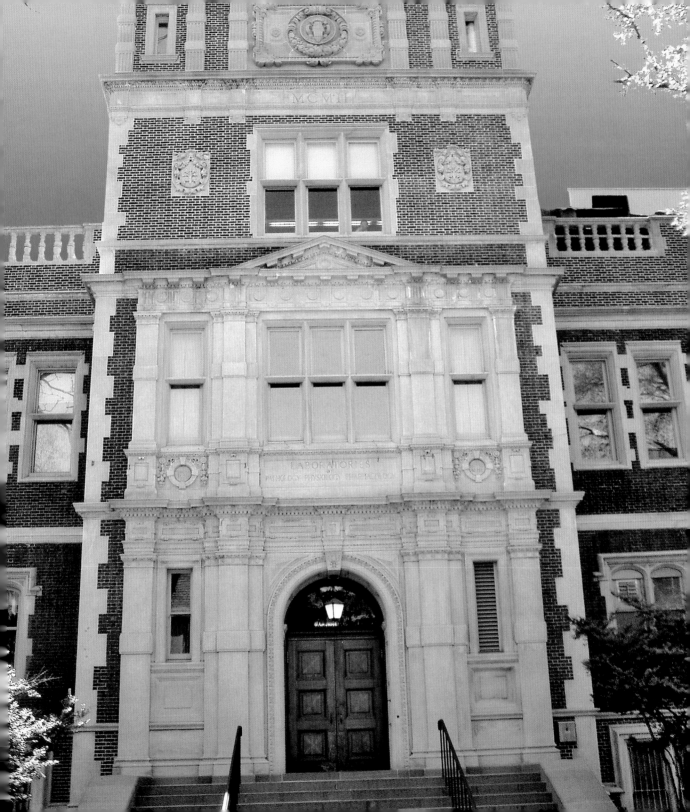

Common Cold

Gaius Plinius Secundus (known as Pliny the Elder; 23–79), Ibn al-Quff (1233–1286), Samuel Auguste Tissot (1728–1797), Walther Kruse (1864–1943)

The common cold is a viral infection of the upper respiratory system. It may be caused by any of more than 100 different viruses, with rhinoviruses and coronaviruses responsible for a majority of all colds. Colds cost Americans billions of dollars every year due to visits to physicians, purchases of drugs, and missed workdays. No practical and effective cure exists, although many drugs are used to decrease the symptoms, which include runny nose, nasal congestion, and a sore throat.

An amazing array of cold "treatments" has existed since antiquity. Roman author Pliny the Elder prescribed jaguar urine and hare feces for fighting coughs. Syrian physician Ibn al-Quff suggested the application of a hot iron to the head until the skull is visible. The Swiss physician Samuel Tissot treated severe colds by **bloodletting**.

In 1914, German bacteriologist Walther Kruse finally demonstrated that viruses caused colds by preparing bacteria-free nasal secretions from cold victims and then showing that volunteers contracted the colds after inhaling the secretions. Normally, transmission of the cold may occur through droplets in the air after a sneeze.

After isolation of the rhinovirus in 1956, physicians recognized this virus as a very common cause of colds. Vaccines for the cold virus are difficult to create because the viruses frequently mutate, changing slightly as they are passed from person to person. Once rhinoviruses infect the lining of the nasopharynx (upper throat), macrophages (a type of white blood cell) come to the body's defense and trigger the production of inflammatory cytokine molecules, which then trigger mucus production. Additionally, the body's bradykinins (small proteins) cause sore throat and nasal irritation.

Influenza, a similar disease, is caused by strains of the influenza virus and tends to be more serious (it is more likely to cause fevers and affect the lower respiratory tract). Severe acute respiratory syndrome (SARS), caused by the SARS coronavirus, is another possibly life-threatening respiratory disease.

SEE ALSO Bloodletting (1500 B.C.), Biological Weapons (1346), Smallpox Vaccination (1798), Discovery of Viruses (1892), Allergies (1906), Stanley's Crystal Invaders (1935), and Antihistamines (1937).

Computer rendering of the human rhinovirus, one of the causes of the common cold.

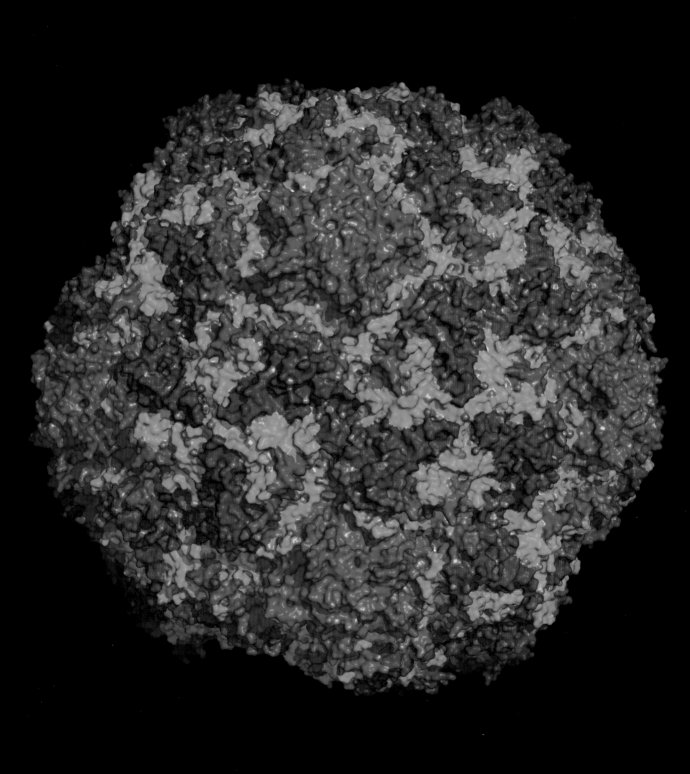

Fluoridated Toothpaste

James Crichton-Browne (1840–1938), **Frederick S. McKay** (1874–1959),
Henry Trendley Dean (1893–1962)

The ancient Greeks, Romans, Chinese, and Indians used toothpastes with an astonishing variety of abrasive materials, ranging from the powder of ox hooves' ashes and burnt eggshells to pumice, crushed bones, powdered charcoal, and oyster shells. Concoctions from nineteenth-century Britain included chalk, pulverized bricks, salt, and burnt bread. In 1892, British physician James Crichton-Browne noted that diets deficient in fluorides (compounds containing the element fluorine) resulted in teeth that were "peculiarly liable to decay." A patent for fluoride toothpaste was filed in 1914.

Today, we know that when sugar is consumed, bacteria on teeth can produce an acidic environment, demineralizing tooth enamel. Fluoride reduces the rate of demineralization. Once the sugar is no longer present, remineralization can take place. Fluoride increases the rate of remineralization and produces a fluoride-containing veneer that is more acid-resistant than the original tooth enamel.

Fluoridation of water supplies in the United States is partly the result of American dentist Frederick McKay, who, while in Colorado Springs, Colorado, in 1901, observed numerous patients' teeth with white or brown spots. Whatever caused this strange effect, McKay noted that people with "Colorado Brown Stain" (now known as fluorosis) had an almost total absence of decay. After years of research, McKay and others demonstrated that this cavity prevention was due to high concentrations of naturally occurring fluoride in the drinking water. In 1945, American dental researcher H. Trendley Dean and colleagues began fluoridating the water in Grand Rapids, Michigan, and the results showed a significant reduction of cavities, as did similar studies in other countries. Fluoridation of drinking water became an official U.S. policy in 1951. When Jamaica fluoridated all table salt in 1987, the occurrence of cavities in citizens declined.

According to the U.S. Centers for Disease Control and Prevention, water fluoridation is one of the "ten great public health achievements" of the twentieth century. However, some view fluoridation to be unethical, suggesting it is a medical treatment given without consent. In the 1950s, some U.S. conspiracists alleged that fluoridation was a Communist plot to sicken U.S. citizens.

SEE ALSO Dental Drill (1864) and Chlorination of Water (1910).

Cross section of tooth, showing enamel (outer surface), dentin (middle layer), and inner pulp with blood vessels and nerves. Dental caries (cavities) may occur where bacteria damage tooth structures such as the enamel, dentin, and cementum, which is the calcified layer around the tooth's root.

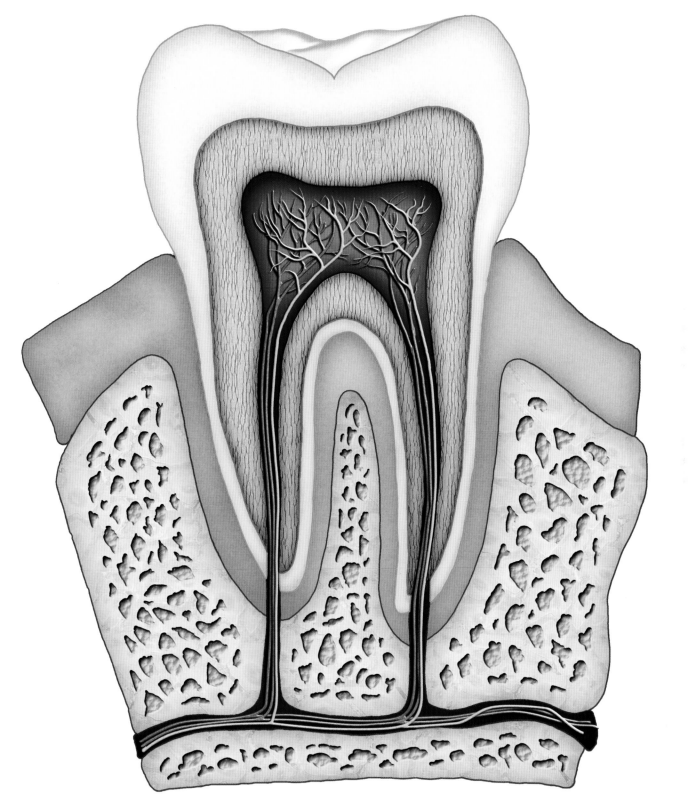

Neurotransmitters

Otto Loewi (1873–1961), Henry Hallett Dale (1875–1968)

Two years after German pharmacologist Otto Loewi won the 1936 Nobel Prize for his discovery of the first neurotransmitter, the Nazis tossed him into jail because he was a Jew. Luckily, Loewi was able to use his Nobel cash to bribe his way out of the country and escape.

In 1921, after dreaming of frog hearts, Loewi rushed into his laboratory and repeatedly stimulated a heart's vagus nerve, which decreased the heart rate. Next, he collected fluid from around the heart and transferred it to a second frog's heart with no attached vagus nerve. The liquid made the second heart beat slower. This suggested to Loewi that some neurochemical (later called acetylcholine and initially studied in 1914 by English physiologist Henry Dale) was released from the vagus nerve to control the heart rate. Loewi correctly concluded that nerves can send "messages" by releasing neurotransmitter chemicals.

Consider two neighboring neurons (nerve cells) separated by a small gap called the synaptic cleft. Electrical activity in the presynaptic neuron triggers this neuron to release neurotransmitter chemicals stored in small sacs (vesicles). These chemicals diffuse across the gap to receptors on the postsynaptic neuron. Depending on the type of receptors, a neurotransmitter may *excite* the postsynaptic neuron (tend to cause it to fire an action potential) or *inhibit* the neuron from sending a signal. The sum of influences on this neuron determines whether it "passes on the message."

Numerous neurotransmitters have been discovered, ranging from nitric oxide (a gaseous molecule) and beta-endorphin (a peptide neurotransmitter that binds to opioid receptors, providing an emotional "high") to glutamate (a form of glutamic acid, an amino acid). Glutamate usually excites postsynaptic neurons. GABA (gamma-aminobutyric acid) usually inhibits neuron firing, and many sedatives or tranquilizers enhance the effects of GABA. Acetylcholine transmits signals from motor neurons to muscles. Dopamine levels play a role in Parkinson's disease and schizophrenia. Cocaine blocks the reuptake (reabsorption) of dopamine into the presynaptic neuron, thus leaving the neurotransmitter in the gap longer and enhancing its effect. Serotonin regulates sleep, memory, and mood. Drugs like Prozac inhibit the reuptake of serotonin, and LSD binds to most serotonin receptors.

SEE ALSO Neuron Doctrine (1891), Discovery of Adrenaline (1893), Nerve Growth Factor (1948), Antipsychotics (1950), Tobacco Smoking and Cancer (1951), and Levodopa for Parkinson's Disease (1957).

Electrical activity in a neuron triggers the release of neurotransmitters stored in small sacs, represented here in yellow-orange. These chemicals diffuse across the gap to receptors on the postsynaptic neuron.

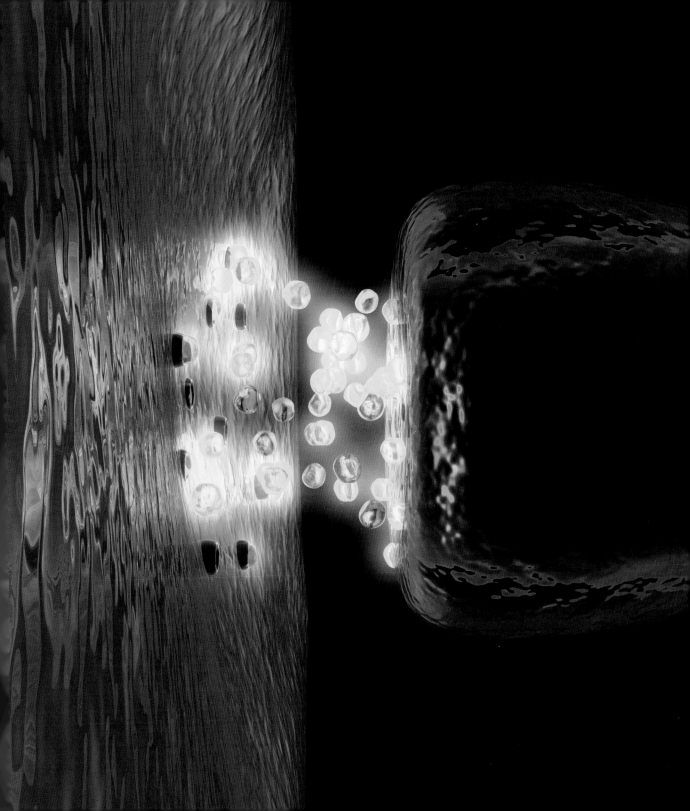

Heparin

William Henry Howell (1860–1945), **Jay McLean** (1890–1957), **Charles Herbert Best** (1899–1978)

Heparin is a powerful blood anticoagulant—a drug that inhibits blood clotting—that has played a major role in clot prevention during open-heart surgery, organ transplants, kidney **dialysis**, and **blood transfusions**. It is also useful in the treatment of thrombosis (formation of blood clots inside a blood vessel). Thrombosis can be deadly when it blocks flow to the lungs. Heparin is sometimes used on surfaces of medical devices that may come in contact with blood. Today, heparin may be derived from tissues such as pig intestines or cow lungs. Interestingly, heparin is found throughout the animal kingdom, even in animals such as lobsters and clams that have no blood clotting systems. This finding suggests that heparin plays additional roles.

Heparin is a carbohydrate polymer (a long molecule composed of repeating structural units) that is naturally produced by certain white blood cells. Although heparin will not dissolve existing clots, it will inhibit them from enlarging and inhibit new clots from forming. One way heparin acts is by binding to antithrombin III, a small protein, causing it to inactivate thrombin, a coagulation protein in the bloodstream.

Heparin is one of the oldest drugs still in widespread use. Early research into the effect of heparin started in 1916, when American researchers Jay McLean and William Howell investigated anticoagulant compounds found in dog livers. Between 1933 and 1936, Canadian researcher Charles Best and colleagues developed a method for producing safe versions of heparin for use in humans.

Today, heparin has a variety of uses, ranging from topical gel treatments for sports injuries, where it blocks histamine and reduces inflammation, to coatings for catheters (thin plastic tubes) and components of **heart-lung machines**. Other anticoagulants in use today include the coumadins (such as warfarin, also used as a rodenticide), which inhibit the action of vitamin K. A famous early user of warfarin was President Dwight Eisenhower, following a heart attack in 1955. Some historians suggest that a high dose of warfarin was used to kill Soviet leader Joseph Stalin in 1953.

SEE ALSO Leech Therapy (1825), Blood Transfusion (1829), Aspirin (1899), Dialysis (1943), and Heart-Lung Machine (1953).

Molecular model of the heparin structure, which consists of a long chain of sugar molecules.

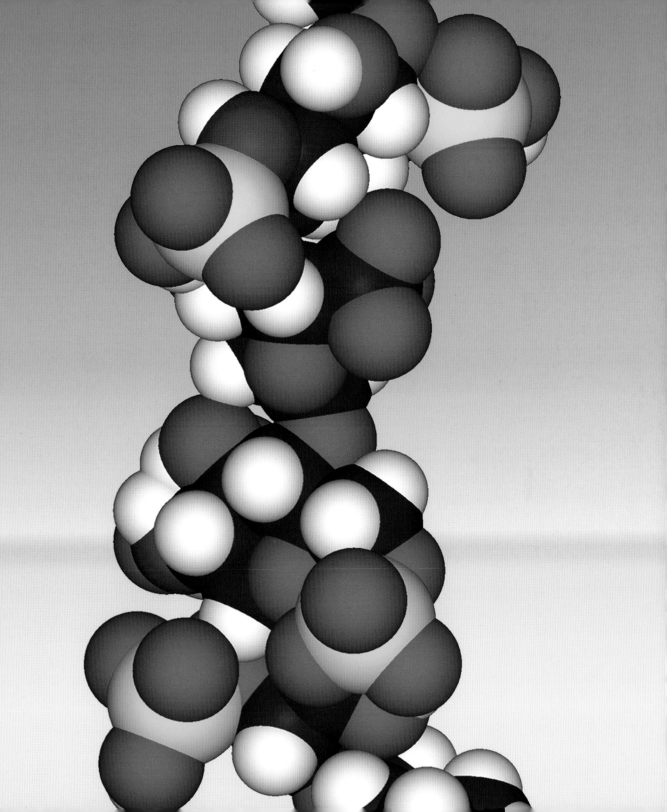

Band-Aid Bandage

Earle Dickson (1892–1961)

In ancient times, healers attempted to treat wounds and cover cuts in the skin by using dressings of various materials, including cloths, cobwebs, honey, and even dung. Physicians were unaware that bacteria and other germs should be kept away from wounds until the development of **germ theory** in the late 1800s. Before surgical dressings of gauze and cotton were commonplace, pressed sawdust was often used to cover wounds in American **hospitals**.

Today, it is impossible to imagine treating our skin cuts without bandages such as Band-Aid adhesive strips, and the amazing ubiquity of Band-Aid strips ensures their place in this history of medicine. Band-Aid is a brand name of the American company Johnson & Johnson (J&J). The bandages were invented in 1920 by J&J employee Earle Dickson, who often applied temporary dressings for the cuts and burns of his accident-prone wife, Josephine, by affixing gauze to her wounds with strips of tape. To make life easier, Dickson developed the idea of placing a series of gauze pads along the center of a roll of adhesive tape. In order to prevent the tape from sticking to itself and to keep the bandages relatively clean, he applied a layer of crinoline fabric to the adhesive surface. Josephine only had to cut bandages from the roll.

Dickson eventually convinced J&J to sell these new bandages. The bandages sold poorly at first, partly because they were sold in inconvenient sections that were three inches (7.6 cm) wide and 18 inches (64 cm) in length. Public interest increased as different sizes of bandages were introduced and after J&J provided free bandages to American Boy Scout troops and butchers in a brilliant publicity stunt. Production increased further during their use in World War II, and in 1958, vinyl bandages were introduced. Dickson eventually rose to become the company's vice president, and today more than 100 billion Band-Aid bandages have been sold!

SEE ALSO Barber Pole (1210), Plaster of Paris Casts (1851), Germ Theory of Disease (1862), Antiseptics (1865), Latex Surgical Gloves (1890), and Maggot Therapy (1929).

The amazing ubiquity of adhesive bandage strips ensures their place in this history of medicine.

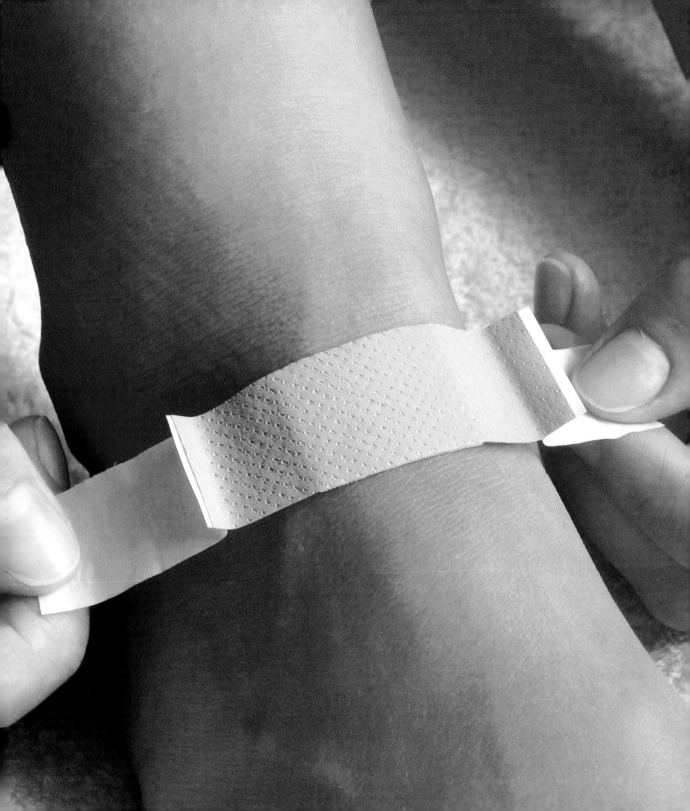

Human Growth Hormone

Oskar Minkowski (1858–1931), **Joseph Abraham Long** (1879–1953), **Herbert McLean Evans** (1882–1971)

The use of human growth hormone (HGH) has raised debates over many decades and, in some applications, is an example of a medical treatment used to solve nonmedical problems. Science journalist Natalie Angier writes, "Men who are considerably shorter than the average American guy height of 5-foot-9½ [inches] . . . are at elevated risk of dropping out of school, drinking heavily, dating sparsely, getting sick or depressed. They have a lower chance of marrying or fathering children than do taller men, and their salaries tend to be as modest as their stature." We are accustomed to modifying our bodies in many ways; thus, is it wrong for parents to provide very expensive injections of HGH to help sons who are simply at the low end of normal height?

HGH is secreted by the pituitary gland, which is about the size of a pea and located at the base of the brain. For individuals who are deficient in HGH, administration of HGH not only can dramatically increase height, but it also can decrease body fat, increase energy levels, and improve immune system functioning. The pituitary releases HGH in pulses throughout the day, with a large pulse occurring about an hour after falling asleep. Vigorous exercise can trigger HGH secretion. HGH stimulates the liver to produce IGF-1 (insulin-like growth factor 1), which stimulates growth in muscles, bones, and other tissues. Too little HGH can result in dwarfism. Too much can produce acromegaly, with symptoms such as excessively thickened jaws and fingers.

In 1887, Lithuanian medical researcher Oskar Minkowski observed that pituitary tumors were associated with acromegaly. In 1921, American researchers Herbert Evans and Joseph Long increased the growth of rats by injecting them with saline extracts of pituitary glands. Children began to be treated with HGH from the pituitary glands of human corpses in the 1960s, and one of the first applications of genetic engineering in the 1980s was the production of HGH grown by bacteria that contained human genes for the hormone.

SEE ALSO Thyroid Surgery (1872), Discovery of Adrenaline (1893), and Pineal Body (1958).

Molecular model of human growth hormone. The spiraling purple ribbons represent alpha-helices made of amino acids.

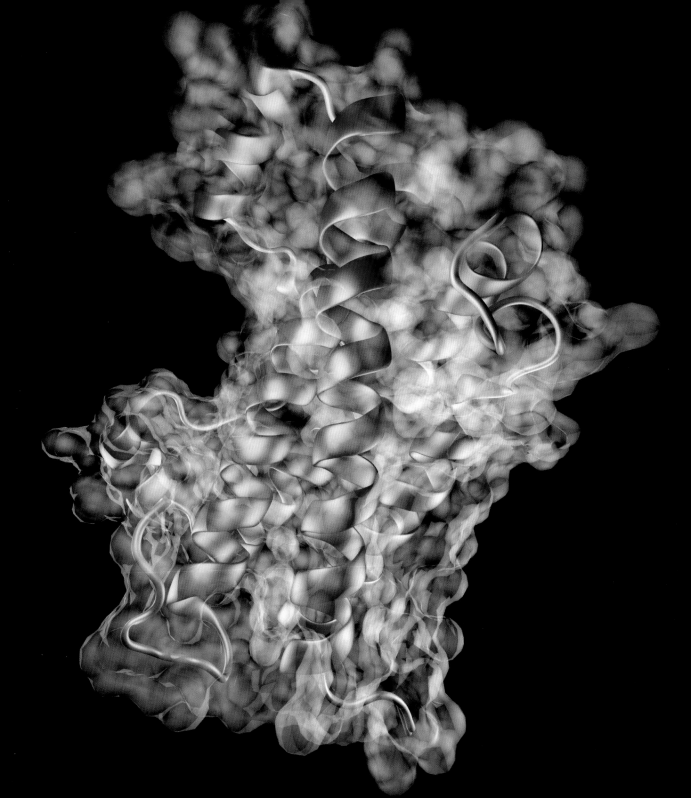

Banishing Rickets

Elmer Verner McCollum (1879–1967), Edward Mellanby (1884–1955)

Rickets is a disease in which soft bones lead to curved legs and increased fractures. In the late nineteenth century, British doctors noticed that as families moved from the countryside to smoggy industrial cities, the incidence of rickets rose dramatically. In one famous study started in 1919, in order to better understand the causes of rickets and to develop cures, British physician Edward Mellanby raised dogs indoors, fed them a monotonous porridge diet, and was able to induce rickets. He then cured the dogs by giving them cod liver oil, suggesting a nutritional cause of rickets. He reasoned that vitamin A, known to be in the oil, was likely to be the essential nutrient.

Soon after Mellanby's work, American biochemist Elmer McCollum and colleagues bubbled oxygen through the oil to inactivate vitamin A, and the oil still cured rickets. In 1922, McCollum named this distinct component present in the oil *Vitamin D*. In 1923, other researchers showed that when a precursor of vitamin D in the skin (7-dehydrocholesterol) was irradiated with sunlight or ultraviolet light, vitamin D was formed.

Technically speaking, because vitamin D can be synthesized by the body when exposed to sunlight, it isn't really an essential vitamin and is more precisely classified as a group of steroid hormones. Darker-skinned babies need to be exposed longer to sunlight for adequate vitamin D production. Within the body, vitamin D in the bloodstream flows to the liver, where it is converted into the prohormone calcidiol. Next, the kidneys or certain white blood cells convert the circulating calcidiol into calcitriol, the biologically active form of vitamin D. When synthesized by the white blood cells, calcitriol assists in the body's immune response. The circulating calcitriol binds to vitamin D receptors (VDRs) in the intestines, bones, kidneys, and parathyroid gland, which leads to beneficial levels of calcium and phosphorous in the blood and to the maintenance of calcium in bones. Vitamin D can also induce the removal of calcium from bone when needed due to a poor calcium diet.

SEE ALSO *A Treatise on Scurvy* (1753), American Medical Association (1847), "Analytic" Vitamin Discovery (1906), and Liver Therapy (1926).

Radiograph of a two-year-old child suffering from rickets and exhibiting bowing of the leg bones.

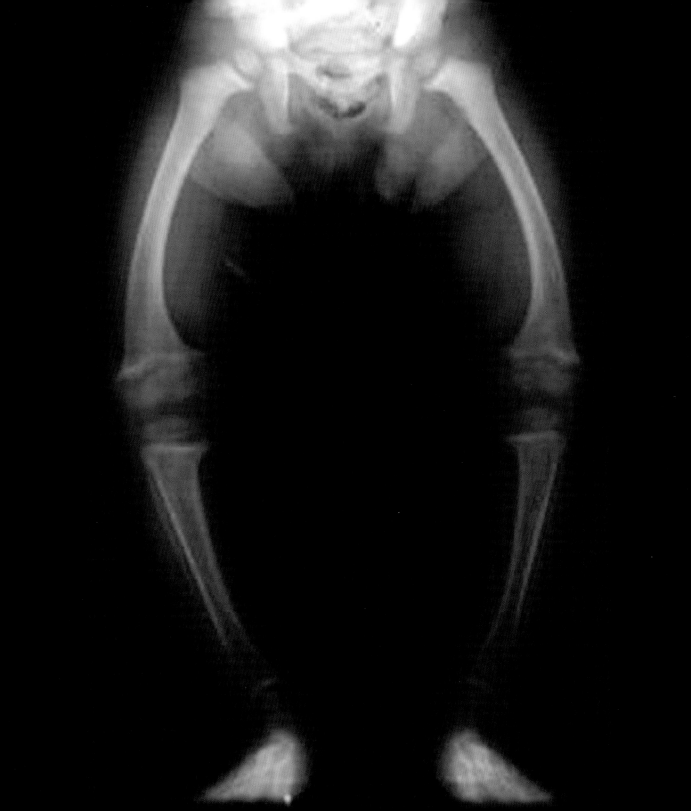

Commercialization of Insulin

Sir Frederick Grant Banting (1891–1941), Charles Herbert Best (1899–1978)

Richard Welbourn, pioneer and historian of endocrine surgery, wrote that the commercial production of insulin in 1922 "was the greatest advance in medical therapy since the introduction of antisepsis fifty years earlier." Insulin is a hormone that controls the ability of cells in our bodies to take in glucose from the blood. Glucose is a simple sugar used by cells as an energy source. The hormone is produced by regions of the pancreas called the islets of Langerhans. Without production of insulin, diabetes mellitus results. Patients with type 1 diabetes require insulin, often in the form of injections. Those with type 2 diabetes exhibit insulin resistance, in which natural insulin becomes less effective at lowering blood sugar. Type 2 diabetes can often be controlled with diet, exercise, and other medications.

In 1921, Canadian physician Frederick Banting and his research assistant Charles Best isolated an extract from dog pancreatic islets and injected it into a dying dog whose pancreas they had removed. Banting described how he would never forget "the joy of opening the door of the cage and seeing the dog, which had been unable to walk previously, jump on the floor and run around the room in a normal fashion following injection of the extract." The dog survived because the extract contained insulin, thus controlling blood glucose levels. In 1922, Banting and Best saved the life of a 14-year-old boy who was dying from diabetes by injecting him with a pure extract. He had been too weak to leave his bed, but just a few weeks later he left the hospital.

Although Banting and Best could have made a fortune, they turned over profits to the University of Toronto for medical research, and the patent was made available without charge. In 1922, the drug firm Eli Lilly produced large quantities of insulin, which were then offered for sale. In 1977, the first genetically engineered insulin was produced by bacteria with the appropriate inserted genes.

SEE ALSO Discovery of Adrenaline (1893), Truth Serum (1922), Antipsychotics (1950), Radioimmunoassay (1959), and Pancreas Transplant (1966).

Depicted here is a molecular model of the form of insulin that is produced and stored in the body, namely a cluster of six insulin molecules, referred to as a hexamer. The biologically active form of insulin is a monomer (a single unit).

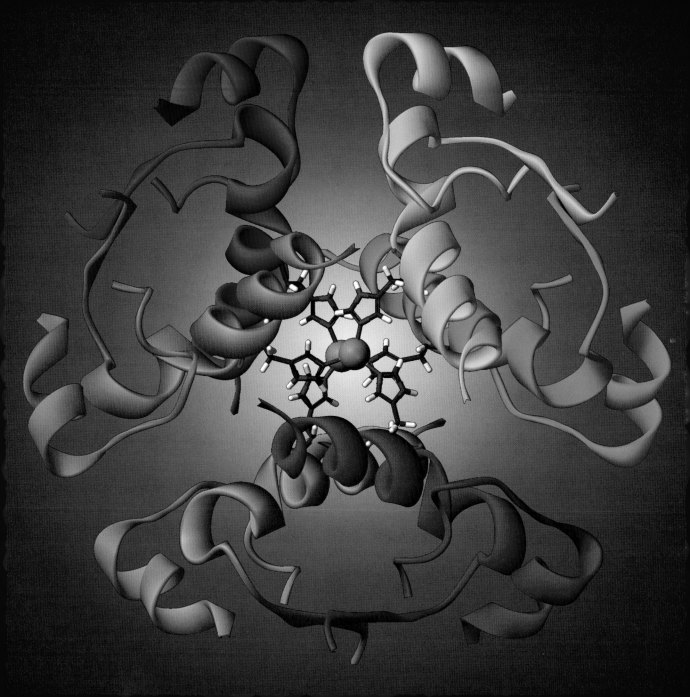

Truth Serum

Robert Ernest House (1875–1930)

The development by U.S. physicians of truth serum, which was tested on criminal suspects, may not be a medical milestone on par with others in this book, but such research is symbolic of a more frightening class of "therapeutic drugs" used as agents of punishment and sometimes torture. Indeed, pharmacological torture, or punitive medicine, became popular in the 1960s and 1970s in such countries as the USSR, where Soviet doctors employed insulin shock treatments and administered haloperidol (to create intense restlessness), promazine (to make a detainee sleepy), and sulfazine (to induce intense fevers and create extreme pain at the injection site). According to author Darius M. Rejali, Soviet doctors also attempted to create loss of inhibition by administering "drug cocktails of sodium amobarbital (amytal) with caffeine or mixes of lysergic acid (LSD_{25}), psilocybin, or peyote (mescaline)."

In 1922, psychoactive compounds were used in U.S. police work, when American obstetrician Robert E. House tested scopolamine on convicted criminals. House was concerned with decreasing the hostility of police interrogations, and after he observed that scopolamine helped reduce the pain of childbirth in his patients and put them into a "twilight sleep," he became convinced that scopolamine could be used as a truth serum, making recipients incapable of lying and thereby freeing innocent prisoners. The drug also led to many confessions, but it induced unreliable confessions involving impossible scenarios and hallucinations. Could the drug be viewed as a form of torture, especially considering that it could make some recipients sick? The CIA investigated the effect of scopolamine and other truth serums during interrogations in the 1950s and determined that no drug consistently elicited truthful statements. However, some recipients believed they had revealed more truth than they did, which often tricked them into later revealing the truth.

Scopolamine is found in the nightshade family of plants and, in minute doses, is used to treat nausea and motion sickness. Scopolamine interferes with acetylcholine, a naturally occurring chemical involved in nerve, gland, and muscle function. Other famous truth serums include sodium amytal and sodium thiopental, which are barbiturates and general **anesthetics**.

SEE ALSO Digitalis (1785), General Anesthesia (1842), Psychoanalysis (1899), Neurotransmitters (1914), Electroconvulsive Therapy (1938), Transorbital Lobotomy (1946), Informed Consent (1947), Antipsychotics (1950), and Thalidomide Disaster (1962).

All Datura *plants, such as the one pictured here, contain alkaloids such as scopolamine and atropine in their flowers and seeds.* Datura *has been used throughout history as a poison and hallucinogen.*

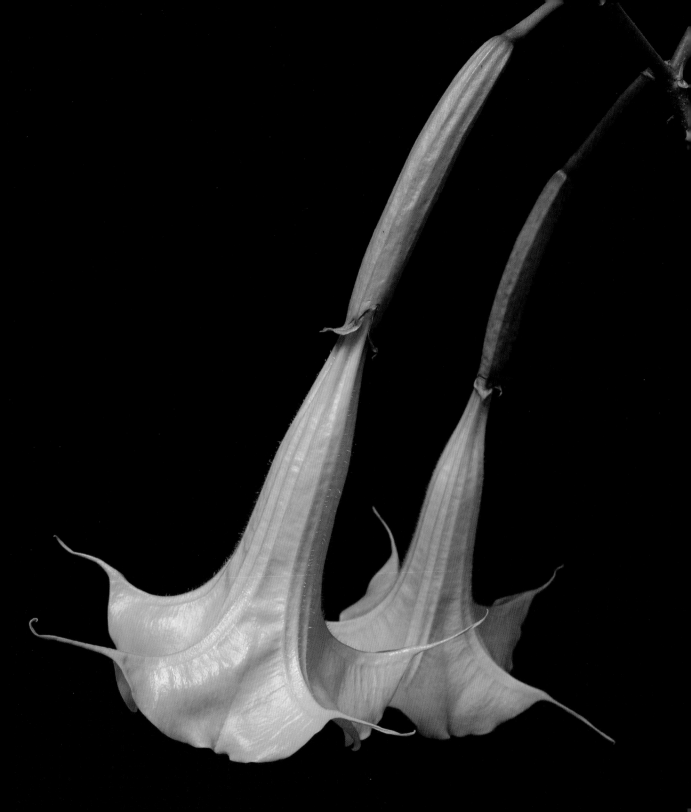

Human Electroencephalogram

Richard Caton (1842–1926), Hans Berger (1873–1941)

"Sometimes the forest is more interesting than the trees," write the authors of *Neuroscience: Exploring the Brain.* "Similarly, we are often less concerned with the activities of single neurons [nerve cells] than with understanding the activity of a large population of neurons. The *electroencephalogram (EEG)* is a measurement that enables us to glimpse the generalized activity of the cerebral cortex [outer layer of brain tissue]."

In 1875, English physiologist Richard Caton used a galvanometer (detector of electric current) to measure electrical activity in rabbit and monkey brains after placing monitoring electrodes directly on brain surfaces. In 1924, German psychiatrist and neurologist Hans Berger observed the first human EEG using sensitive galvanometers and discovered that EEGs from awake and sleeping subjects were different. Berger gave the term *alpha waves* to a particular rhythmic EEG pattern that corresponded to a relaxed state when patients closed their eyes. Berger's research grew out of his interest in psychic phenomena and telepathy, and his early work was performed in secrecy. In 1937, the first clinical department in the United States to perform and charge for EEG services was opened at Massachusetts General Hospital.

Today, the EEG is still used for a variety of research purposes, including the study of sleep patterns. It also provides an indication of brain death and helps diagnose tumors and **epilepsy**, a neurological disorder characterized by recurrent seizures. EEGs may also be used in the study of evoked potentials, brain signals triggered by a stimulus (e.g., a sound or a visual pattern).

During recordings, electrodes are affixed to the scalp at standard regions, and many readings are taken simultaneously. Because nerve signals must penetrate several tissue layers and the skull, the electrical activity associated with a single nerve cell is not read; rather, the EEG corresponds to the collective activity of numerous underlying neurons after their activity is amplified by electrical circuits. Functional **magnetic resonance imaging** (fMRI), a special form of MRI used to measure changes in blood flow related to neural activity, may be used to provide more information on location. With electrocorticography, electrodes are placed directly on the brain to help detect higher-frequency, lower-voltage components.

SEE ALSO Treatment of Epilepsy (1857), Neuron Doctrine (1891), Electrocardiograph (1903), and Magnetic Resonance Imaging (MRI) (1977).

EEG caps can be used to position electrodes near the subject's head during EEG tests.

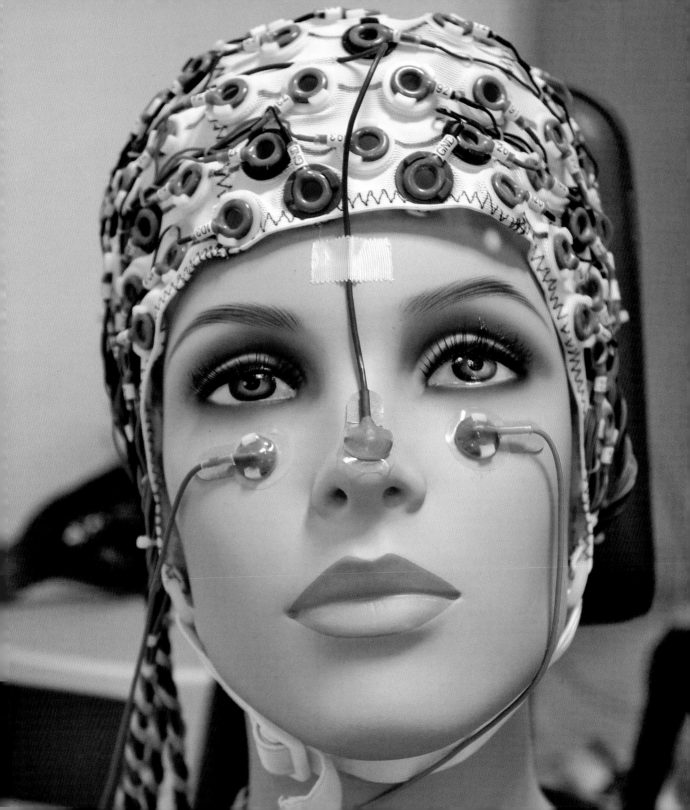

Modern Midwifery

Mary Breckinridge (1881–1965)

Midwife Nancy Sullivan writes, "In ancient times and in primitive societies, the work of the midwife had both a technical or manual aspect and a magical or mystical aspect. Hence, the midwife was sometimes revered, sometimes feared, sometimes acknowledged as a leader of the society, sometimes tortured and killed." **Hospital** chaplain Karen Hanson writes, "Midwives were among those, mostly women, condemned as witches [and] regarded suspiciously, for they mediated the mysteries of birth, illness, and death." The use of midwives declined dramatically during the late Middle Ages and the European Renaissance due to fears of witchery and the growing use of surgeons.

Today, midwifery is a health-care profession in which providers care for women during their pregnancies, labor, and birth, as well as provide education relating to breastfeeding and infant care. In the United States, Certified Nurse-Midwives (CNMs) have specialized education in both **nursing** and midwifery. Midwives practice in hospitals and homes, referring pregnant women to obstetricians when additional care is needed.

In 1925, the American nurse-midwife Mary Breckinridge introduced midwifery to the United States after her training in England, when she founded the Kentucky Committee for Mothers and Babies, which soon became the Frontier Nursing Service. During its first several years of operation, mothers and babies of eastern Kentucky experienced substantially lower mortality rates than the rest of America. In 1939, Breckinridge started the first nurse-midwifery school in the United States.

Hanson writes, "The demise of the midwife and other lay healers in America was mostly a by-product of the ascendancy of heroic medicine and the rise of the physicians as the official healer in the community. Medicine in the nineteenth century was being drawn into the market place. . . . Whereas the midwives . . . provided a neighborly service, the physicians made healing a commodity and a source of wealth in itself." In 1900, midwives delivered half of the babies born in the United States, but by 1939, only 15 percent of births were attended by midwives.

SEE ALSO Burning of Dr. Wertt (1522), Mary Toft's Rabbits (1726), Hunter's *Gravid Uterus* (1774), Women Medical Students (1812), Nursing (1854), and Cesarean Section (1882).

Birth of Esau and Jacob. Figure by artist François Maitre (c. 1475), illustrating St. Augustine's La Cité de Dieu.

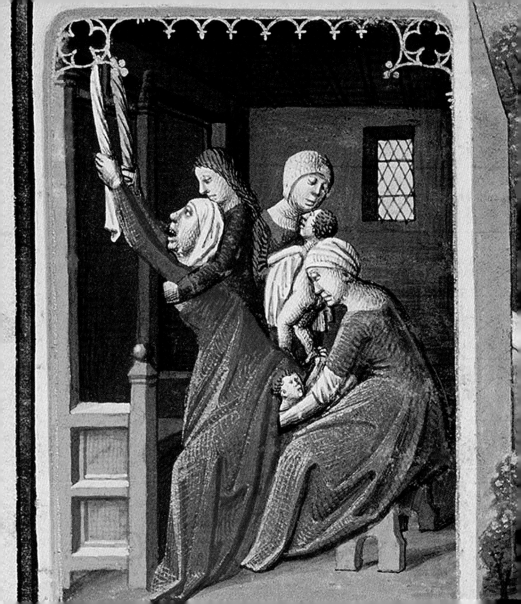

Liver Therapy

George Richards Minot (1885–1950), **George Hoyt Whipple** (1878–1976), **William Parry Murphy** (1892–1987), **William Bosworth Castle** (1897–1990)

In the mid-1920s, pernicious anemia (PA) killed about 6,000 Americans per year. Symptoms included personality changes, clumsy movements, and eventual death. Anemias come in many forms but generally involve a decrease in the number of red blood cells (RBCs) and the hemoglobin that they contain. Hemoglobin is an iron-containing molecule that can carry oxygen for use by tissues in the body.

In 1925, American physician George Whipple showed that iron played an essential role in canine anemia, which he caused by draining blood from dogs. When he fed liver to the anemic dogs, their symptoms eased, and it was soon determined that the iron in liver played a key role in their recovery. In 1926, American physicians George Minot and William Murphy showed that when PA patients ate huge quantities of raw liver, symptoms decreased, and "liver therapy" was subsequently often prescribed. Some patients were so weak from PA that they had to be fed liquefied raw liver through stomach tubes inserted in nostrils.

American physician William Castle wondered exactly why so much liver was necessary to elicit an effect in PA patients. It turned out that the PA patients also lacked hydrochloric acid in the stomach. Castle found that if he gave raw hamburger to PA patients after he regurgitated the meat by self-induced vomiting, the PA symptoms diminished. He suggested that something in the liver and some "intrinsic factor" related to the gastric juices were likely both needed to avoid PA.

Today, we know that the needed factor in liver is vitamin B_{12}, which is required for the production of hemoglobin. Additionally, normal parietal cells of the stomach secrete both acid and intrinsic factor (IF, a protein), the latter of which is necessary for the absorption of vitamin B_{12} in the small intestine. PA is an autoimmune disease in which IF and parietal cells are destroyed. In some sense, it was a happy coincidence that Whipple's liver therapy to replace iron in iron-deficient anemia also led to a cure for PA, which involved B_{12} deficiency.

SEE ALSO *A Treatise on Scurvy* (1753), "Analytic" Vitamin Discovery (1906), Banishing Rickets (1922), Cause of Sickle-Cell Anemia (1949), and Autoimmune Diseases (1956).

Artistic model of vitamin B_{12}, visually highlighting the vitamin's central metal atom, cobalt, with a beetle, a reminder that trace amounts of dietary cobalt are essential for all animals.

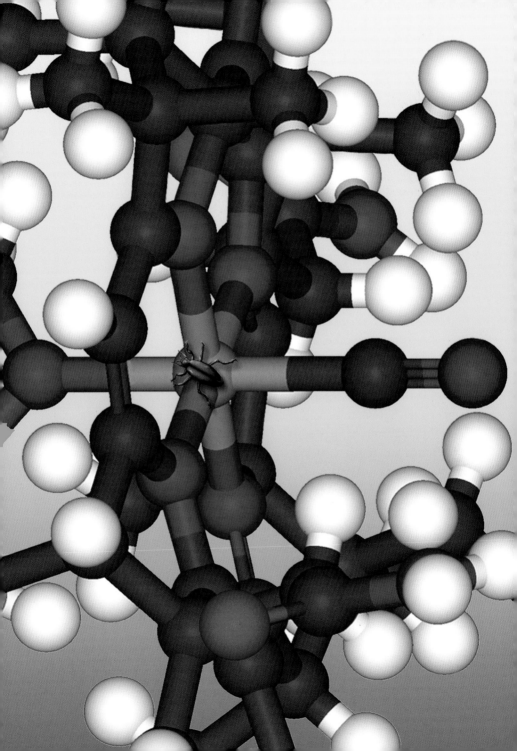

Sterilization of Carrie Buck

Francis Galton (1822–1911), **Oliver Wendell Holmes Jr.** (1841–1935),
Carrie Buck (1906–1983)

The practice of eugenics often includes the improvement of the human species by discouraging reproduction of individuals who have genetic defects or undesirable traits. The ancient Spartans practiced a form of eugenics when a council of elders tossed puny or deformed newborns into a chasm. English statistician Francis Galton contemplated the creation of a "highly gifted race of men by judicious marriages" and coined the word *eugenics* in 1883.

In modern times, the United States was the first country among many to undertake compulsory sterilization for the purpose of eugenics. One famous case concerns Carrie Buck of Virginia, who was raped at age 17 by a nephew of her foster mother. In 1924, her foster parents committed Carrie to the Virginia Colony for **Epileptics** and Feeble-Minded, supposedly because of her "feeblemindedness" and "promiscuity," but in reality out of embarrassment over the rape and pregnancy. Carrie was ordered to undergo sterilization.

The U.S. Supreme Court found that the Virginia Sterilization Act did not violate the U.S. Constitution, and Carrie was sterilized in 1927. To help convince the judges that sterilization was appropriate, lawyers argued that both Carrie's mother and her daughter, Vivian, were feebleminded. In 1927, Supreme Court Justice Oliver Wendell Holmes Jr. wrote of Carrie: "It is better . . . if instead of waiting to execute degenerate offspring for crime . . . society can prevent those who are manifestly unfit from continuing their kind. . . . Three generations of imbeciles are enough." However, by all accounts, Vivian was of average intelligence and had been on the school honor roll. Carrie's sister Doris was also sterilized without being told the nature of her operation and, for years, wondered why she was unable to have children with her husband. Carrie herself was an enthusiastic reader until her death in 1983.

From the early 1900s to the 1970s, more than 65,000 individuals were sterilized in the United States. By the end of World War II, the Germans had sterilized around 400,000. Partly in reaction to Nazi abuses, the eugenics movement was largely discredited by the international community of politicians and scientists.

SEE ALSO Abortion (70), Salpingectomy (1883), Imprisonment of Typhoid Mary (1907), Truth Serum (1922), Informed Consent (1947), HeLa Cells (1951), and Birth-Control Pill (1955).

Map from The Passing of the Great *(1916), a book by American eugenicist Madison Grant (1865–1937). Grant believed that the "Nordic race" was responsible for human development, and he suggested that "worthless race types" be segregated and their traits eliminated from the human gene pool.*

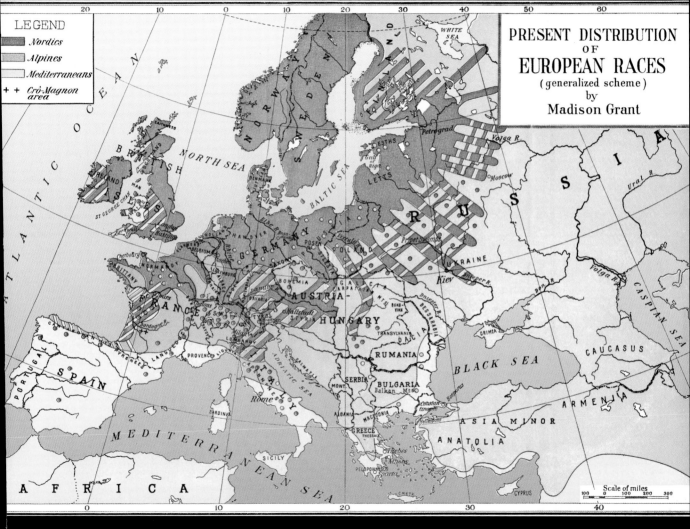

PRESENT DISTRIBUTION
OF
EUROPEAN RACES
(generalized scheme)
by
Madison Grant

LEGEND

- Nordics
- Alpines
- Mediterraneans
- + + Crô-Magnon area

Scale of miles
100 0 100 200 300

"The Rabbit Died"

Selmar Aschheim (1878–1965), Bernhard Zondek (1891–1966)

"Am I pregnant?" The answer to this question has concerned women, their families, and their doctors for millennia, and many inaccurate but creative tests involving urine have been used to gain insights. In ancient Egypt, women urinated on bags of wheat and barley. Supposedly, if barley or wheat grew, a male or female child, respectively, would be born. If nothing grew, she was not pregnant. In more modern times, a woman's urine was injected into rabbits to test for pregnancy, which led to the use of the phrase "the rabbit died" as a popular euphemism for a positive pregnancy test.

Today, many pregnancy tests are used to detect the presence of human chorionic gonadotropin (HCG), a hormone that is produced by the early embryo after the fertilized egg has implanted in the uterus (about six to 12 days after ovulation). HCG is later also secreted by the placenta. In 1928, German gynecologists Selmar Aschheim and Bernhard Zondek developed a pregnancy test in which an immature female mouse was injected with urine from a woman and later dissected. When HCG was present in the urine, the mouse showed signs of ovulation, and the woman would be told she was pregnant. A similar test was developed using young rabbits, which were also killed to check their ovaries a few days after urine injection. Note that the phrase "the rabbit died" is misleading because all rabbits died in order to have their ovaries examined. Later, tests on frogs were developed, in which female frogs produced eggs within about a day in response to HCG. In the 1970s, more accurate tests were developed that used antibodies against HCG to indicate pregnancy. These tests could be used at home, and a colored band or a + symbol indicated pregnancy.

SEE ALSO Urinalysis (4000 B.C.), Abortion (70), Discovery of Sperm (1678), Discovery of Adrenaline (1893), IUD (1929), and Birth-Control Pill (1955).

Woman awaiting results of pregnancy determination, oil on panel (c. 1660), by Dutch artist Jan Steen (1626–1679).

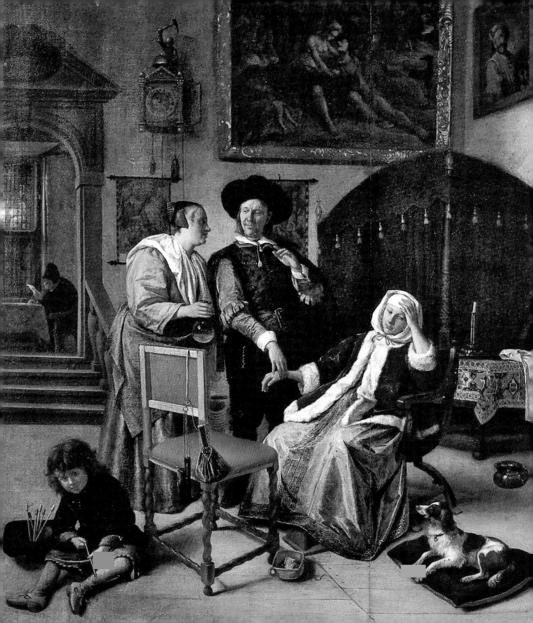

Iron Lung

Louis Agassiz Shaw (1886–1940), **Philip Drinker** (1894–1972)

The iron lung is among the first mechanical devices that could substitute for an essential function of the human body. It was also one of the early examples of biomedical engineering, a field devoted to using engineering approaches in medicine. In particular, the iron lung enables a person to breathe when muscle control is lost. The lung resembles a steel cylinder that surrounds a patient, whose head protrudes from one end through a rubber collar. A pump periodically changes the air pressure within the cylinder to inflate and deflate the person's lung while the person breathes through the mouth. When the pressure is low, the chest expands, and air is drawn into the patient's lungs.

Invented by Americans Philip Drinker and Louis Shaw in 1928, the device became famous for its use in the treatment of polio-virus victims in the 1940s and 1950s, some of whom became paralyzed and could not breathe on their own. Despite the lifesaving features of the iron lung, physician Robert Eiben wrote that it was "unlikely that there was ever a polio patient who was not fearful of the 'iron lung.' . . . A number of patients acknowledged that they thought going in . . . meant almost certain death, and others equated the machine with a coffin." While some individuals remained in an iron lung for the rest of their lives, most polio patients were weaned off the lung within a month of their acute attack. One person lived in a lung for 60 years. Tiny iron lungs were designed for infants.

Eventually, positive-pressure ventilators (e.g., devices that blow air into the patient's lungs via an airway tube) replaced most of the iron lungs—but even today, some patients linger within a lung. Author Ruth DeJauregui writes of the importance of the iron lung and later devices: "From assisting paralyzed patients to breathe, to supplying air-borne medications, and from helping workers avoid hazardous fumes to supplying air to premature babies in a controlled environment, the respirator is essential to modern medicine."

SEE ALSO Spirometry (1846), Dialysis (1943), Heart-Lung Machine (1953), Polio Vaccine (1955), and Lung Transplant (1963).

Photo (mirrored) of the famous polio-patient iron-lung room of the Rancho Los Amigos Hospital, California (1953). The hospital was started around 1888, when poor patients from the Los Angeles County Hospital were relocated to the "Poor Farm," the old nickname for the facility.

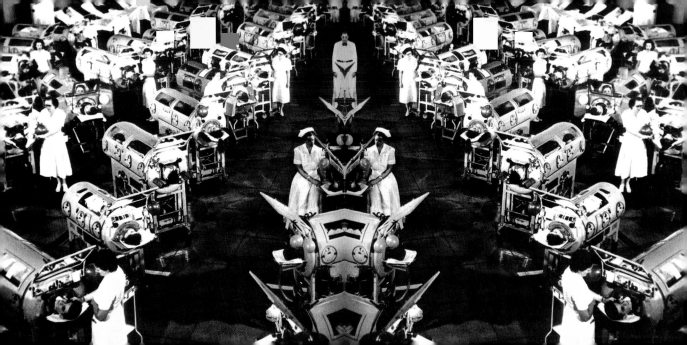

Pap Smear Test

Georgios Nicholas Papanikolaou (1883–1962)

Prior to the invention of the Pap smear test around 1928, cervical **cancer** killed more women in the United States than any other kind of cancer. When the test finally became commonly used in the 1950s, death rates dropped dramatically, and the Pap test was hailed as the most successful and widely used cancer screening method in history. In the 1800s, physicians had noted that cancer of the cervix (the lower, narrow portion of the uterus where it joins with the vagina) seemed to spread like a sexually transmitted disease and was extremely rare in celibate nuns. However, it was not until the 1980s that the human papillomavirus (HPV) was identified in cervical cancer tissues and has since been implicated in virtually all such cancers.

The Pap test, named after Greek pathologist Georgios Papanikolaou, allows physicians to take samples from the cervix in order to detect precancerous and cancerous cells. Samples may be obtained by using a spatula on the outer opening of the cervix, and a brush may be rotated in the cavity of the cervix. The cells are then smeared on a glass slide, stained, and examined using a microscope. Alternatively, samples may first be placed in a vial of liquid that preserves the cells for later study. If suspicious cells are found, a physician can perform colposcopy, using a scope to illuminate and magnify the cervix and taking biopsies for further examination.

Cancers may be treated by local surgical methods such as a loop electrical excision procedure, in which an electrical current quickly cuts away the affected cervical tissue in the immediate area of a wire loop. Very advanced stages of cervical cancer may require removal of the uterus, along with **radiation** and chemotherapy.

Today, women may be vaccinated against HPV but should still have Pap tests, because the vaccine does not protect against all forms of HPV or HPV acquired before vaccination. Only a very small percentage of women infected with HPV develop cancer.

SEE ALSO Condom (1564), *Micrographia* (1665), Causes of Cancer (1761), Smallpox Vaccination (1798), Hysterectomy (1813), Discovery of Viruses (1892), Mammography (1949), HeLa Cells (1951), and Reverse Transcriptase and AIDS (1970).

Micrograph of a Pap test result, indicating abnormal cells (lower left), which may lead to invasive cervical cancer. A Pap stain was applied and the negative image used to highlight features.

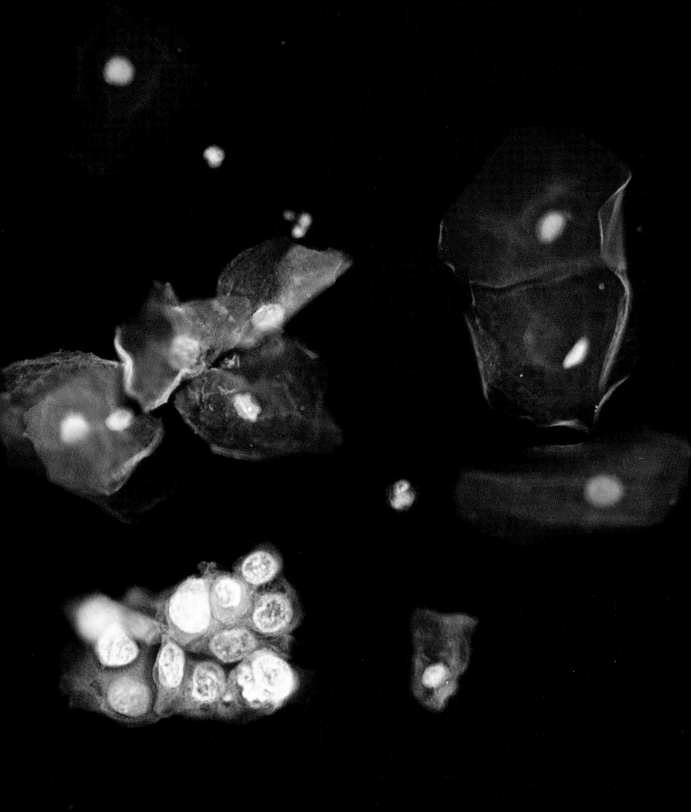

Penicillin

John Tyndall (1820–1893), **Alexander Fleming** (1881–1955), **Howard Walter Florey** (1898–1968), **Ernst Boris Chain** (1906–1979), **Norman George Heatley** (1911–2004)

Reflecting on his discovery later in life, Scottish biologist Alexander Fleming recalled, "When I woke up just after dawn on September 28, 1928, I certainly didn't plan to revolutionize all medicine by discovering the world's first antibiotic, or bacteria killer. But I suppose that was exactly what I did."

When Fleming returned from a vacation, he noticed that mold had developed on his contaminated culture plate of the bacterium *Staphylococcus*. He also noticed that the bacterial growth was inhibited near the mold, so he concluded that the mold was releasing a substance that repressed bacterial growth. He soon grew a pure mold culture in broth, determined the mold to be of the *Penicillium* genus, and referred to the antibiotic substance in the broth as penicillin. Interestingly, many ancient societies had noticed that mold could serve as a remedy, and Irish physicist John Tyndall even demonstrated the antibacterial action of the *Penicillium* fungus in 1875. However, Fleming was probably the first to suggest that this mold secreted an antibacterial substance and then isolate it. Later studies showed that penicillin works by weakening the cell walls of bacteria.

In 1941, Australian pharmacologist Howard Florey, German biochemist Ernst Chain, and English biochemist Norman Heatley, while working together in England, were finally able to turn penicillin into a usable drug, showing that it cured infections in mice and people. The U.S. and British governments were determined to produce as much penicillin as possible to help their soldiers during World War II, and a moldy cantaloupe in Peoria, Illinois, produced more than two million doses before 1944. Penicillin was soon used to defeat major bacterial diseases, such as blood poisoning, pneumonia, diphtheria, scarlet fever, gonorrhea, and syphilis. Unfortunately, antibiotic-resistant bacterial strains have evolved, necessitating the quest for additional antibiotics.

Molds are not the only producers of natural antibiotics. For example, the bacterium *Streptomyces* was the source of streptomycin and the tetracyclines. Penicillin and these later-discovered antibiotics triggered a revolution in the battle against disease.

SEE ALSO Antiseptics (1865), Ehrlich's Magic Bullets (1910), Sulfa Drugs (1935), and Peptic Ulcers and Bacteria (1984).

Close-up image of the Penicillium *fungus, which produces penicillin.*

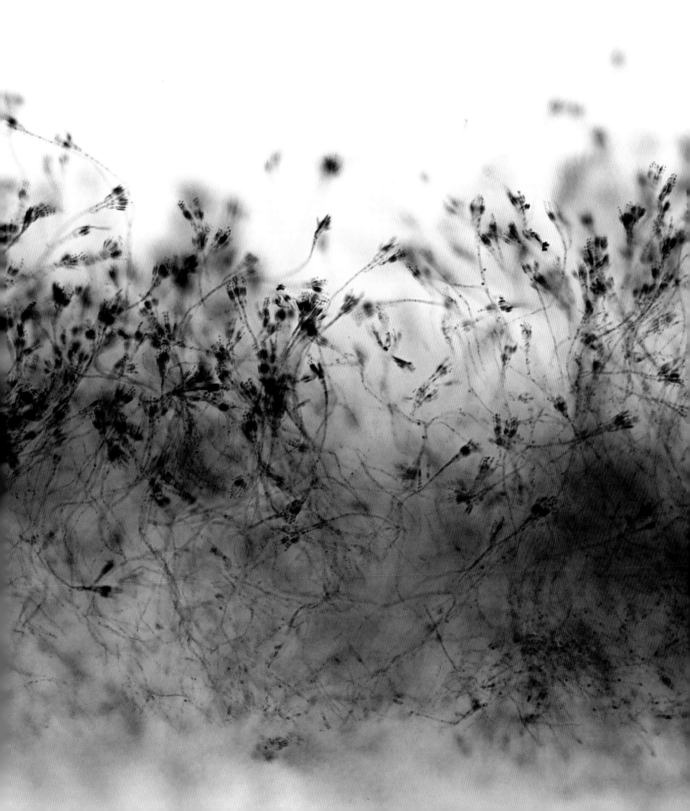

IUD

Ernst Gräfenberg (1881–1957)

In 1929, German physician Ernst Gräfenberg published a report on an IUD (intrauterine device) made from a flexible ring of silk that could be inserted into a woman's uterus to prevent pregnancy. A year later, he reported on an improved ring wrapped in silver wire that was even more effective. Unknown to Gräfenberg, the silver had copper contaminants that increased its efficacy.

Alas, in 1933, as Nazis gained power, Gräfenberg, a Jew, was forced to relinquish his position as head of the department of gynecology and obstetrics at the Britz-Berlin municipal **hospital**. In 1937, he was in jail but finally escaped to New York after U.S. supporters paid a large ransom for his release.

Although research continues into the precise mechanism of IUD action, the copper ions appear to kill **sperm**. Also, the mere presence of the device triggers the release of prostaglandins (hormonelike substances) and white blood cells by the endometrium (inner lining of the uterus), both of which are hostile to sperm and eggs. Perhaps the most famous IUD is the Dalkon Shield, produced in the 1970s, which had several design flaws that made it unsafe—including a multifilament string that unfortunately acted as a wick, encouraging bacteria to enter the uterus. This led to sepsis, miscarriage, and death.

Today, the modern IUD is the most widely used method of reversible birth control. Several varieties of the IUD are popular as forms of birth control, including T-shaped IUDs with copper wire wrapped around a plastic frame. The upper arms of the T hold the IUD in place near the top of the uterus. Other forms resemble the letter U or have copper beads on a plastic string. Also available are IUDs that release hormones such as a synthetic progestogen. In addition to the leukocyte/prostaglandin mechanism of birth control, these IUDs also inhibit pregnancy by reducing the frequency of ovulation and thickening the cervical mucus to obstruct sperm.

SEE ALSO Abortion (70), Condom (1564), Discovery of Sperm (1678), Hysterectomy (1813), Latex Surgical Gloves (1890), "The Rabbit Died" (1928), and Birth-Control Pill (1955).

Image of the Mirena IUD, indicating proper positioning in the uterus. Sometimes referred to as an intrauterine system, this device contains a cylinder that releases a synthetic progestogen hormone.

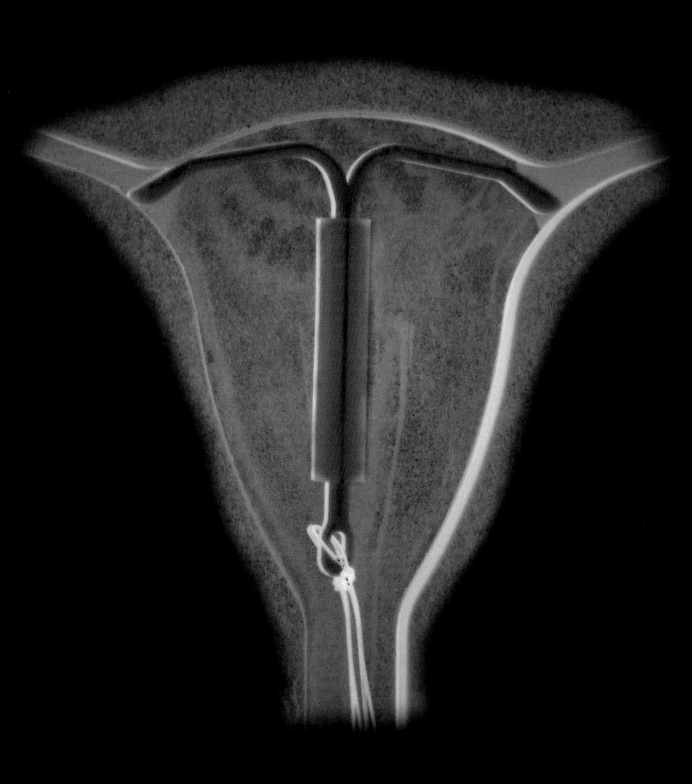

Maggot Therapy

John Forney Zacharias (1837–1901), William Stevenson Baer (1872–1931)

Imagine visiting a friend with a wound that has trouble healing. It crawls with maggots (fly larvae)—tiny natural surgeons that physicians have determined have extraordinary powers of healing. Welcome to the world of maggot therapy (MT).

American surgeon William Baer was among the first American doctors to carefully study the deliberate application of larvae for wound healing. During World War I, Baer had observed a soldier who remained on the battlefield for days with many serious wounds. Back at the **hospital**, when the soldier's clothes were removed, Baer saw "thousands and thousands" of maggots in the wounds. Surprisingly, the soldier exhibited no fever and had healthy pink tissue in the wounds. These experiences led Baer, in 1929, to apply maggots to the tissue of patients with intractable chronic osteomyelitis (infection of the bone). The maggots worked minor miracles, and Baer noticed rapid debridement (removal of dead, damaged, or infected tissues), reduction in the number of disease-causing organisms, reduced odor, and rapid rates of healing. In fact, maggots

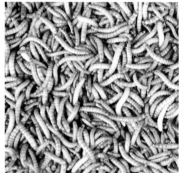

have been observed to promote wound healing since antiquity. During the American Civil War, physician John Zacharias noted, "Maggots . . . in a single day would clean a wound much better than any agents we had at our command. . . . I am sure I saved many lives by their use."

Today, MT is an approved method for cleaning out necrotic (dead) wound tissue. For effective results, care must be taken to use cleaned eggs of appropriate flies—for example, the green bottle fly, or *Phaenicia* (*Lucilia*) *sericata*, which selectively eats dead tissue and avoids healthy tissue. The maggots disinfect the wound by consuming bacteria and also liquefy dead tissue by secreting a broad range of enzymes, which also kill bacteria. Maggots can operate on wounds with greater precision than a surgeon, and their secretions stimulate the host to produce useful tissue growth factors. The maggots' movements may further stimulate the formation of healthy tissue and a cleansing serous exudate (fluid).

SEE ALSO Tissue Grafting (1597), Zoo Within Us (1683), Leech Therapy (1825), Antiseptics (1865), and Band-Aid Bandage (1920).

LEFT: *A variety of maggots.* RIGHT: *Green bottle fly, whose maggots selectively eat dead tissue and avoid healthy tissue.*

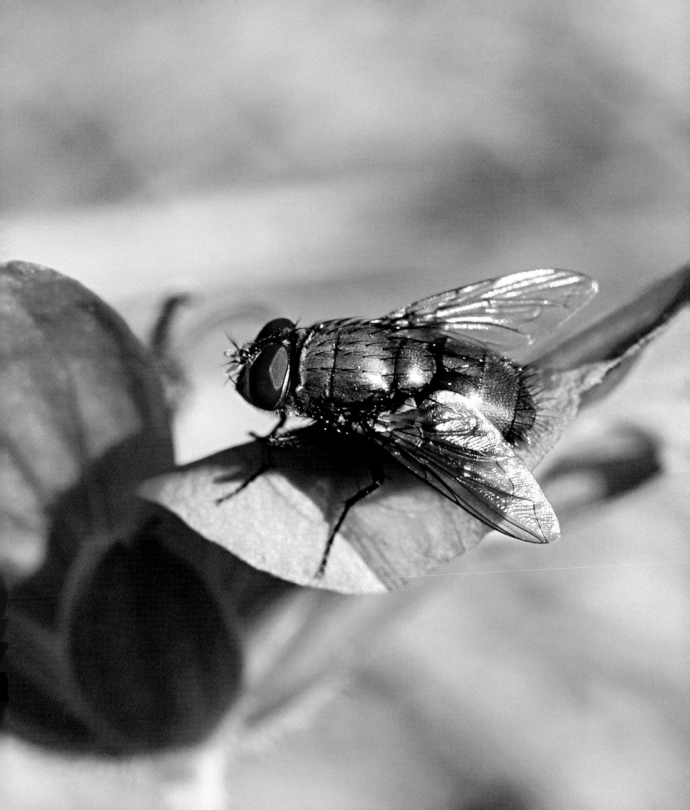

Medical Self-Experimentation

Walter Reed (1851–1902), **Werner Theodor Otto Forssmann** (1904–1979), **John Robin Warren** (b. 1937), **Barry James Marshall** (b. 1951)

Medical self-experimentation (MSE) by physicians has a long history, some of which has been touched upon in the SEE ALSO entries listed below. For example, medical acceptance of the bacterial cause of stomach ulcers is due to the pioneering efforts of Australian researchers Robin Warren and Barry Marshall. In 1984, to help convince his skeptical colleagues, Marshall actually drank the contents of a petri dish containing the bacterium *H. pylori*, and five days later he developed gastritis (inflammation of the stomach lining).

One of the most famous cases of MSE involves German physician Werner Forssmann, who hypothesized that a catheter could be inserted into the heart to deliver drugs and dyes useful for **X-ray** studies. However, no one knew if this would kill a person, so in 1929 he inserted a cannula into his arm, through which he passed a catheter until it reached his heart. Interestingly, Warren, Marshall, and Forssmann all won Nobel Prizes.

As another example, beginning in 1900, physicians working under U.S. Army surgeon Walter Reed allowed mosquitoes to feast on their bodies in order to prove that **yellow fever** was transmitted by the insects. One physician died from the experiments.

Today, patients also perform MSE in order to obtain insight into their conditions. Such experiments, of course, can be risky and range from serious attempts to decrease the severity of inflammatory bowel diseases (by patients deliberately infecting themselves with whipworms in helminthic therapy to modulate the immune system) to less justifiable experiments performed by self-trepanners who, in the late 1960s, drilled holes into their skulls in order to determine the effect on their consciousness.

Physician David L. J. Freed eloquently explains physician MSE: "Why do we do it? Because we are . . . more representative of human beings than a hundred laboratory rats; because we are better informed of the risks and possible benefits than probably anyone else in the world; because we are impatient of bureaucratic delays and burning with our need to know the answer; because we believe that the potential benefits to mankind are great."

SEE ALSO Trepanation (6500 B.C.), Zoo Within Us (1683), Cocaine as Local Anesthetic (1884), Cause of Yellow Fever (1937), Self-Surgery (1961), and Peptic Ulcers and Bacteria (1984).

In 1929, Forssmann inserted a catheter into his heart, which led to future studies that used catheters to supply useful dyes in X-ray studies of other organs. Shown here is an angiogram of the head, revealing blood vessels.

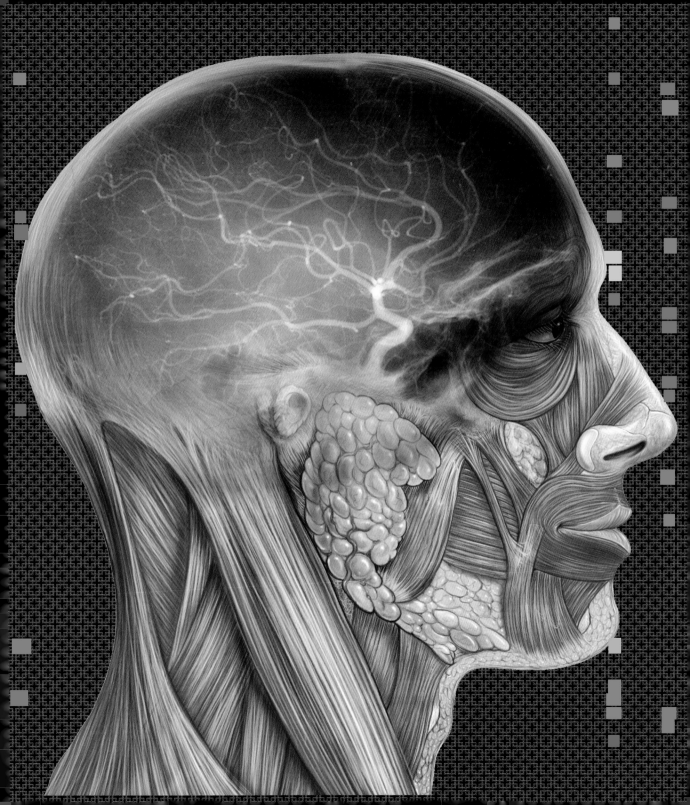

Jung's Analytical Psychology

Sigmund Freud (1856–1939), Carl Gustav Jung (1875–1961)

Swiss psychiatrist Carl Jung once wrote, "Your vision will become clear only when you can look into your own heart. Who looks outside, dreams; who looks inside, awakens." Somewhat like Austrian physician Sigmund Freud, who emphasized the importance of unconscious mental processes in shaping human behavior and emotions, Jung encouraged his patients to discuss and draw images from their fantasies and dreams. In fact, Jung was a close collaborator with Freud until about 1912. While Freud focused on a psychosexual explanation for human behavior, Jung's approach became more spiritual and mystical.

Jung postulated two layers to the unconscious. The first layer, the personal unconscious, is similar to Freud's unconscious; it includes content from one's life that is not immediately obvious because it is forgotten or difficult to access. The second layer is the collective unconscious, a realm of latent memories somehow inherited from our ancestors and shared with the human race. He called certain common images

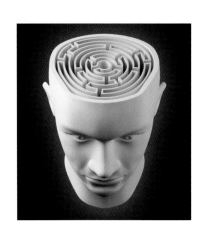

and themes across cultures archetypes, which, in his view, tend to have a universal meaning for all people. According to Jung, these archetypes often appear in dreams and are made obvious in a culture's use of symbols in myths, religion, art, and literature. In Jung's analytical psychology, individuals can take steps toward self-realization and enhance their well-being if they contemplate such dream symbols.

Although Jung had many unusual ideas that did not have a direct impact on medical treatments, many of his ideas still persist. For example, he was the first to consider the personality dimensions of extraversion and introversion, which people still find useful today. He also had an indirect influence on the founding of Alcoholics Anonymous when he suggested that recovering alcoholics place themselves in a religious atmosphere of "their own choice." This spiritual approach appeared to positively transform some alcoholics when other approaches did not work. Jung also proposed that patients draw in order to ameliorate fear or anxiety.

SEE ALSO *De Praestigiis Daemonum* (1563), Psychoanalysis (1899), Searches for the Soul (1907), Electroconvulsive Therapy (1938), Transorbital Lobotomy (1946), Antipsychotics (1950), Cognitive Behavioral Therapy (1963), and Near-Death Experiences (1975).

Jung often advised his patients to draw or paint images from their dreams. According to Jung, these vision collections formed a kind of "cathedral, the silent places of your spirit where you will find renewal."

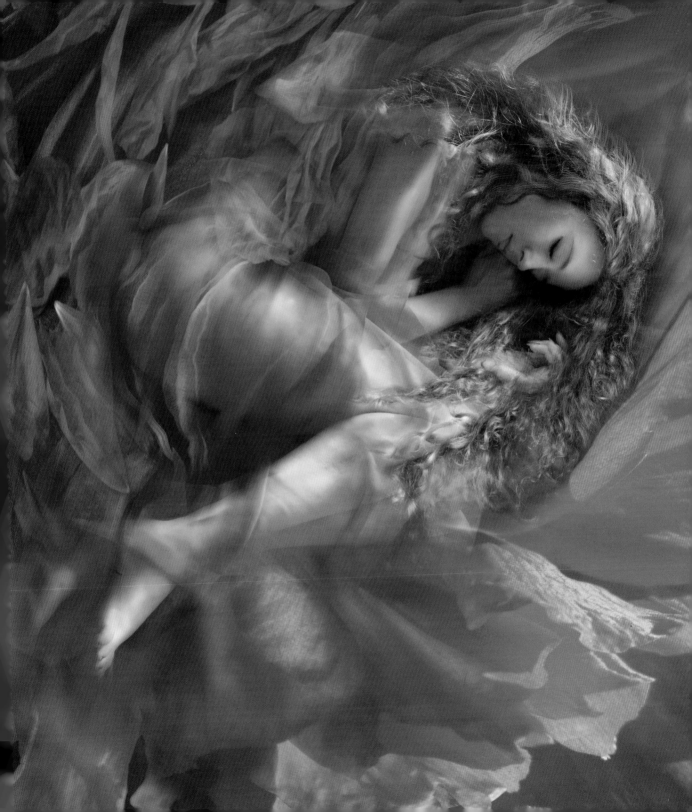

Stanley's Crystal Invaders

Friedrich Wöhler (1800–1882), Wendell Meredith Stanley (1904–1971)

In 1935, American biochemist Wendell Stanley stunned the scientific world when he created crystals from the tobacco mosaic virus (TMV), the first virus ever discovered. Scientists wondered how something that appeared to be living could also be crystalline; TMV, it seemed, straddled the ghostlike edge between the living and nonliving realms.

Today we know that viral shapes range from icosahedra (20-sided symmetrical objects) to long helices. Rodlike TMVs have a protein overcoat that surrounds a single strand of RNA, which carries its genetic code. Once inside a plant cell, the RNA replicates, and more coat proteins are generated in the plant cell. New TMV particles spontaneously assemble from the various pieces.

TMV causes a mottled browning of tobacco leaves and infects other vegetables, such as tomatoes. Like most other viruses, TMV is too small to be seen directly with a light microscope. The entry "**Discovery of Viruses**" provides a sampling of virus-caused diseases. The 1918 Spanish flu was caused by a particularly deadly virus that killed more than 25 million people within six months of the initial outbreak.

Other historical examples highlight the blurry line between the organic and inorganic realms. For example, scientists once believed that organic material had some kind of "vital force" and could not be synthesized by scientists in a lab. However, in 1828, German chemist Friedrich Wöhler demonstrated this to be false when he combined inorganic chemicals in his laboratory to create urea, an organic compound normally produced by the liver.

Science historian Angela Creager writes, "TMV was a protagonist in debates about the origin of life, a crucial tool in research on biological macromolecules, and an unlikely major player in the development of commercial instrumentation in science. In the midcentury campaigns to fight poliomyelitis and **cancer**, the state of knowledge about TMV helped to justify large-scale funding for virus research and provided a pragmatic guide for the investigation of human pathogens."

SEE ALSO Smallpox Vaccination (1798), Discovery of Viruses (1892), Common Cold (1914), Polio Vaccine (1955), Reverse Transcriptase and AIDS (1970), and Oncogenes (1976).

Tobacco mosaic virus particles (rods) stained with heavy metal to make them visible in the transmission electron microscope. Additional image processing is performed to visually highlight the viruses.

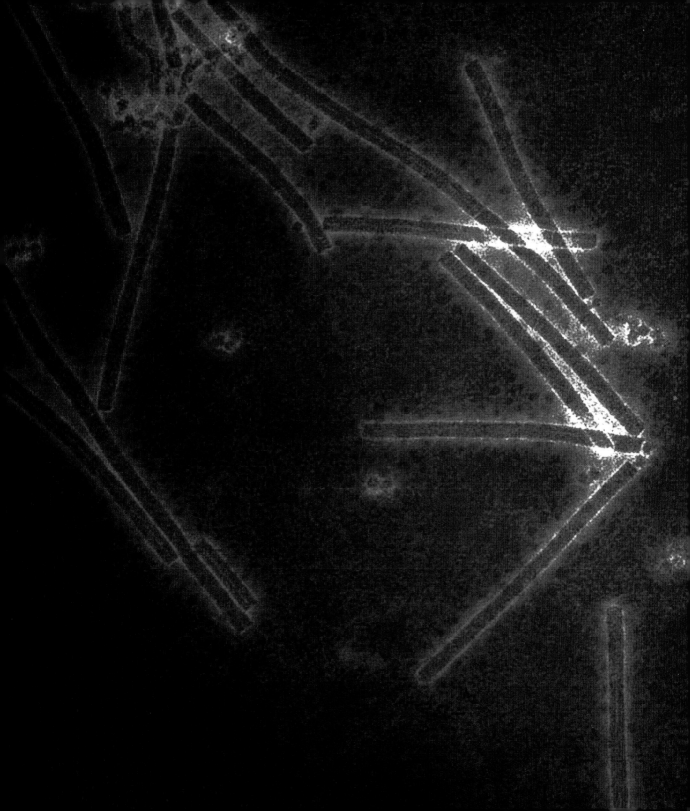

Sulfa Drugs

Gerhard Johannes Paul Domagk (1895–1964), Daniel Bovet (1907–1992)

"With Gerhard Domagk, a medicine-historical era of undreamed-of conquests of infectious diseases began," writes author Ekkehard Grundmann. "The change of scenery is hardly imaginable for us nowadays. Before the introduction of sulfonamides, 30% of all patients suffering from meningitis died; about the same number applies to pneumonia and tonsillitis, and every seventh woman died of puerperal sepsis. That changed from 1935 on."

Sulfonamides (sometimes called sulfa drugs) consist of a class of chemical compounds, some of which have antibacterial properties. In 1932, German bacteriologist Domagk discovered the first drug that could be used to systematically treat a range of bacterial infections in humans, including infections caused by *Streptococcus* bacteria, while testing Prontosil, a dye-based sulfa drug. It was fortuitous that Domagk had the largely untested drug in hand when he rushed to prevent infection and amputation of his daughter's arm, which recovered completely. The results of successful clinical trials were published in 1935. Interestingly, Prontosil did not display antibacterial properties in a test tube. Around 1936, the Swiss-born pharmacologist Daniel Bovet discovered that chemical reactions in the body broke the sulfonamide into two pieces: an inactive dye portion and a colorless active compound called sulfanilamide.

In the early 1940s, researchers discovered that sulfanilamide worked by suppressing the synthesis of folic acid in bacteria, thereby preventing further multiplication of the bacteria and giving the body's immune system a better chance of fighting the infection. Sulfa drugs were the only effective antibiotics available in the years before treatment with **penicillin**, saving countless lives during World War II and beyond. Today, although other antibiotics are generally preferred, sulfa drugs still play a role, for example, in cases in which bacteria develop resistance to other antibiotics.

In 1939, Domagk was awarded the Nobel Prize in Medicine for his discoveries involving the sulfonamide Prontosil. However, the Nazi authorities prohibited him from accepting the prize because a 1935 recipient had been a pacifist and critical of the Nazi regime.

SEE ALSO Semmelweis's Hand Washing (1847), Ehrlich's Magic Bullets (1910), and Penicillin (1928).

Before the introduction of sulfonamides, 30 percent of all patients suffering from meningitis died. Meningococcus bacteria, shown in this colorized rendition, can infect membranes that envelop the central nervous system.

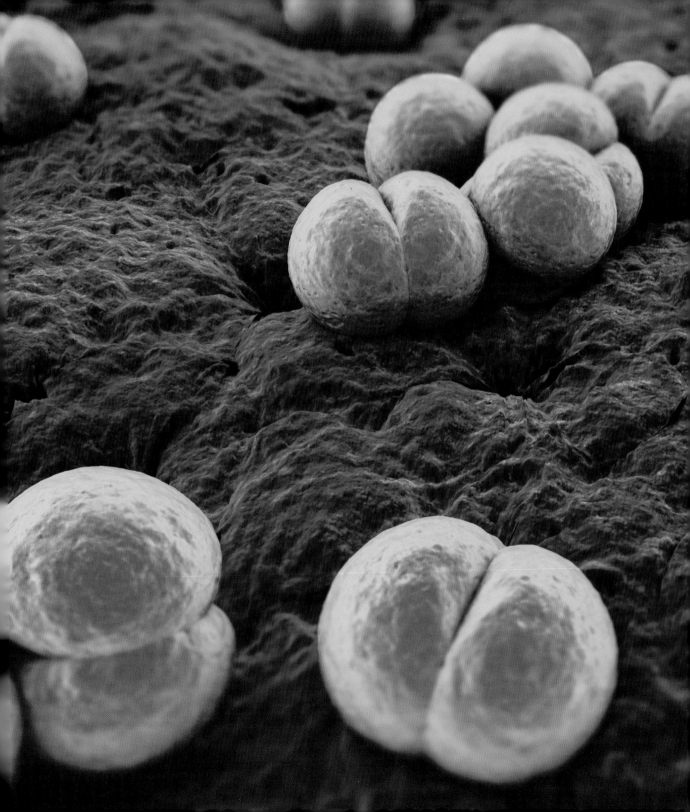

Antihistamines

Henry Hallett Dale (1875–1968), **George Barger** (1878–1939), **Daniel Bovet** (1907–1992), **Anne-Marie Staub** (b. 1914)

"From a technical point of view," writes physician David Healy, "the development of the antihistamines marked a watershed in the development of drugs." Early research on these simple chemicals led scientists beyond drugs that combated allergies into such far-flung realms as antipsychotic medicines and treatments for stomach ulcers.

Histamines are found in many plants and insect venoms. In humans, histamine is present in most tissues and stored in white blood cells (mast cells and basophils, specifically), where it participates in the immune response, including allergic reactions and inflammation. Histamine increases the permeability of capillaries to white blood cells so that they can fight foreign invaders, and fluid that escapes from the capillaries also flushes the area, which can lead to a runny nose. Histamine also acts as a **neurotransmitter** in certain neurons (brain cells). In the stomach, histamine-secreting cells stimulate acid production.

In 1910, British chemists George Barger and Henry Dale first isolated histamine from ergot, a fungus that grows on plants. The nettle plant has stinging hairs that act like hypodermic needles, injecting histamine upon being touched. In humans, histamine works by binding to four kinds of histamine receptors on the surface of cells. The two most well-known receptors are H_1 (found on smooth muscle, cells lining interior walls of blood vessels, and in central nervous system tissue) and H_2 (located on the stomach's parietal cells).

In 1937, Swiss pharmacologist Daniel Bovet and his student Anne-Marie Staub produced the first antihistamine, but it was too toxic for humans. Bovet and colleagues persevered and, in 1944, produced Neo-Antergan (pyrilamine), which was useful in humans. The first-generation antihistamines, used for nasal allergies and insect stings, functioned by binding to H_1 receptors and also caused drowsiness. Later-generation antihistamines did not cross the blood-brain barrier and avoided sedation. The structure of the antipsychotic drug chlorpromazine differs only slightly from the antihistamine promethazine. Several neurological diseases (e.g., **Alzheimer's** and multiple sclerosis) are associated with significant changes in the brain's histamine system.

SEE ALSO Phagocytosis Theory (1882), Allergies (1906), Alzheimer's Disease (1906), Cortisone (1948), and Antipsychotics (1950).

Bee venom contains melittin (a toxin), histamine, and other substances that cause pain and itching.

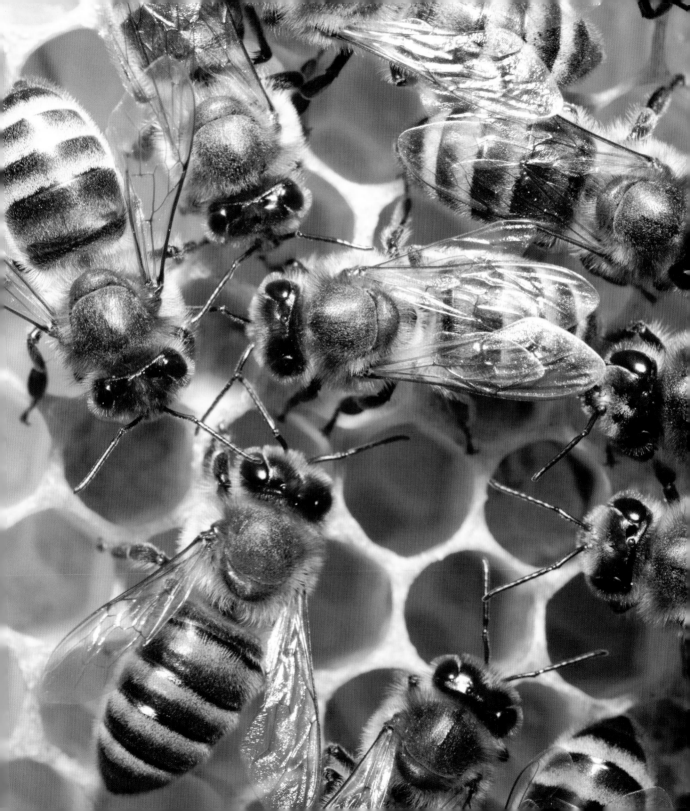

Cause of Yellow Fever

Carlos Juan Finlay (1833–1915), **Walter Reed** (1851–1902), **Max Theiler** (1899–1972)

Science writer Mary Crosby writes of yellow fever, "The virus attacks every organ [and] the patient grows delirious. The body . . . hemorrhages, running red from the eyes, nose and mouth. Vomit, black with blood, roils. Then, the fever leaves its mark, tinting the skin and whites of the eyes a brilliant yellow, giving the virus its infamous name: yellow fever."

Several species of female mosquito, including *Aedes aegypti*, transmit the virus, which is most prevalent in South America and Africa. The majority of cases involve fever and vomiting and leave the victims alive. However, 15 percent of cases enter a second stage with jaundice (a yellowing of the skin due to liver damage) and bleeding, which can be fatal. In 1881, Cuban physician Carlos Finlay first suggested that mosquitoes might transmit yellow fever. In 1900, U.S. Army surgeon Walter Reed began experiments with human subjects to confirm this hypothesis, thus making yellow fever the first virus shown to be transmitted by mosquitoes. In 1937, South Africa–born virologist Max Theiler finally developed a weakened live virus by growing many generations in chicken eggs until the virus lost its harmful properties but retained its capacity to replicate and thereby cause the human immune system to mount a defense after vaccination. In 1951, Theiler received the first Nobel Prize ever given for the development of a virus vaccine.

Yellow fever shaped the history of the United States in profound ways. For example, in 1793, a major outbreak in Philadelphia (the capital of the United States at this time) caused George Washington and the U.S. administration to flee the city. In 1802, yellow fever killed many thousands of Napoleon's troops in the Caribbean, thus causing him to relinquish claims to New Orleans and other territories in the United States and sell them to Thomas Jefferson for a low price. The French effort to build the Panama Canal was thwarted by **malaria** and yellow fever.

SEE ALSO Smallpox Vaccination (1798), Discovery of Viruses (1892), Cause of Malaria (1897), Cause of Rocky Mountain Spotted Fever (1906), Medical Self-Experimentation (1929), and Stanley's Crystal Invaders (1935).

"The Fever Districts of the United States and W. Indies" (1856). Note the intense yellow rim indicating yellow fever.

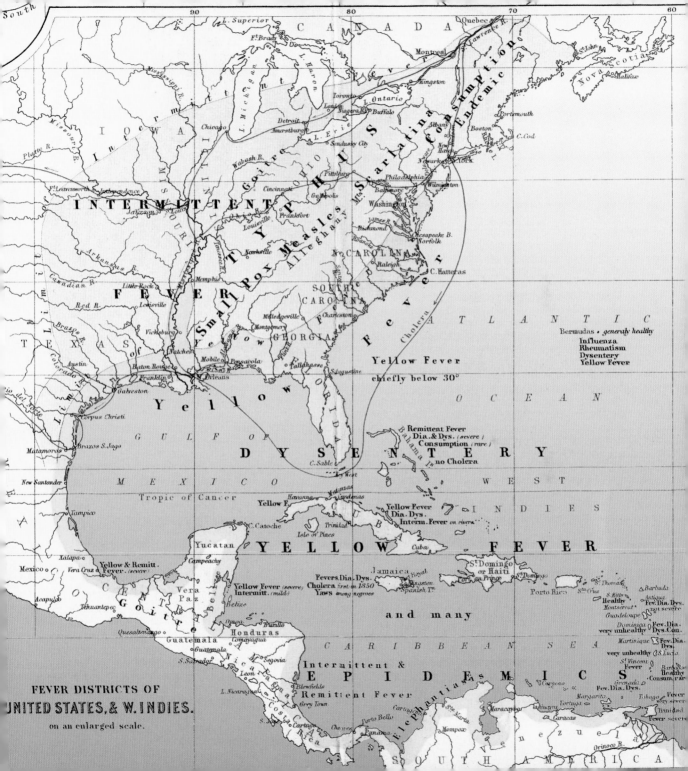

FEVER DISTRICTS OF
UNITED STATES, & W. INDIES.
on an enlarged scale.

Electroconvulsive Therapy

Ugo Cerletti (1877–1963), **Lucio Bini** (1908–1964)

Lawyer Curtis Hartmann writes of his experiences with electroconvulsive therapy (ECT), in which brain seizures were electrically induced to treat his crushing depression: "I awaken about 20 minutes later, and . . . much of the hellish depression is gone. . . . It is a disease that for me, literally steals me from myself—a disease that executes me and then forces me to stand and look down at my corpse. . . . Thankfully, ECT has kept my monster at bay, my hope intact."

In 1938, Italian medical researchers Ugo Cerletti and Lucio Bini got the idea for their experiments concerning human ECT after Cerletti watched the "electric execution" of pigs at a slaughterhouse in Rome. In the early days of ECT, patients received no **anesthesia** or muscle relaxants, as they do today. So strong were their seizures that patients often broke their own bones.

Today, ECT is used to painlessly treat severe depression and other disorders that have not responded to medications. Treatments are often administered several times. ECT is usually considered to provide a temporary "cure" and is often followed up with medications and periodic use of ECT. One common side effect is memory loss with respect to events immediately prior to or after the ECT application. Such effects are reduced with the brief pulse currents used today instead of the sine-wave currents of the past. In rats, ECT increases the level of growth-factor chemicals that encourage the formation of new nerve synapses.

Despite the lives saved by ECT, recipients have sometimes reported significant side effects, particularly when ECT is administered by inexperienced staff. Nurse Barbara Cody writes of her ECTs in the 1980s: "Fifteen to 20 years of my life were simply erased; only small bits and pieces have returned. I was also left with . . . serious cognitive deficits. . . . Shock 'therapy' took my past, my college education, my musical abilities, even the knowledge that my children were, in fact, my children. I call ECT a rape of the soul."

SEE ALSO Unchaining the Lunatics (1793), Treatment of Epilepsy (1857), Truth Serum (1922), Human Electroencephalogram (1924), Transorbital Lobotomy (1946), and Informed Consent (1947).

American author Ernest Hemingway poses while on safari in Africa, 1953. According to biographer Jeffrey Meyers, Hemingway received ECT as many as 15 times in December 1960 and was "released in ruins." In 1961, Hemingway killed himself with his shotgun.

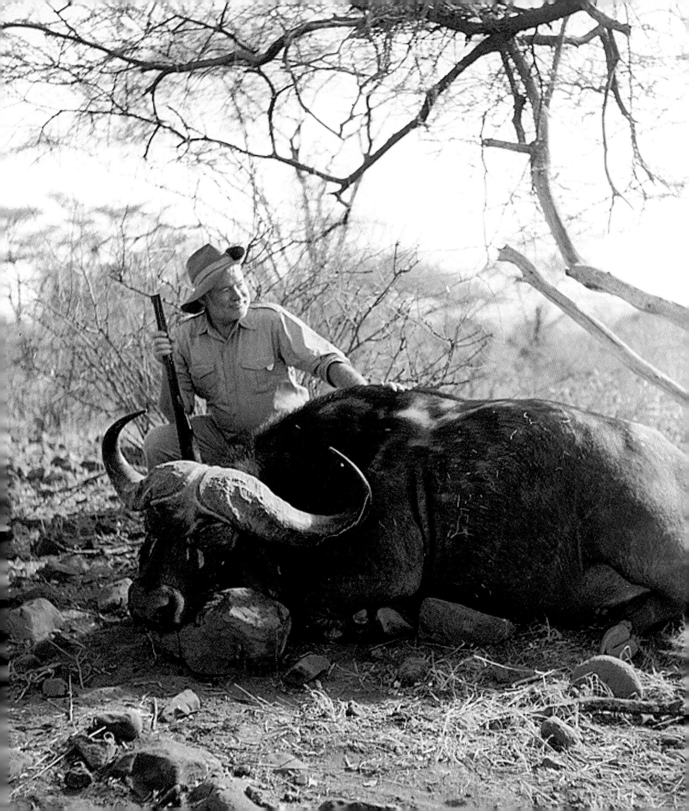

"Autistic Disturbances"

Leo Kanner (1894–1981), **Bruno Bettelheim** (1903–1990), **Hans Asperger** (1906–1980)

"He wandered about smiling, making stereotype movements with his fingers. . . . He shook his head from side to side. . . . When taken into a room, he completely disregarded the people and instantly went for objects." These and other descriptions from the 1943 paper "Autistic Disturbances of Affective Contact" by Austrian psychiatrist Leo Kanner mark an important milestone in the history of autism research and contain the first use of the term *autism* in its modern sense. Most of the characteristics that Kanner described in 11 children, such as language deficit and a desire for sameness before 30 months of age, are still regarded as components of the autistic spectrum of disorders.

Autism is a behavioral disorder characterized by impaired social-interaction and communication skills that can be identified before a child is three years old. Autism is one disorder within the autism spectrum, which also includes Asperger's syndrome, named after German pediatrician Hans Asperger, who wrote about similar behaviors in 1944. Asperger's syndrome is similar to classical autism, but language and cognitive skills are generally better in children with Asperger's.

The number of individuals diagnosed with autism has increased dramatically since the 1980s, due in part to changes in diagnostic practices and increased public attention. Children with autism also often exhibit repetitive behaviors, restricted interests, and atypical eating. Alas, in the late 1960s, Austrian-born child psychologist Bruno Bettelheim erroneously promoted the idea that autism was caused by cold, unsupportive parents, especially mothers whom he referred to as "refrigerator mothers." Numerous other proposed causes, such as childhood vaccination, have not been proven. Today, we know that autism is a complex neurological disorder with a strong genetic basis that may involve disturbances in the timing of the development of brain systems. Boys are at higher risk than girls. Intensive behavioral therapy early in life can help some autistic children develop skills that enable them to better cope and interact. Some individuals are incapable of any communication, while a small percentage of individuals display "savant syndrome," with amazing skills associated with memory, art, or calculations.

SEE ALSO Psychoanalysis (1899), Prosopagnosia (1947), and Cognitive Behavioral Therapy (1963).

Individuals with autism sometimes exhibit the need to repetitively stack or line up objects. For example, as children, they may spend hours lining up their toy cars in certain patterns rather than using them for more common forms of play.

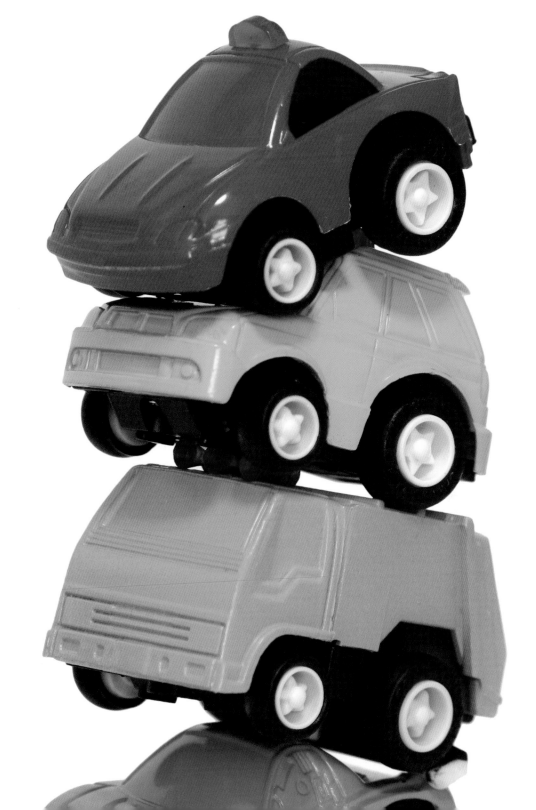

Dialysis

Georg Haas (1886–1971), **Willem Johan Kolff** (1911–2009), **Belding Hibbard Scribner** (1921–2003)

Our kidneys serve many functions, including hormone secretion and the removal of wastes that are diverted to the urinary bladder. When diseases such as diabetes cause kidney failure, the lost kidney function can be replaced by dialysis machines that employ an artificial membrane to filter the blood. In the process of hemodialysis, larger substances, such as red blood cells and large proteins, are trapped on the side of the membrane in contact with the blood. Toxins from the patient's blood pass through the membrane by diffusion into a liquid called the dialysate. This dialysate is discarded, along with the toxins, and the purified blood is returned to the body. Excess fluid in the blood is also removed.

Around 1924, German physician Georg Haas was the first to perform dialysis on a patient, but his equipment was not able to save patients' lives. Dutch physician Willem Kolff is considered the father of dialysis; he constructed the first full-scale dialysis machine in 1943. His original version used sausage skins and various spare parts. The first patient to be saved by Kolff's dialysis machine was a woman in acute renal failure who had entered a coma. In 1945, she was dialyzed for 11 hours before regaining consciousness. Her first intelligible words on leaving the coma were, "I'm going to divorce my husband!"

Not until the early 1960s were connection devices—such as the Teflon shunt invented by physician Belding Scribner—available to reduce clotting and stay in place, so that dialysis could be repeatedly performed without injury to blood vessels. Around this time, as a result of the limited numbers of dialysis machines, anonymous committees decided who lived and died.

The physician John Maher writes, "Survival rates with dialysis treatment that approach those of matched control patients with good renal functions represent one of the outstanding technological achievements. . . . Yet, dialysis is an imperfect substitution for renal function compared to the divine prototype. It is expensive [and] time consuming [and] fails to substitute for renal hormonal and metabolic activities."

SEE ALSO Urinalysis (4000 B.C.), Iron Lung (1928), Heart-Lung Machine (1953), and Kidney Transplant (1954).

A hemodialysis machine with rotating pumps may be used by people who wait for kidney transplants. Note that with dialysis, bicarbonate ions and other substances from the dialysate can enter the blood. Hemodialysis typically involves four-hour sessions three times a week.

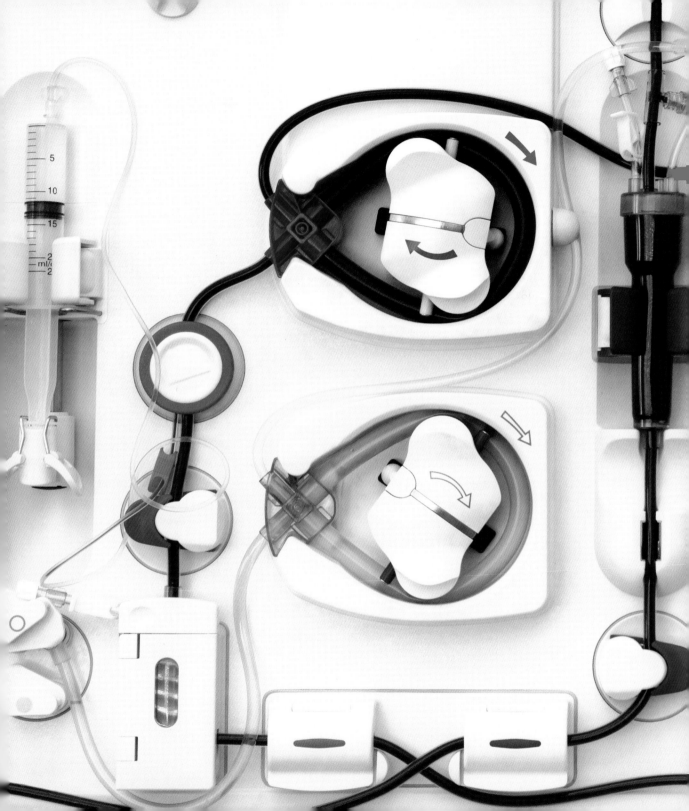

Blalock-Taussig Shunt

Helen Brooke Taussig (1898–1986), **Alfred Blalock** (1899–1964), **Vivien Theodore Thomas** (1910–1985)

The physician Sherwin B. Nuland writes of the desperate nature of blue baby syndrome at Johns Hopkins **Hospital** in the 1930s, before surgical cures were available: "An afternoon spent in the Pediatric Cardiology Clinic was a test for even the most stoic physicians. Underdeveloped children, so short of breath that they had spells of unconsciousness with the most minimal exertion, came in large numbers. With nose, ears, extremities, and sometimes entire bodies ink-blue with cyanosis [blood with lack of oxygen], they squatted on the floor or lay still on the examination tables so as not to worsen their air-hunger."

The Tetralogy of Fallot refers to one common cause of blue baby syndrome. Babies with this heart defect have a low level of oxygen in the blood because of the mixing of oxygenated and deoxygenated blood in the heart's left ventricle, which is caused by a hole in the wall that normally separates the left and right ventricles. Additionally, a narrowing near the pulmonary valve decreases blood flow from the heart to the pulmonary arteries that carry blood from the heart to the lungs.

American cardiologist Helen Taussig approached American surgeon Alfred Blalock and his technician and assistant Vivien Thomas about the possibility of rerouting blood in blue babies in such a way that additional blood from the heart would be oxygenated by the lungs. In 1944, the operation was performed on a 15-month-old girl and has since saved thousands of lives. In particular, Blalock joined the subclavian artery to the pulmonary artery (today the procedure may make use of artificial tubing). Thomas had performed the operation on more than 200 dogs before it was first tried on the little girl.

The Blalock-Taussig shunt marked the start of the modern era of cardiac surgery. Once the era of open-heart surgery began, the shunt was performed with decreasing frequency because surgeons could open the heart directly and repair its defects, for example, by closing the hole in the internal heart wall with a Gore-Tex patch.

SEE ALSO Al-Nafis's Pulmonary Circulation (1242), Digitalis (1785), Ligation of the Abdominal Aorta (1817), Artificial Heart Valves (1952), and Heart-Lung Machine (1953).

Diagram depicting a ventricular septal defect (the hole between the right and left sides of the heart, marked by the yellow dot), one of the features of the Tetralogy of Fallot.

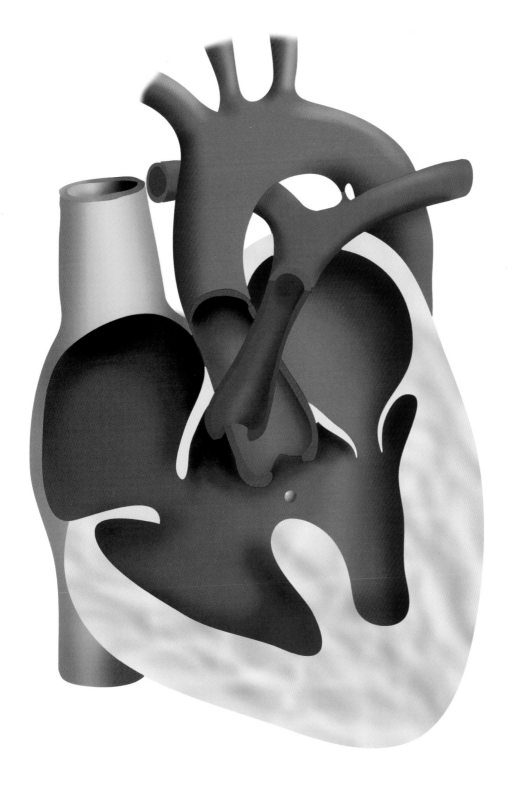

Cancer Chemotherapy

Sidney Farber (1903–1973), **Louis S. Goodman** (1906–2000), **Alfred Gilman** (1908–1984)

Many **cancer** chemotherapies work by killing cells that divide rapidly—one of the characteristics of cancer cells. Alas, this means that such agents also destroy healthy cells that divide rapidly, including cells in hair follicles, the digestive tract, and bone marrow. Surprisingly, one of the first effective anticancer drugs was discovered when American pharmacologists Alfred Gilman and Louis Goodman performed research, under the cloak of wartime secrecy, after more than 1,000 people were accidentally exposed to American-made mustard gas bombs. This chemical warfare agent was found to damage rapidly growing white blood cells, and scientists reasoned that this might be useful for treating certain lymphomas (cancers of certain white blood cells). When a patient with non-Hodgkin's lymphoma was injected with a related nitrogen compound in 1943, Gilman and Goodman observed a dramatic but temporary shrinkage of the tumor masses. The government gave Gilman and Goodman permission to publish their findings in 1946.

In 1948, American pathologist Sidney Farber discovered that methotrexate—a drug that blocked the action of enzymes requiring the folate vitamin—triggered remission in children afflicted with acute lymphoblastic leukemia. In 1951, chemists synthesized 6-mercaptopurine (6-MP), a drug that inhibits **DNA** synthesis and is useful in the treatment of childhood leukemia. In 1956, methotrexate was used to effectively treat the first solid cell tumor in a woman with choriocarcinoma. Various combinations of anticancer drugs were found to be useful in 1965, and platinum-based drugs that cause cross-linking of DNA, which ultimately triggers apoptosis (programmed cell death), were reported in 1969.

Several main categories of chemotherapy drugs that affect cell division and DNA synthesis exist: alkylating agents (which link DNA strands to prevent DNA replication), antimetabolites (which prevent the assembly of DNA from its building blocks), plant alkaloids (which block microtubule function needed for cell division), topoisomerase inhibitors (which disrupt normal DNA coiling patterns), and antitumor antibiotics (which block proper DNA and RNA function). Targeted therapies include monoclonal antibodies, which can bind to precise targets, and inhibitors of certain kinase enzymes. Many previously fatal cancers are now generally curable.

SEE ALSO Causes of Cancer (1761), Cell Division (1855), Radiation Therapy (1903), Ehrlich's Magic Bullets (1910), DNA Structure (1953), Oncogenes (1976), and Telomerase (1984).

Vinblastine and vincristine drugs, extracts from the Catharanthus roseus *plant, are used as chemotherapeutic agents to treat leukemia and other cancers. Substances from the plant can also be hallucinogenic.*

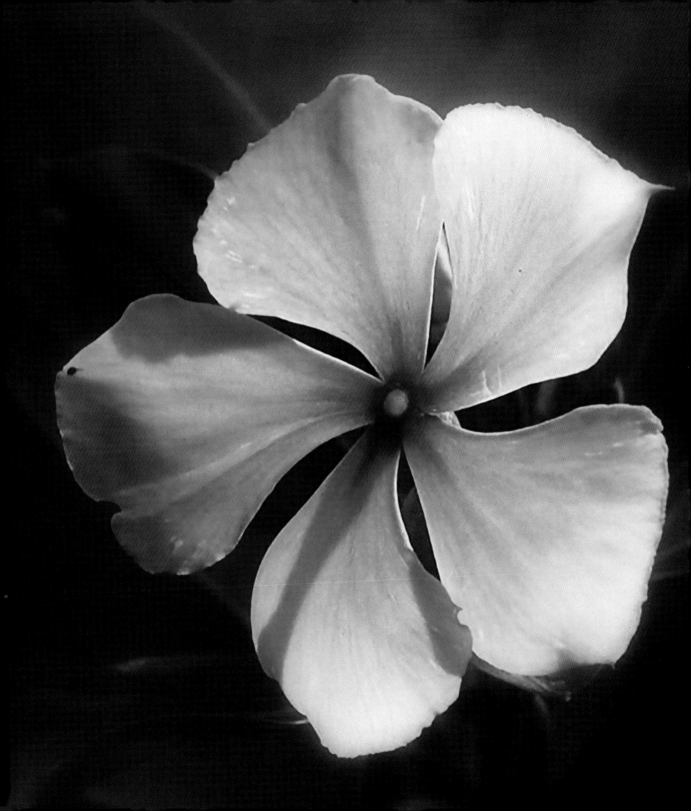

Transorbital Lobotomy

Egas Moniz (1874–1955), **Walter Jackson Freeman II** (1895–1972), **James Winston Watts** (1904–1994), **Rosemary Kennedy** (1918–2005)

Scientists had known since the mid-1800s that particular regions of the brain were specialized for different functions. Thus, the idea that brain surgery might be used to control madness was not far-fetched. However, the lobotomies performed in the 1900s, in which connections to and from the prefrontal cortex were severed, seem quite crude today. This cortex at the front part of the brain controls personality expression, decision making, social inhibition, and more.

Prefrontal leukotomy or lobotomy involves the drilling of holes in the skull, followed by the use of wire loops or blades to cut the brain. Portuguese neurologist Egas Moniz received the Nobel Prize for some of the early work in leukotomies, and in 1936 American neurosurgeon James Watts and physician Walter Freeman performed the first prefrontal leukotomy in the United States. However, Freeman desired a faster approach, and in 1946 he began performing transorbital lobotomies, placing an ice pick–like instrument into the eye socket beneath the upper eyelid and hammering the pick into the brain. The instrument was then pivoted from side to side to sever nerve fibers.

Medical historian Ole Enersen writes that Freeman performed lobotomies "with a recklessness bordering on lunacy, touring the country like a travelling evangelist. . . . Between 1948 and 1957, he alone lobotomized 2,400 patients. In most cases this procedure was nothing more than a gross and unwarranted mutilation." Lobotomies were performed in order to "cure" disorders ranging from obsessive-compulsive disorder to schizophrenia and depression, although the results often included blunted emotions and an inability to make plans. In the 1940s and 1950s, about 40,000 people in the United States were lobotomized. The use of lobotomies diminished after the invention of **antipsychotic** drugs such as chlorpromazine.

Rosemary Kennedy, sister of President John F. Kennedy, was one of the most famous failures of lobotomy surgery. At age 23, her moody, rebellious behavior caused her father to order a lobotomy that left her paralyzed, incontinent, incoherent, and institutionalized for the remainder of her life.

SEE ALSO Unchaining the Lunatics (1793), Phrenology (1796), Cerebral Localization (1861), Truth Serum (1922), Electroconvulsive Therapy (1938), and Antipsychotics (1950).

Before intentional lobotomies, there was the famous case of Phineas Gage (1823–1860), shown here holding the large iron rod that was accidentally driven completely through his head, destroying much of his brain's left frontal lobe. He survived with some changes in personality.

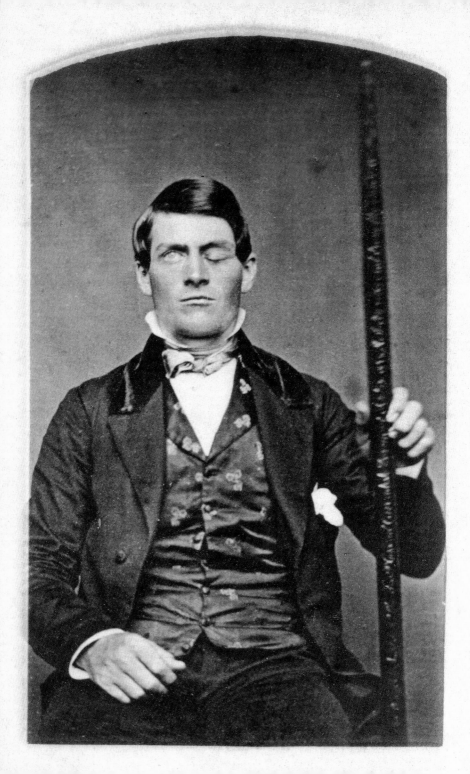

Informed Consent

The ancient **Hippocratic Oath** demonstrates that physicians have long desired to keep patients from harm. However, the oath never mentions human experimentation and the need to obtain informed consent—permission to perform tests and procedures from patients to whom the tests and risks of tests are adequately explained. In fact, through most of the history of medicine, physicians often found it appropriate to deliberately deceive their patients.

The need for obtaining informed consent from subjects of medical research became particularly apparent at the end of World War II, when Nazi doctors were brought to trial in Nuremberg, Germany, for their horrific experiments on humans. These studies, often performed on Jews and other prisoners, include the cooling of naked subjects in ice, injecting chemicals into the eyes of twins to change eye color, and sewing twins together in an attempt to create **conjoined twins**.

The Nuremberg Code of medical ethics, developed in 1947, stresses the need for voluntary consent of human subjects who must understand the proposed research, which should be designed to benefit society. The subject should also be free to terminate the experiment, which should be conducted in ways to avoid all unnecessary physical and mental suffering. Both the Nuremberg Code and ethical guidelines proposed in the 1964 Declaration of Helsinki helped to shape U.S. regulations governing federal funding of research.

In order for subjects to give informed consent, they must have adequate reasoning faculties at the time consent is given. Children are usually considered "incompetent" to consent, and legal guardians may act on their behalf. Physicians are often permitted to provide emergency treatments to unconscious patients who cannot give consent.

A famous example of lack of informed consent is the Tuskegee syphilis experiment, conducted between 1932 and 1972 in Tuskegee, Alabama, in which men with syphilis were not treated properly and not told they had syphilis so that U.S. researchers could study the progression of the disease. Some men died of syphilis, and wives often contracted the disease.

SEE ALSO Hippocratic Oath (400 B.C.), Persecution of Jewish Physicians (1161), Separation of Conjoined Twins (1689), Truth Serum (1922), Sterilization of Carrie Buck (1927), Randomized Controlled Trials (1948), Placebo Effect (1955), Hospice (1967), and Do Not Resuscitate (1991).

As part of the 1953 project MK-ULTRA, the CIA administered LSD without people's consent in order to study the effects of LSD. LSD may cause users to experience radiant colors, rippling and crawling geometric patterns, and other sensory distortions.

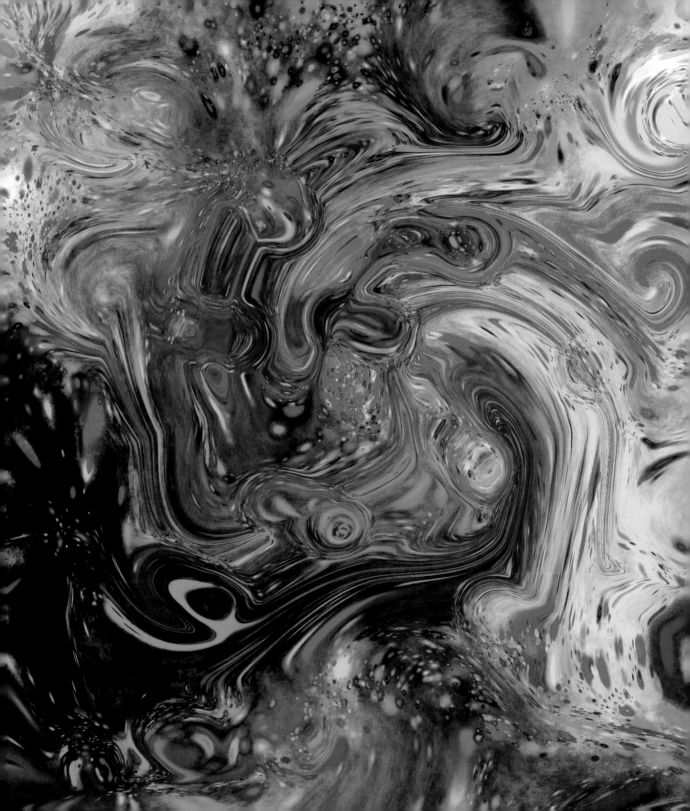

Prosopagnosia

Joachim Bodamer (1910–1985)

Imagine looking at your spouse, your child, or your own reflection in a mirror and seeing a stranger. People with extreme versions of prosopagnosia, or "face blindness," suffer from these symptoms, which can make ordinary social interactions quite difficult.

Originally thought to be triggered by sudden brain damage, such as caused by an accident or a stroke, a congenital form of the disorder also exists. In 1947, the German neurologist Joachim Bodamer coined the term *prosopagnosia* when discussing symptoms of a young man who, after being shot in the head, could not recognize family members or even his own face. The specific brain area often associated with prosopagnosia is the fusiform gyrus, located in the lower part of the cerebral cortex. In many instances, an afflicted person is able to normally distinguish objects not associated with human faces. In one famous case, a prosopagnosiac farmer could distinguish his sheep from their faces better than he could distinguish human faces.

Research on prosopagnosia is important in the history of medicine, not only because it provides insight on theories of face perception, but because it illuminates the manner in which perceptual representations are organized and stored in the brain. The disorder also forces us to continually question our fundamental notions of awareness, familiarity, and knowledge, as well as how these concepts are managed in the brain. Moreover, this affliction is representative of numerous uncommon disorders of the mind. For example, when people afflicted with Capgras syndrome see a friend, spouse, or themselves in a mirror, they believe they are seeing an identical impostor. Also, consider Fregoli syndrome, in which the patient insists that he or she knows someone who is actually unfamiliar. People with Cotard's syndrome mistakenly believe that they have lost organs or that they are walking corpses. In the syndrome of subjective doubles, the patient believes that he or she has a double, with the same appearance, who is leading a separate life.

SEE ALSO Cerebral Localization (1861), Alzheimer's Disease (1906), Searches for the Soul (1907), "Autistic Disturbances" (1943), and Face Transplant (2005).

Prosopagnosiacs have great difficulty recognizing and distinguishing faces, even the faces of family members and close friends.

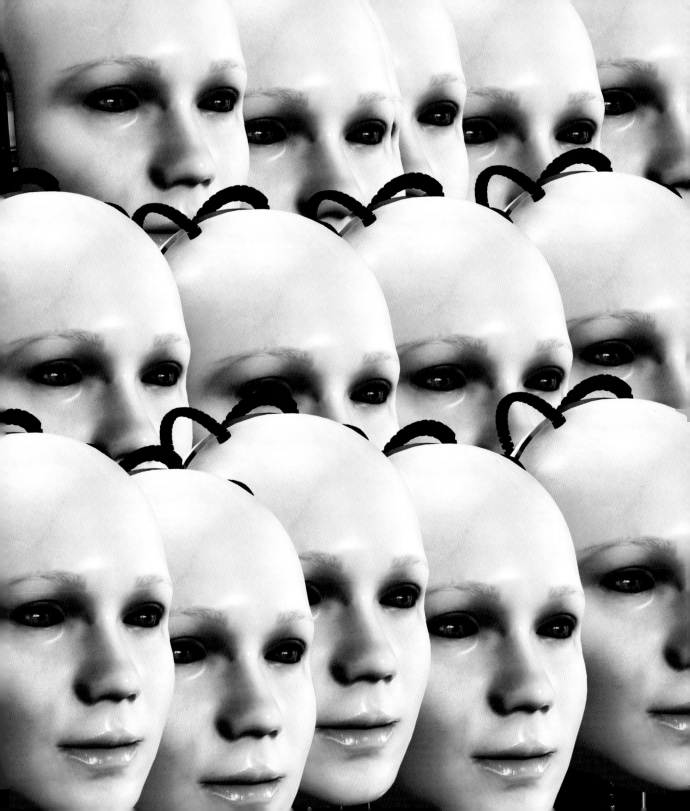

Cortisone

Edward Calvin Kendall (1886–1972), **Philip Showalter Hench** (1896–1965), **Tadeusz Reichstein** (1897–1996), **Lewis Hastings Sarett** (1917–1999)

In 1948, American physician Philip Hench and colleagues administered cortisone, a steroid hormone, to Mrs. Gardner, a wheelchair-bound 29-year-old who was crippled with rheumatoid arthritis and looked twice her age. This form of arthritis is a chronic inflammatory disease characterized by pain, swelling, and damage to the joints. Gardner had not been able to get out of bed without help for five years. However, after just three days of injections, she recovered and walked with a slight limp. A day later, she went on a three-hour shopping spree in downtown Rochester, New York. It was as if a medical miracle had just occurred!

Cortisone works its "miracles" by suppressing the immune system and reducing inflammation. The adrenal glands, which sit atop the kidneys, produce cortisone and cortisol (also known as hydrocortisone) from cholesterol. Enzymes in the body can convert hydrocortisone to cortisone, and vice versa. Hydrocortisone is the more active of the two substances, in that it has a greater effect on cells and tissues.

Cortisone treatments have many applications, such as decreasing inflammation, suppressing rejection of organs in transplants, and treating asthma. During his presidential campaign in 1960, President John F. Kennedy was given large doses of hydrocortisone to treat his Addison's disease, a condition in which the adrenal glands fail to make cortisone. In fact, the symptoms of various autoimmune diseases, in which the body attacks its own cells and tissues, can be reduced using cortisone-like drugs. Unfortunately, long-term use of cortisone or hydrocortisone can produce significant side effects, including high blood pressure.

Other key researchers involved in the discovery, isolation, testing, or chemical synthesis of cortisone include Polish-born Swiss chemist Tadeusz Reichstein and American chemists Lewis Sarett and Edward Kendall. In 1950, cortisone production processes were still very limited—one ton of cattle adrenal glands yielded only 25 grams (0.06 pound) of pure cortisone! Prednisone, which has a structure very similar to the naturally occurring cortisone molecule, is also used to treat inflammatory diseases.

SEE ALSO Discovery of Adrenaline (1893), Allergies (1906), Antihistamines (1937), Autoimmune Diseases (1956), and Statins (1973).

Cortisone molecule featuring five oxygen atoms (in red) and four ringlike structures.

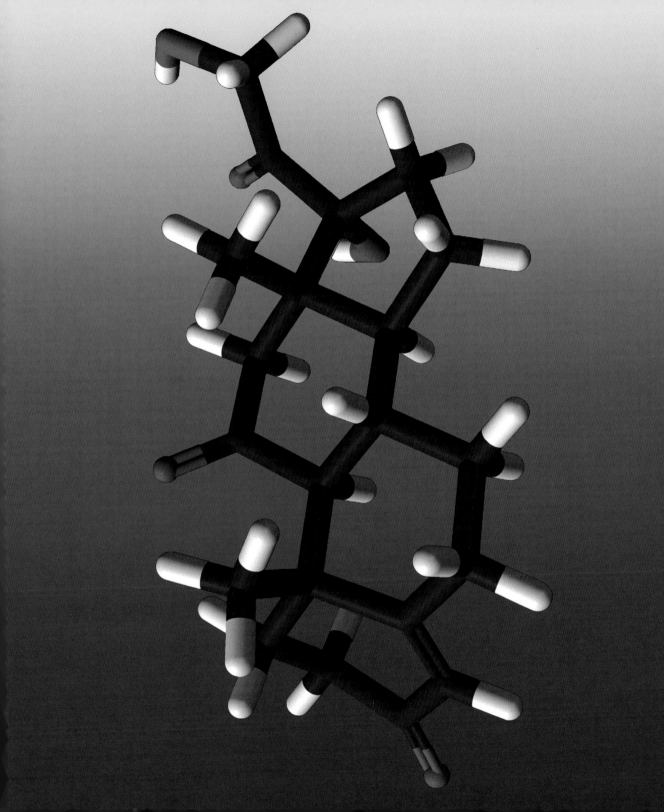

Nerve Growth Factor

Elmer Daniel Bueker (1903–1996), **Rita Levi-Montalcini** (b. 1909), **Stanley Cohen** (b. 1922)

Italian neurologist Rita Levi-Montalcini once said she was more artist than scientist, using intuition to help guide her thinking about the behavior of the nervous system and the nerve growth factor (NGF) she discovered. After Italian Fascist leader Benito Mussolini passed a law that deprived Jews of academic jobs, she had to perform some of her earliest research in her bedroom laboratory. Levi-Montalcini became the first Nobel Laureate to live beyond 100 years of age.

NGF is a small secreted protein that plays a role in the growth and survival of certain target neurons (nerve cells). In 1948, American scientist Elmer Bueker discovered that implantation of a mouse tumor in the body wall of a chick embryo caused a large outgrowth of nerve fibers from the chick's sensory ganglia (masses of nerve cell bodies). Levi-Montalcini and colleagues subsequently found that a mouse tumor was invaded by the chick embryo's sensory nerve fibers and sympathetic nerve fibers, which are part of the autonomic nervous system concerned especially with preparing the body to react to situations of stress. Sympathetic ganglia at a distance from the tumor also grew in size, suggesting that the tumor secreted NGF into the bloodstream of the chick embryo. American biochemist Stanley Cohen and Levi-Montalcini also found that if an antibody to the factor was injected into newborn rats, thus depriving the rat of NGF, the rat's sympathetic nervous system did not develop properly.

Interestingly, NGF levels are higher when people first fall in love. NGF also increases the survival times for mice after heart attacks and reduces movement disturbances in rats with Parkinson's disease. In 1983, Levi-Montalcini and colleagues determined that NGF could affect nerves in the brain and spinal cord. Cohen also discovered epidermal growth factor (EGF), which triggered early eyelid opening and tooth eruption in newborn animals. Today, we know of many factors that affect cell proliferation and that often promote differentiation into the various kinds of cells in the human body.

SEE ALSO Neuron Doctrine (1891), Alzheimer's Disease (1906), Neurotransmitters (1914), and Levodopa for Parkinson's Disease (1957).

Dorsal root ganglion (mass of nerve cell bodies) from a chicken embryo after incubation for several hours in NGF growth medium. Growing out of the ganglion are numerous axons, shaded pink in this colorized rendering.

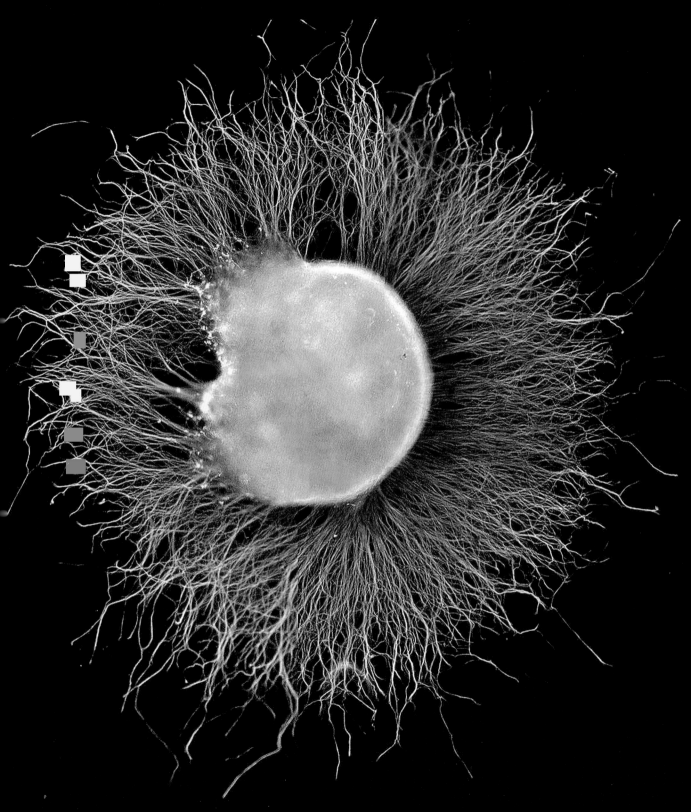

Randomized Controlled Trials

Austin Bradford Hill (1897–1991)

The design of tests for determining the efficacy of a medical treatment can be surprisingly difficult for many reasons. For example, physicians and test subjects may view results in a biased and nonobjective fashion. Treatment effects may be subtle, and patients may respond favorably simply due to the **placebo effect**, in which a patient thinks her condition is improving after taking a fake "treatment" (such as an inert sugar pill) that she *believes* should be effective.

Today, one of the most reliable approaches for testing possible medical treatments is the randomized controlled trial (RCT). The nature of a treatment should be chosen at random, so that each patient has the same chance of getting each of the treatments under study. For example, each participant in the trial may randomly be assigned to one of two groups, with one group scheduled to receive medicine X and the other scheduled to receive medicine Y. RCTs may be double-blind, which implies that neither the primary researchers nor the patients know which patients are in the treated group (receiving a new drug) or the control group (receiving a standard treatment). For reasons of ethics, RCTs are usually performed when the researchers and physicians are genuinely uncertain about the preferred treatment.

The most famous early clinical study involving RCT is English statistician Bradford Hill's "Streptomycin Treatment of Pulmonary Tuberculosis," published in 1948 in the *British Medical Journal.* In this study, patients randomly received a sealed envelope containing a card marked S for streptomycin (an antibiotic) and bed rest, or C for control (bed rest only). Streptomycin was clearly shown to be effective.

Clinical epidemiologist Murray Enkin writes that this trial is "rightly regarded as a landmark that ushered in a new era of medicine. [Hundreds of thousands] of such trials have become the underlying basis for what is currently called 'evidence-based medicine.' The [RCT] concept has rightly been hailed as a paradigm shift in our approach to clinical decision making."

SEE ALSO Avicenna's *Canon of Medicine* (1025), *A Treatise on Scurvy* (1753), Alternative Medicine (1796), Koch's Tuberculosis Lecture (1882), Informed Consent (1947), and Placebo Effect (1955).

Public health campaign poster, trying to halt the spread of tuberculosis. In 1948, Bradford Hill published a study using RCTs to demonstrate the effectiveness of streptomycin to treat tuberculosis.

PREVENT DISEASE

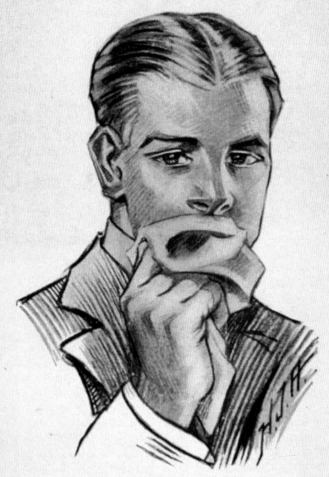

CARELESS
SPITTING, COUGHING, SNEEZING,
SPREAD INFLUENZA
and TUBERCULOSIS

✟ RENSSELAER COUNTY TUBERCULOSIS ASSOCIATION, TROY, N. Y. ✟

Cause of Sickle-Cell Anemia

James Bryan Herrick (1861–1954), **Ernest Edward Irons** (1877–1959), **Linus Carl Pauling** (1901–1994)

African tribal populations often created their own names for sickle-cell anemia (SCA), a painful blood disease that can kill afflicted children. In one West African tribe, such children might be referred to as *ogbanjes*, meaning "children who come and go." According to some legends, these children died in order to save their families from demons.

SCA is notable as being the first disease in which a specific protein abnormality was shown to be the definitive cause, and as the first genetic disorder whose molecular basis was fully elucidated. People with SCA have red blood cells with defective hemoglobin proteins that normally carry oxygen through the bloodstream to tissues. SCA occurs when a child inherits one defective hemoglobin gene from one parent and another defective gene from the other parent. A child who inherits one normal and one defective gene has sickle-cell trait (SCT), which is usually asymptomatic. SCT has provided an evolutionary advantage in malaria-stricken regions because people with SCT are resistant to **malaria** infection.

In SCA, the red blood cells (RBCs) can assume an inflexible sickle (crescent) shape that can obstruct capillaries and restrict blood flow. Symptoms include pain, increased blood pressure in the pulmonary artery, stroke, and kidney failure. Anemia (low numbers of RBCs) is caused by destruction of the sickle cells in the spleen. However, if a malaria parasite invades an RBC in a person with SCT, the RBC can rupture more quickly than in a normal individual, thus making it difficult for the parasite to reproduce.

In 1910, American physician James Herrick and his intern Ernest Irons reported on a patient's sickle-shaped blood cells. In 1949, American chemist Linus Pauling and colleagues showed that SCA resulted from a defective hemoglobin molecule. SCA can be treated with blood transfusions, bone-marrow transplants, and hydroxyurea, the last of which reactivates the production of normal and beneficial fetal hemoglobin.

SEE ALSO Blood Transfusion (1829), Mendel's Genetics (1865), Cause of Malaria (1897), Inborn Errors of Metabolism (1902), Liver Therapy (1926), Amniocentesis (1952), and Gene Therapy (1990).

Normal and sickle-shaped red blood cells.

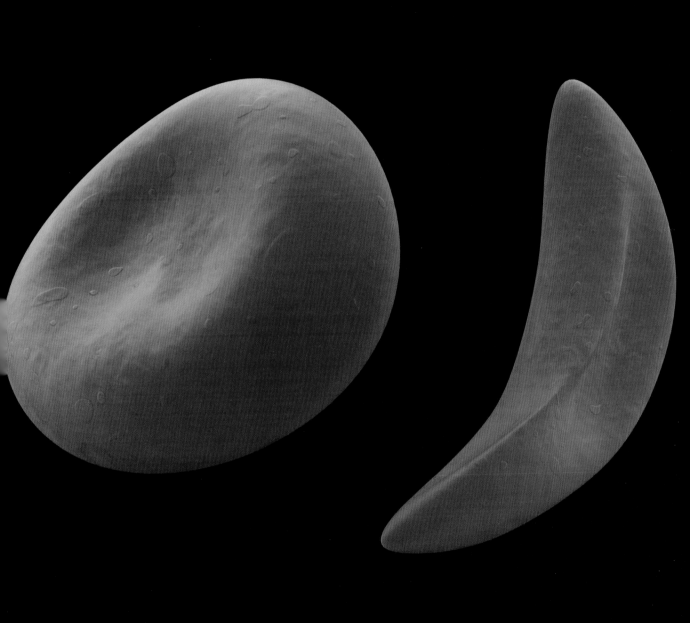

Mammography

Albert Salomon (1883–1976), **Raul Leborgne** (1907–1986), **Robert L. Egan** (1920–2001)

In 1913, German surgeon Albert Salomon became the first physician to describe the usefulness of **X-ray** studies of breast **cancers**. During his impressive career, he studied thousands of mastectomy specimens, comparing X-ray images with microscopic tissue samples, and he was the first person to observe, on X-ray images, microcalcifications associated with malignancy. Microcalcifications are tiny specks of calcium that may indicate the presence of small benign cysts or early breast cancer.

In 1949, Uruguayan physician Raul Leborgne emphasized the need for breast tissue to be compressed between plates of the mammography device to obtain clear pictures. Such compression reduces the thickness of tissue that X-rays must penetrate and reduces the dosage of X-rays needed. In 1960, American radiologist Robert Egan became well known for achieving clear and reproducible mammograms with appropriate voltages and films.

Today, full-field digital mammography (FFDM) makes use of digital electronic detectors instead of traditional film cassettes. The resultant digital information is easily enhanced, magnified, and stored. **Ultrasound**, **MRI**, and **PET** scans can be used as adjuncts to mammography. Mammography can miss some cancers, especially in younger women who have denser tissues than older women that may obscure cancerous tissues. Computer-aided diagnosis (CAD) employs computer software to search for possible cancers that a physician might miss.

If a possible cancer is detected during a mammography, a biopsy may be performed to allow a pathologist to view actual tissue from a particular site in the breast under study. Unfortunately, mammograms can sometimes suggest the presence of breast cancers that do not actually exist, leading to unnecessary biopsies.

Cancers can result when genetic mutations inhibit the ability of cells to stop dividing. A woman's risk of developing breast cancer increases with age. Also, women who inherit a defective BRCA1 or BRCA2 gene have increased risks for breast and ovarian cancers. Treatment for breast cancer includes surgery, chemotherapy, monoclonal antibodies, and **radiation**. Some breast cancers may be treated by blocking the effect of hormones like estrogen.

SEE ALSO Causes of Cancer (1761), Mendel's Genetics (1865), X-rays (1895), Radiation Therapy (1903), Pap Smear Test (1928), Cancer Chemotherapy (1946), Medical Ultrasound (1957), Positron Emission Tomography (PET) (1973), and Magnetic Resonance Imaging (MRI) (1977).

Mammography images of a normal (left) and cancerous breast (right).

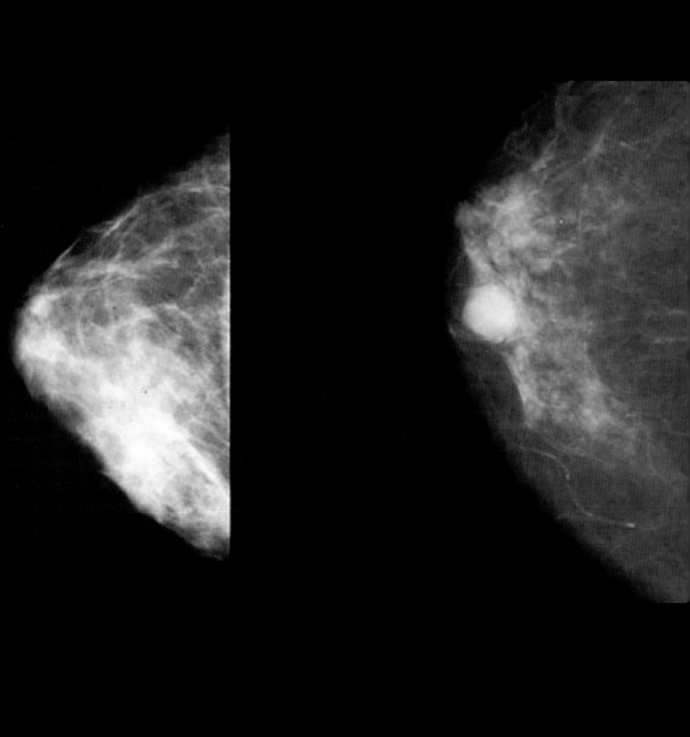

Antipsychotics

Jean Delay (1907–1987), **Henri Laborit** (1914–1995), **Pierre Deniker** (1917–1998)

According to British psychiatrist Trevor Turner, the antipsychotic drug chlorpromazine should be considered one of the greatest medical breakthroughs. He writes, "Without the discovery of chlorpromazine, we might still have the miserable confinements [in asylums in which] the attendant's role was akin to a zookeeper's. . . . It is hard not to see chlorpromazine as a kind of 'psychic penicillin,' enabling patient and carer to communicate."

Antipsychotic drugs are used to treat people with psychoses, abnormal thought processes that may include delusions or hallucinations exhibited in schizophrenia and extreme manic episodes in bipolar disorder. The first antipsychotic, chlorpromazine, was discovered nearly by accident. After it was synthesized in 1950 by French chemist Paul Charpentier, French surgeon Henri Laborit tested it as an **anesthetic** and found that it helped remove the anxiety of surgical patients. Laborit's work came to the attention of French psychiatrists Pierre Deniker and Jean Delay, who used the drug on some of their most agitated, uncontrollable patients. Many patients with delusions and hallucinations showed astonishing improvements. In 1954, chlorpromazine (brand name Thorazine) was approved for use in the United States, and by 1964 around 50 million people worldwide had taken the drug. The number of people confined to psychiatric asylums began to fall dramatically, and the older schizophrenia treatments, such as insulin shock therapy and **electroconvulsive therapy**, were used with less frequency. Unfortunately, some chlorpromazine users developed movement disorders such as muscle tremors. Clozapine, a newer antipsychotic, reduces the risk of movement disorders but may dangerously reduce the number of white blood cells. All antipsychotics tend to block receptors in the central nervous system for dopamine (a **neurotransmitter** that plays a role in motivation and voluntary movement).

Medical experts Joe and Teresa Graedon write, "Hundreds of years ago, people with mental illness might be burned at the stake. . . . In the early twentieth century, some patients with schizophrenia were lobotomized with an ice pick. . . . It was in this barbaric context that the first antipsychotic drugs were developed."

SEE ALSO Unchaining the Lunatics (1793), Psychoanalysis (1899), Alzheimer's Disease (1906), Neurotransmitters (1914), Truth Serum (1922), Antihistamines (1937), Electroconvulsive Therapy (1938), Transorbital Lobotomy (1946), and Cognitive Behavioral Therapy (1963).

Cat paintings by English artist Louis Wain (1860–1939). Some psychologists have suggested that Wain's schizophrenia influenced some of his wilder cat illustrations.

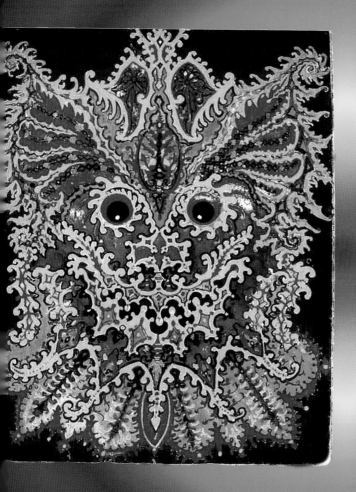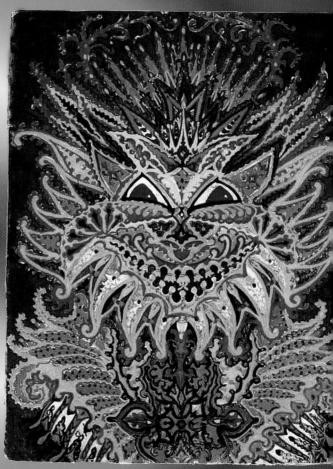

HeLa Cells

George Otto Gey (1899–1970), Henrietta Lacks (1920–1951)

Medical researchers use human cells grown in the laboratory to study cell functions and to develop treatments for diseases. Such cells can be frozen and shared among different researchers. However, most cell lines divide only a limited number of times and then die. A breakthrough occurred in 1951, when American biologist George Gey cultured cells removed from a cancerous tumor of the cervix and created the first immortal human cells. These HeLa cells, named after the unwitting donor, Henrietta Lacks, continue to multiply to this day. Gey freely gave the cells to any scientists who requested them, and more than 60,000 scientific articles and 11,000 patents have since been published relating to research performed on the cells.

Author Rebecca Skloot writes, "If you could pile all HeLa cells ever grown onto a scale, they'd weigh more than 50 million metric tons—as much as a hundred Empire State Buildings. HeLa cells were vital for developing the **polio vaccine**; uncovered secrets of **cancer**, viruses, and the effects of the atom bomb; helped lead to important advances like in vitro fertilization, **cloning**, and gene mapping; and have been bought and sold by the billions."

HeLa cells contain an active **telomerase** enzyme that continually repairs the ends of chromosomes that would normally become too damaged after multiple cell divisions to permit the cells to continue propagating. The genetic makeup of HeLa cells is far from ordinary, as they contain genes from human papillomavirus 18 and extra copies of several human chromosomes. Because the cells are so prolific and can even be spread on particles through the air, they have contaminated many other cell cultures in laboratories.

Lacks died at age 31 from the spread of her cancer, and her family did not learn of her "immortality" until decades later. The cells have since been launched into space to test the effects of low gravity and have been used in research topics ranging from AIDS to the testing of toxic substances.

SEE ALSO Causes of Cancer (1761), Sterilization of Carrie Buck (1927), Pap Smear Test (1928), Polio Vaccine (1955), Reverse Transcriptase and AIDS (1970), Oncogenes (1976), Telomerase (1984), and Human Cloning (2008).

Scanning electron micrograph of HeLa cells dividing.

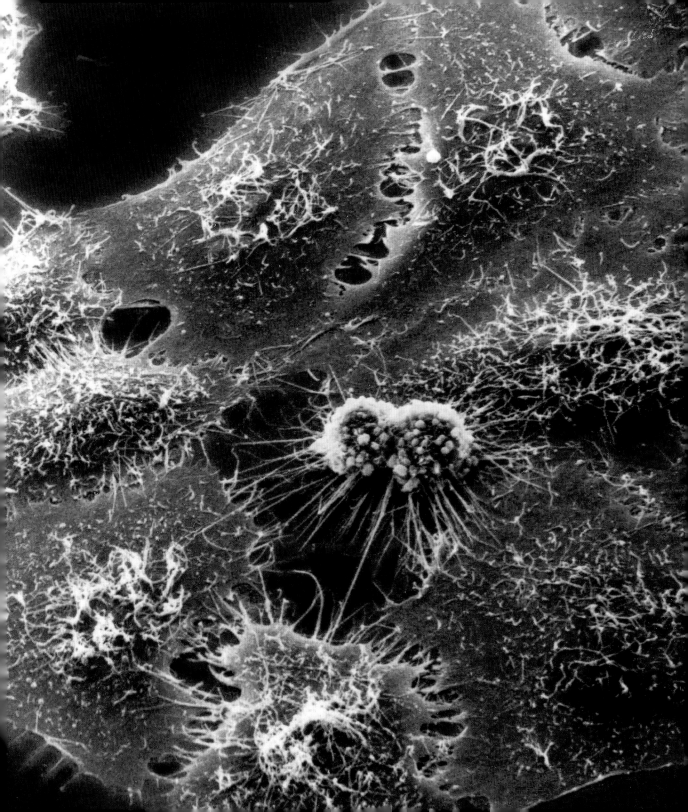

Tobacco Smoking and Cancer

Austin Bradford Hill (1897–1991), **William Richard Shaboe Doll** (1912–2005), **Iain Norman Macleod** (1913–1970)

In the early 1500s, tobacco came to Europe from its native soils in the New World, and it was actually touted as a healthful treatment for various ailments, ranging from gonorrhea to gunshot wounds. By the late 1500s, tobacco was a popular recreational drug. Today, some Native American nations grow tobacco for ceremonial use since its smoke is believed to carry prayers to the heavens.

One of the important early studies finding a strong relationship between cigarette smoking and lung **cancer** was conducted by British physiologist Richard Doll and British statistician Bradford Hill. Published in 1951, their study relied on interviews with around 700 patients from 20 London **hospitals**. They found that "heavy smokers were 50 times as likely as nonsmokers to contract lung cancer." Doll found the correlation to be so frightening that he gave up his own smoking habit midway through the study. Their subsequent study focused on more than 30,000 physicians and confirmed the relationship. In 1954, Iain Macleod, Health Minister for the United Kingdom, spoke at a news conference announcing, "It must be regarded as established there is a relationship between smoking and cancer of the lung." Macleod chain-smoked throughout his speech.

Today, tobacco is the single largest cause of preventable deaths. Tobacco use increases the risk of various cancers (e.g., lung, kidney, larynx, neck, breast, bladder, esophagus, pancreas, and stomach cancer), as well as heart attacks, strokes, chronic obstructive pulmonary disease (e.g., difficulty breathing caused by emphysema and chronic bronchitis), miscarriages, premature births, atherosclerosis, and high blood pressure. In the twentieth century alone, tobacco use resulted in the deaths of approximately 100 million people.

Tobacco smoke contains several cancer-causing substances that bind to **DNA** (a cell's genetic material) and that cause mutations (changes in the genetic sequence). Mutations may inhibit programmed cell death and make cells cancerous. Tobacco also contains nicotine, an addictive substance that, when smoked, increases the release of dopamine (a **neurotransmitter**) in the nucleus accumbens, a part of the brain that plays a role in pleasure, addiction, and various emotions.

SEE ALSO Causes of Cancer (1761), *The Sanitary Condition of the Labouring Population of Great Britain* (1842), Spirometry (1846), Neurotransmitters (1914), Stanley's Crystal Invaders (1935), and DNA Structure (1953).

In 1881, James Bonsack (1859–1924) patented the cigarette rolling machine, shown in this patent diagram, to speed the production of cigarettes. This complex and revolutionary machine could produce 120,000 cigarettes in ten hours.

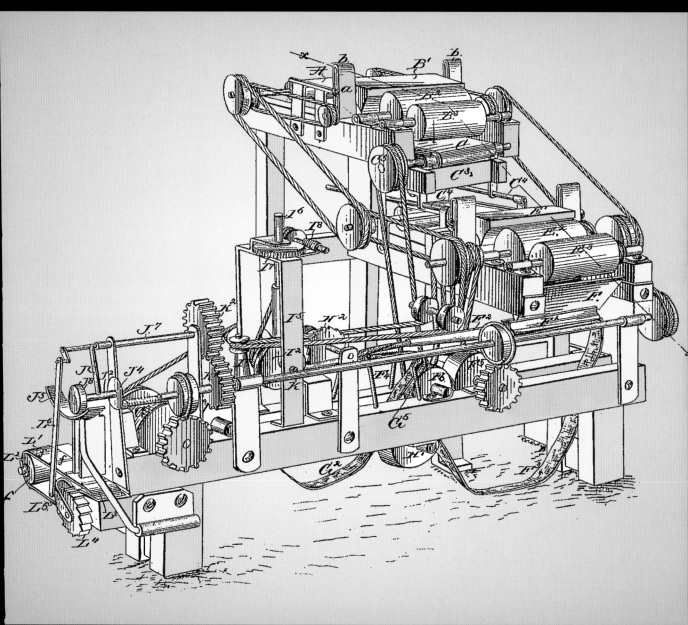

Amniocentesis

Douglas Charles Aitchison Bevis (1919–1994)

According to author Frank N. Magill, "For thousands of years, the inability to see or touch a fetus in the uterus was a staggering problem in obstetric care and in the diagnosis of the future mental and physical health of human offspring. A beginning to the solution of this problem occurred on February 23, 1952, when *The Lancet* published a study called 'The Antenatal Prediction of a Hemolytic Disease of the Newborn.'" In this research, British obstetrician Douglas Bevis described the use of amniocentesis to determine the possibility of the fetus having a potentially fatal blood disorder due to a blood factor incompatibility between the fetus and mother.

Amniocentesis refers to a medical test, usually performed between the fourteenth and twentieth weeks of pregnancy, in which a small amount of amniotic fluid is removed from the sac surrounding the developing fetus. Amniotic fluid contains fetal proteins and skin cells that are shed during fetal growth. The fetal chromosomes and **DNA** are examined for genetic abnormalities such as Down syndrome, which is caused by the presence of all or part of an extra twenty-first chromosome. During amniocentesis, **ultrasound** is used to help the physician guide a long needle through the mother's abdominal wall, uterus, and amniotic sac to collect fluid. Possible neural tube defects (including spina bifida, caused by incomplete closure of the embryonic neural tube) can be assessed by measuring the level of alpha-fetoprotein.

Amniocentesis may be performed on women who have significant risks of genetic diseases, such as those with a family history of certain birth defects or who are over 34 years of age. Amniocentesis can also be used to test for **sickle-cell anemia**, cystic fibrosis, muscular dystrophy, and Tay-Sachs disease, or to determine if a baby's lungs are sufficiently mature for birth. Another fetal diagnostic method, chorionic villus sampling, involves removal of a small piece of the placenta, a temporary organ joining the mother and fetus.

SEE ALSO Abortion (70), Chromosomal Theory of Inheritance (1902), Inborn Errors of Metabolism (1902), Cause of Sickle-Cell Anemia (1949), Mammography (1949), DNA Structure (1953), Fetal Monitoring (1957), Medical Ultrasound (1957), and Fetal Surgery (1981).

Human fetus surrounded by amniotic sac.

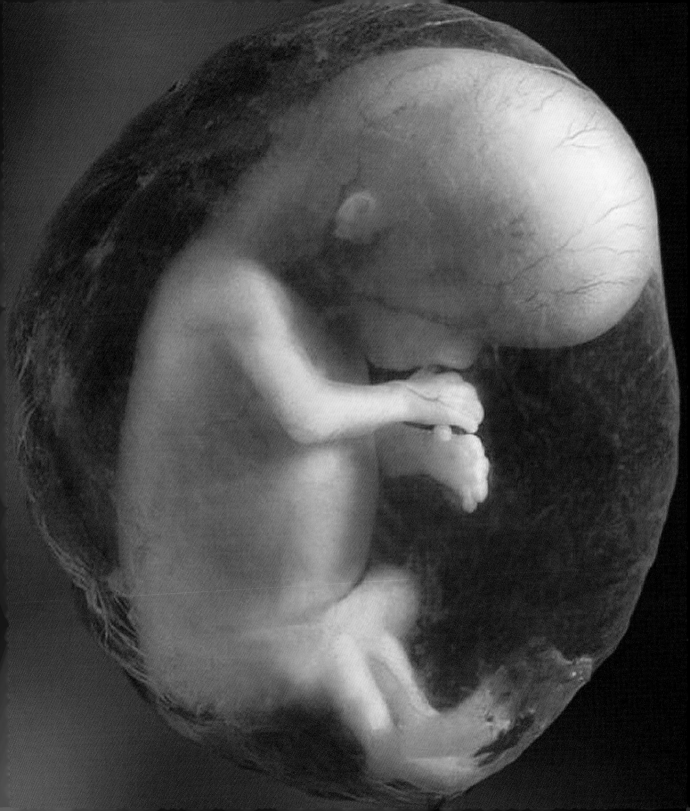

Artificial Heart Valves

Miles Lowell Edwards (1898–1982), Charles A. Hufnagel (1916–1989), Albert Starr (b. 1926)

The human heart has four one-way valves that control the movement of blood through the heart. When functioning properly, all valves ensure that the blood flows in one direction and they prevent backflow. The mitral valve and the tricuspid valve open and close between the atria and ventricles, while the aortic valve and the pulmonary valve reside in arteries leaving the heart. The valve flaps open and close in response to the pressures on each side.

When valves do not function properly—for example, when the mitral valve becomes thickened as a complication of rheumatic fever—the valves may need to be replaced by artificial ones. Stenosis refers to a narrowing in the valve orifice that impedes the forward flow of blood, and regurgitation refers to backflow through the valve. Modern mechanical valves can last a patient's normal lifetime, but they require the use of anticoagulants (blood thinners) to reduce blood clotting resulting from damage to red blood cells and platelets. Less durable heart valves made of tissue, such as those from a pig or from a cow's pericardial sac, cause less damage and do not require anticoagulants, but they may require replacement.

The first artificial heart valve employed a silicone ball in a metal cage. As the ball moved back and forth due to pressure changes, it served as a one-way valve. In 1952, American surgeon Charles Hufnagel implanted a caged-ball valve in a patient with a damaged aortic valve. American surgeon Albert Starr and engineer Lowell Edwards invented a similar valve, which was implanted in 1960. Later valves replaced the moving ball with either a tilting disc or semicircular leaflets, and the use of pyrolytic carbon reduces the formation of blood clots. When animal tissues are used to form biological valves, biological markers are removed so as to reduce tissue rejection.

SEE ALSO Circulatory System (1628), Morgagni's "Cries of Suffering Organs" (1761), Digitalis (1785), Blalock-Taussig Shunt (1944), Heart-Lung Machine (1953), Heart Transplant (1967), and Fetal Surgery (1981).

Starr-Edwards mitral valve with moving ball.

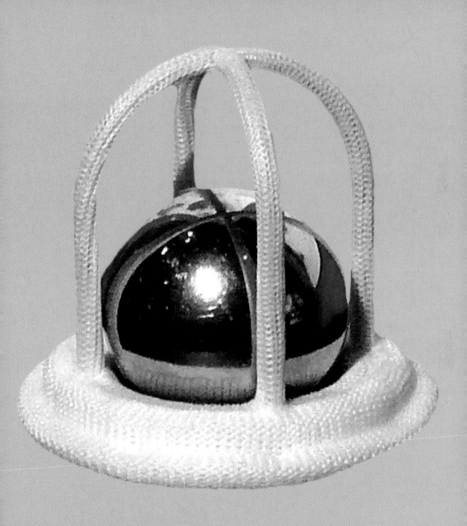

DNA Structure

Maurice Hugh Frederick Wilkins (1916–2004), **Francis Harry Compton Crick** (1916–2004), **Rosalind Elsie Franklin** (1920–1958), **James Dewey Watson** (b. 1928)

The British journalist Matt Ridley writes, "The double helix [structure of DNA] has been a shockingly fecund source of new understanding—about our bodies and minds, our past and future, our crimes and illnesses." The DNA (deoxyribonucleic acid) molecule may be thought of as a "blueprint" that contains hereditary information. It also controls protein production and the complex development of cells starting from a fertilized egg. Just as an error in an architectural blueprint for a building might lead to home collapses or leaks, errors in the DNA, such as changes in the sequence caused by mutagens, might lead to disease. Thus, an understanding of the messages in the DNA can lead to cures for disease, including the development of new drugs.

At a molecular level, DNA resembles a twisted ladder in which the different rungs of the ladder (referred to as bases) represent a code for protein production. DNA is organized into structures called chromosomes, and the **human genome** has approximately three billion DNA base pairs in the 23 chromosomes of each **sperm** cell or egg. Generally speaking, a gene is a sequence of DNA that contains a "chunk" of information that, for example, specifies a particular protein.

In 1953, molecular biologists James Watson and Francis Crick discovered the double helical structure of DNA using molecular-modeling methods, along with **X-ray** and other data from scientists such as Maurice Wilkins and Rosalind Franklin. Today, with recombinant DNA technology, genetically modified organisms can be created by inserting new DNA sequences that force the organism to create desirable products, such as **insulin** to be used by humans. Forensic detectives can study DNA left at crime scenes to help identify potential criminals.

In December 1961, the *New York Times* reported on breakthroughs in understanding of the genetic code in DNA by explaining that "the science of biology has reached a new frontier," leading to "a revolution far greater in its potential significance than the atomic or hydrogen bomb."

SEE ALSO Mendel's Genetics (1865), Chromosomal Theory of Inheritance (1902), Inborn Errors of Metabolism (1902), Genes and Sex Determination (1905), Commercialization of Insulin (1922), Epigenetics (1983), Polymerase Chain Reaction (1983), Telomerase (1984), RNA Interference (1998), and Human Genome Project (2003).

Molecular model of a portion of a DNA strand.

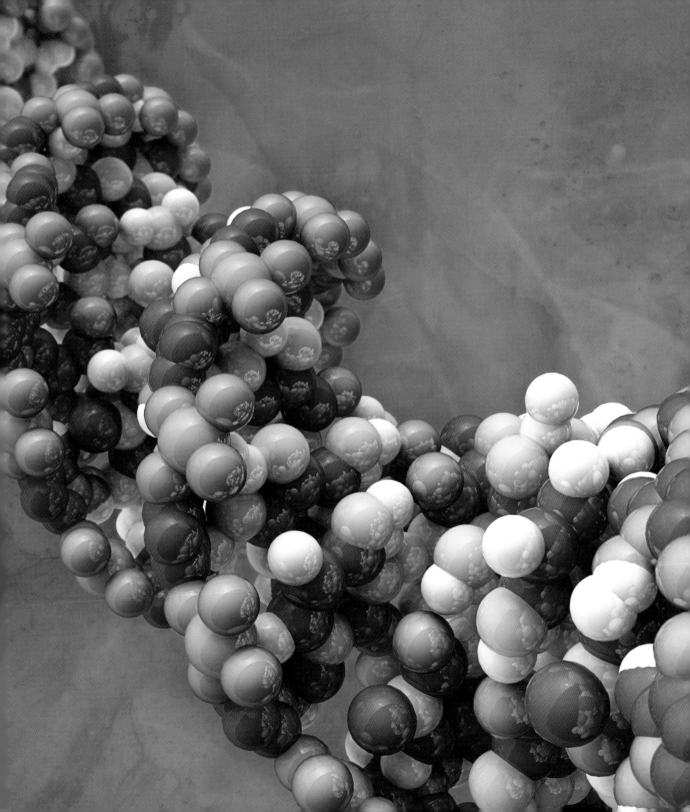

Heart-Lung Machine

John Heysham Gibbon Jr. (1903–1973)

The heart-lung machine (HLM) is a device that circulates blood and ensures adequate blood oxygen content during operations, such as those that involve repairing heart valves or holes in the heart's inner walls. Referred to as cardiopulmonary bypass, the process bypasses the heart and lungs and, along with chemicals that temporarily stop the heart, allows the surgeon to operate in a relatively bloodless and motionless environment. **Heparin** is used to reduce clotting in the circulating blood, and the blood may be cooled to slow the body's metabolism, thereby decreasing the need for oxygen.

In 1953, American surgeon John Gibbon became the first to successfully use an HLM when he repaired a hole in the inner heart wall of an 18-year-old woman. During the repair, her heart and lungs were stopped for 27 minutes.

Innovative approaches were required to reduce potential damage to the red blood cells caused by an artificial pump. For example, scientists experimented with roller pumps that gently propel the blood through tubing or centrifugal pumps that spin the blood in order to create a pumping action. More difficult than replacing the beating of the heart was the need to temporarily replace the lung's oxygenation function. Various historical solutions have been used, including the bubbling of oxygen (followed by filtration of the bubbles) and the use of membranes. In a natural lung, the complicated surfaces where oxygen and carbon dioxide are exchanged have about the same surface areas as one side of a tennis court! Gibbon's initial design, developed with IBM, involved a revolving drum that incorporated a metal grid to create turbulence for oxygenation.

Some patients report loss of intellectual ability after HLM, but this decline may also occur in patients with similar risk factors for cardiovascular disease and, thus, may not actually result from the HLM. According to author Autumn Stanley, the HLM is "one of the most important apparatus inventions in recent medical history, making possible all open-heart surgery, and lengthier surgical procedures in general, to say nothing of heart and heart-lung transplants."

SEE ALSO Al-Nafis's Pulmonary Circulation (1242), Circulatory System (1628), Heparin (1916), Iron Lung (1928), Dialysis (1943), Blalock-Taussig Shunt (1944), Cardiopulmonary Resuscitation (1956), Lung Transplant (1963), and Heart Transplant (1967).

Life-size reconstruction of heart surgery in a 1980s-era operating theater; a heart-lung machine is in the foreground. This realistic model is on exhibit in the Lower Wellcome Gallery of London's Science Museum. (Photo by Nina Recko.)

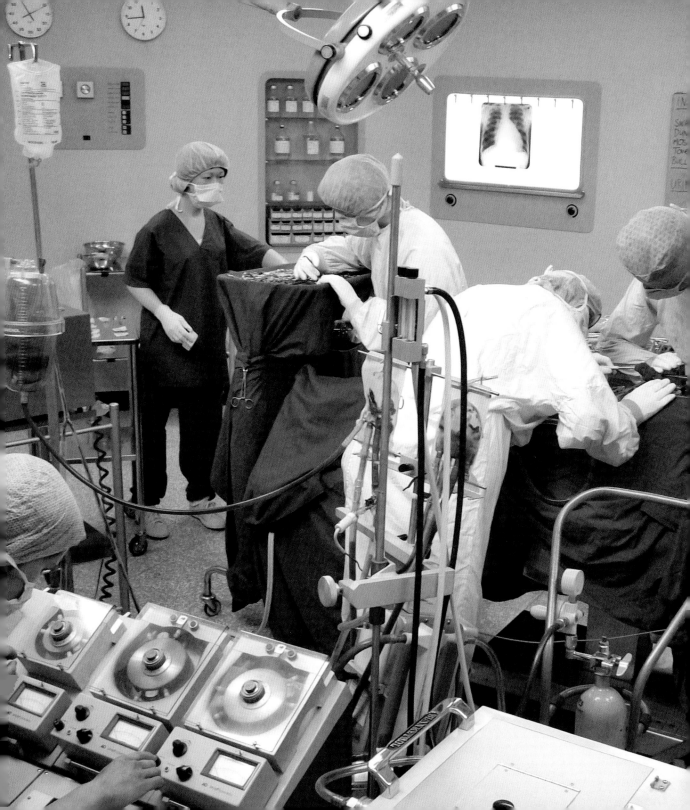

Endoscope

Philipp Bozzini (1773–1809), **Harold Horace Hopkins** (1918–1994), **Basil Isaac Hirschowitz** (b. 1925)

The endoscope is a tubelike device used by physicians to peer within the body. Endoscopes can illuminate the tissue under study with a light in an optical-fiber system and transmit the image back to the observer. Another tube channel may allow the physician to insert medical instruments such as cutting tools to take tissue samples or cauterizing (heating) tools to stop bleeding.

Numerous specialized endoscopes exist today, including colonoscopes (for examining the large intestine), bronchoscopes (for the lower respiratory tract), and cystoscopes (for the urinary tract). Sometimes, endoscopes are inserted into the body through small incisions during the process of **laparoscopy** or arthroscopy, the latter of which is used to explore joints.

Around 1806, German physician Philipp Bozzini developed a tube, mirror, and candle system that directed light into "the canals and cavities" of the body (such as the mouth and rectum) and redirected the light back to the eye. The Vienna Medical Society promptly scolded him for his "undue curiosity." In 1954, British physicist Harold Hopkins designed fiber-optic endoscopes using an array of flexible glass fibers to transmit light. South African physician Basil Hirschowitz and collaborator Larry Curtiss improved the illumination and image quality of this scope. Hirschowitz recalled, "I looked at this rather thick, forbidding but flexible rod, took the instrument and courage in both hands and swallowed it over the protest of my unanesthetized pharynx [throat]." A few days later, he snaked the instrument into his first patient with a duodenal ulcer. Physician James Le Fanu writes, "Hopkins' fiber-optic instrument changed the practice of medicine . . . [enabling] the doctor to travel much further and deeper than ever before into previously uncharted territory."

Today, videoscopes utilize tiny digital cameras (with a charge-coupled device, or CCD) at the tip of the scope and display images of tissues on a TV screen. Optical fibers transmit light for illuminating tissues, but the images are transmitted electronically. Capsule endoscopy wirelessly transmits images from a swallowed capsule. Endoscope ultrasonography makes use of **ultrasound** to visualize tissue structures.

SEE ALSO Medical Ultrasound (1957), Angioplasty (1964), Fetal Surgery (1981), Laparoscopic Surgery (1981), Robotic Surgery (2000), and Telesurgery (2001).

A typical flexible endoscope has control mechanisms for suctioning, moving the endoscope tip, introducing air or water, and more.

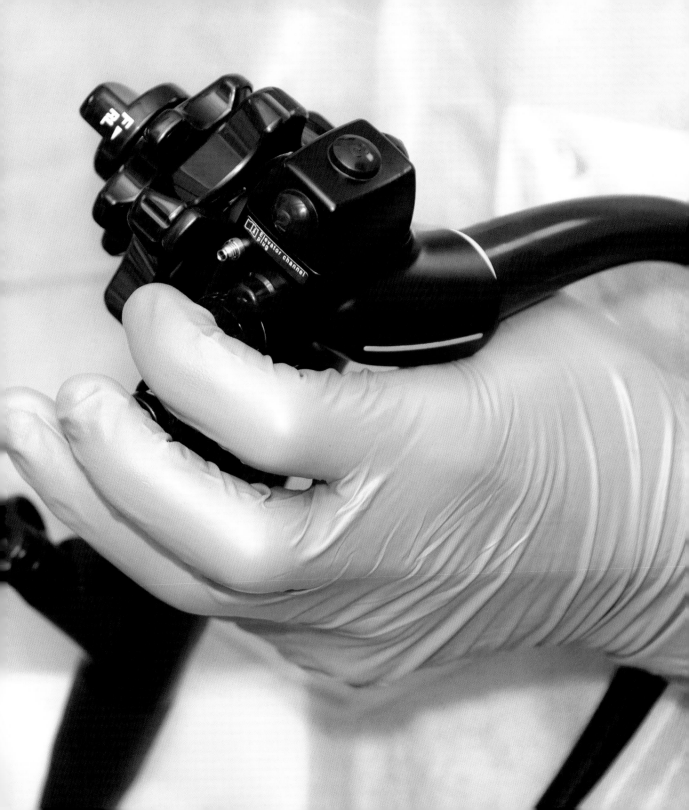

Kidney Transplant

Alexis Carrel (1873–1944), Peter Brian Medawar (1915–1987), Joseph Edward Murray (b. 1919)

Centuries ago, our kidneys were treated with special awe. According to the Talmud of the Jews, "Man has two kidneys, one of which prompts him to good, the other to evil" (Berakhoth 61a). In the Bible, animal kidneys are reserved for burnt offerings to God (Leviticus 3:4).

In 1954, American surgeon Joseph Murray and colleagues performed the first truly successful kidney transplant between donor and recipient men who were twins. Prior to the surgery, Murray was told that kidney transplants "were impossible" and that he was "playing God and shouldn't do it." In 1990, Murray won the Nobel Prize for his transplant achievements.

The groundbreaking organ transplants in the 1950s relied upon prior work of as French surgeon Alexis Carrel, who pioneered **vascular suturing**, and British surgeon Peter Medawar's research on the immune-system rejection of skin grafts. Success of organ transplants between unrelated individuals did not become safe until immunosuppressant drugs became available so that the recipient's immune system did not reject the tissue of the foreign organ. For example, azathioprine and **cyclosporine** were two immunosuppressive compounds discovered in 1962 and 1972, respectively.

Kidneys may fail for many reasons, including high blood pressure and diabetes. **Dialysis** can be used to replace kidney function, but patients tend to live longer with a transplanted kidney. When transplants are performed, the original, weaker kidneys are often left in place. The new kidney is transplanted in a lower abdominal position and attached to the iliac artery and vein, and the donor's ureter is connected to the bladder.

Kidneys are involved in the removal of waste, which flows as urine to the bladder, as well as in the regulation of the concentration of blood electrolytes. Additionally, kidneys release the hormones erythropoietin (which stimulates the bone marrow to make red blood cells), renin (which regulates blood pressure), and calcitriol (the active form of vitamin D, which helps maintain calcium levels).

SEE ALSO Tissue Grafting (1597), Vascular Suturing (1902), Corneal Transplant (1905), Dialysis (1943), Bone Marrow Transplant (1956), Liver Transplant (1963), Lung Transplant (1963), Hand Transplant (1964), Pancreas Transplant (1966), Heart Transplant (1967), Cyclosporine (1972), Small Bowel Transplant (1987), Face Transplant (2005), and Growing New Organs (2006).

During transplants, the original, weaker kidneys are often left in place, and the new kidney is transplanted in a lower position. The donor's ureter (yellow in this diagram) is then connected to the bladder.

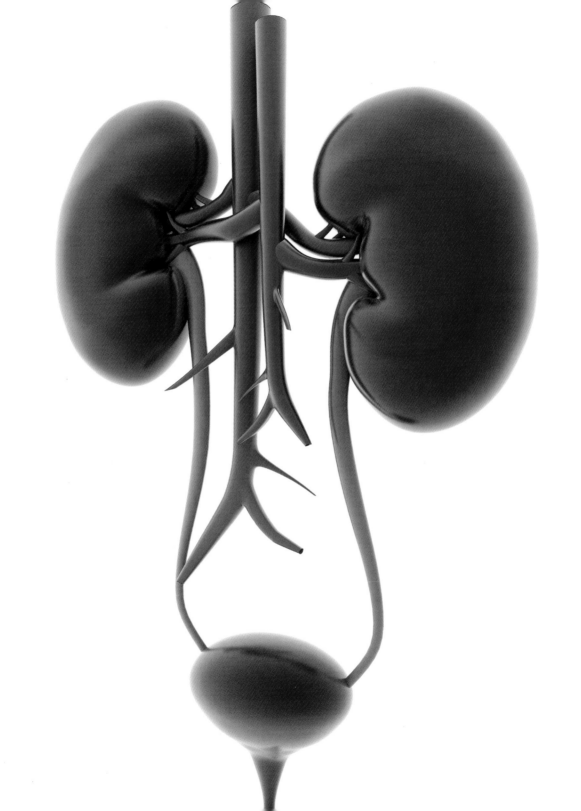

Birth-Control Pill

Margaret Higgins Sanger Slee (1879–1966), **Pope Paul VI** (**Giovanni Montini**; 1897–1978), **Gregory Pincus** (1903–1967), **Frank Benjamin Colton** (1923–2003), **Carl Djerassi** (b. 1923)

Oral contraceptives, or birth-control pills, were among the most socially significant medical advances of the twentieth century. Supplied with an easy and effective means to prevent pregnancies, more women graduated from college and entered the work force. In the 1930s, researchers had determined that high concentrations of the hormone progesterone, which is normally present during pregnancy, also tricks a nonpregnant body into behaving as if it were pregnant and thus prevent the monthly release of an egg. In the early 1950s, American chemists Carl Djerassi and Frank Colton, working independently, discovered ways to manufacture chemical compounds that mimicked natural progesterone. American biologist Gregory Pincus confirmed that shots of progesterone prevent egg release from the ovary of mammals.

Margaret Sanger, a famous advocate for birth control, helped Pincus obtain the necessary funding to develop a hormonal birth-control pill for humans. Pincus selected Colton's formula, and in 1955 he and colleagues announced clinical-trial results demonstrating the efficacy of the pill. In addition to inhibiting ovulation, contraception is enhanced by changes in the cervical mucus that inhibit **sperm** entrance to the uterus, and by changes in the lining of the uterus that inhibit egg implantation. U.S. regulators approved the pill for contraception in 1960, and the Searle drug company named it Enovid.

The original formulation, which also contained the hormone estrogen, had some undesirable side effects; however, modern formulations contain much reduced doses of hormones and have been shown to decrease ovarian, endometrial, and colon **cancers**. Generally speaking, women smokers who take the pill have an increased risk of heart attacks or strokes. Today, different hormonal formulations are available (including pills only with progestin, a type of progesterone) that supply hormone doses that are constant or that change from one week to the next.

In 1968, Pope Paul VI condemned artificial birth control, including the pill. Although adoption of the pill was rapid in the United States, distribution of contraceptives to unmarried women was not legal in Connecticut until 1972!

SEE ALSO Abortion (70), Condom (1564), Discovery of Sperm (1678), Salpingectomy (1883), Sterilization of Carrie Buck (1927), "The Rabbit Died" (1928), IUD (1929), and Amniocentesis (1952).

A psychedelic portrait of a "post-pill paradise" in a new era for women. In the 1960s, many women achieved greater personal control over contraception, which contributed to the sexual revolution.

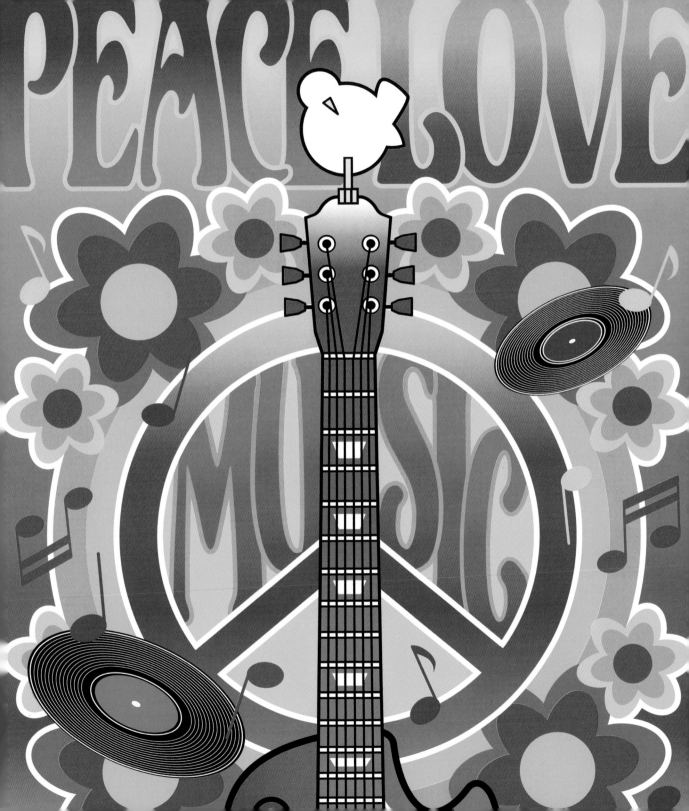

Placebo Effect

Henry Knowles Beecher (1904–1976)

Medical experts Arthur and Elaine Shapiro write, "The panorama of treatment since antiquity provides ample support for the conviction that, until recently, the history of medical treatment is essentially the history of the placebo effect. . . . For example, the first three editions of the *London Pharmacopoeia* published in the seventeenth century included such useless drugs as usnea (moss from the skull of victims of violent death) and Vigo's plaster ([including] viper's flesh, live frogs, and worms)."

Today, the term *placebo* often refers to a fake "drug" (such as a sugar pill) or a sham surgery (such as cutting the skin but going no deeper to treat a condition) that nevertheless produces a perceived or actual improvement in those patients who believe the medical intervention will turn out to be effective. The placebo effect suggests the importance of patient expectations and the role of the brain in physical health, particularly for subjective outcomes such as levels of pain.

In 1955, American physician Henry Beecher documented the famous case of

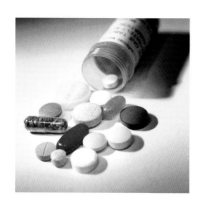

soldiers in World War II who experienced significant pain relief when given injections of saline solutions when the morphine supplies were not available. One mechanism of the placebo effect appears to involve endogenous opioids—natural painkillers produced by the brain—as well as the activity of the **neurotransmitter** dopamine.

In one study, mice given a compound that suppresses the immune system along with a sweet-tasting chemical became conditioned over time, so that immune suppression occurred when given only the sweetener. Thus, conditioning may play a role in human placebos. A placebo administered to people as a stimulant can increase blood pressure, and alcohol placebos can cause intoxication. Color and size of pills often make a significant difference in perceived effectiveness. The placebo effect also tends to work to varying degrees depending on the society and country tested. A nocebo response refers to a negative response to a placebo, such as the feeling of pain when the patient believes that the inert drug may have unpleasant side effects.

SEE ALSO Witch Doctor (10,000 B.C.), Mithridatium and Theriac (100 B.C.), Acupuncture *Compendium* (1601), Patent Medicines (1906), Informed Consent (1947), and Randomized Controlled Trials (1948).

Because a person's expectations influence the placebo effect, the pill color, size, and shape all affect the placebo response. Red pills work better as stimulants, while "cool"-colored pills work better as depressants. Capsules are often perceived to be particularly effective.

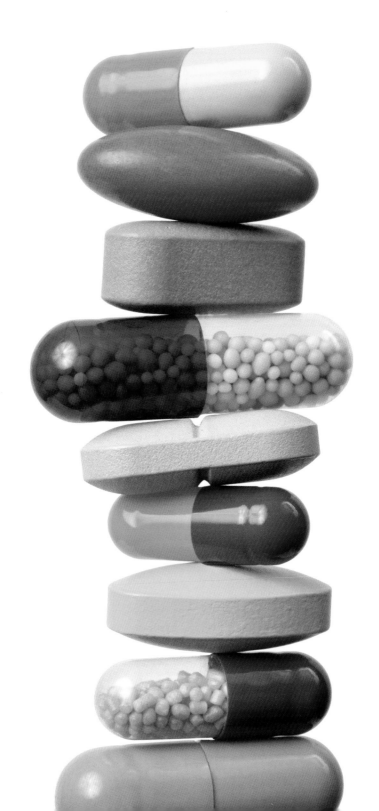

Polio Vaccine

Albert Bruce Sabin (1906–1993), Jonas E. Salk (1914–1995)

Polio is a viral disease that can cause crippling muscle paralysis. In 1952, nearly 58,000 cases were reported in the United States, with 3,145 deaths and 21,269 suffering from mild to disabling paralysis. At this time, Americans ranked only the atomic bomb above polio in terms of their worst nightmares. According to physician Paul Offit, on April 12, 1955, when the existence of an injectable vaccine was finally announced on radio and TV, "church bells were ringing across the country, factories were observing moments of silence, synagogues and churches were holding prayer meetings, and parents and teachers were weeping."

Polio has afflicted humanity since prehistoric times, as suggested by ancient Egyptian carvings and paintings depicting children with withered limbs and walking with canes. Three different varieties of the polio virus can cause paralysis by colonizing the gastrointestinal tract from contaminated food or water and then spreading to the central nervous system. Depending on the nerves infected, the virus can cause paralysis of just the legs or virtually the entire body, preventing a person from breathing without the aid of a machine (see entry "**Iron Lung**").

Two types of vaccines are used today to combat the virus. One is based on the inactivated virus developed in 1952 by American medical researcher Jonas Salk, who cultured polio in monkey kidney tissue cells and chemically inactivated it with formalin. When inactivated forms of the three viral varieties are injected, the body develops antibodies to combat the three live forms later on. Subsequent to the Salk vaccine, American medical researcher Albert Sabin developed an *oral* polio vaccine (OPV) based on "weakened" forms of the three polio viruses that replicate in the gut but not the nervous system, producing a similar kind of immunity. Today, because the weakened virus in the OPV can, on very rare occasions, actually revert to the paralyzing viral form, many industrial nations make use of the injectable vaccine. A widespread vaccination effort has now made polio very rare in the Western world.

SEE ALSO Smallpox Vaccination (1798), Discovery of Viruses (1892), Iron Lung (1928), Stanley's Crystal Invaders (1935), HeLa Cells (1951), and Structure of Antibodies (1959).

Molecular model of polio virus (top) binding to CD155, a polio virus receptor protein (bottom, colored purple) that spans cellular membranes.

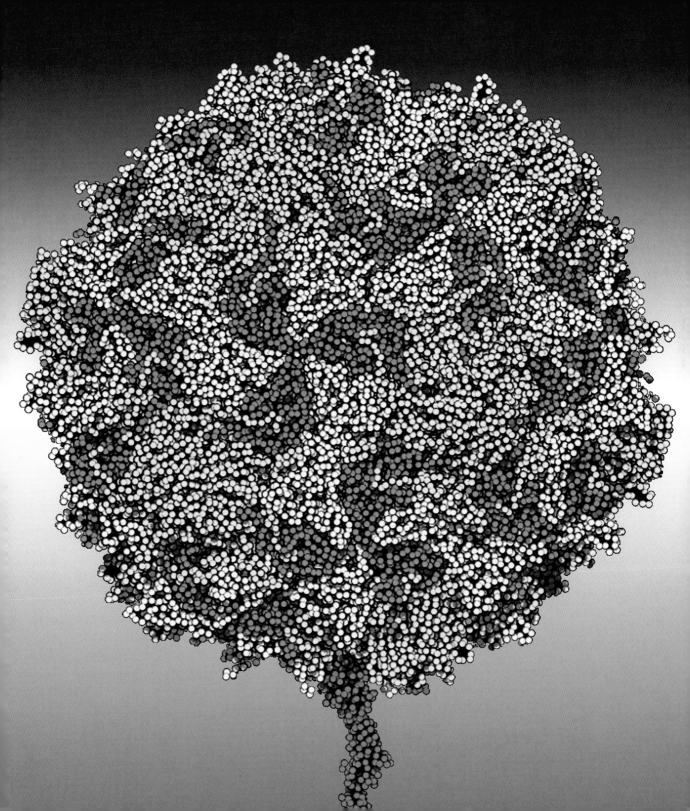

Autoimmune Diseases

Hashimoto Hakaru (1881–1934), **Ernest Witebsky** (1901–1969), **Deborah Doniach** (1912–2004), **Peter Campbell** (1921–2005), **Ivan Maurice Roitt** (b. 1927), **Noel Richard Rose** (b. 1927)

Autoimmune diseases occur when the immune system attacks and destroys healthy body cells and tissues, as if the body does not properly recognize itself. In 1956, Hashimoto's thyroiditis was the first glandular disease demonstrated to be an autoimmune disease. At this time, British researchers Ivan Roitt, Deborah Doniach, and Peter Campbell discovered circulating autoantibodies to thyroglobulin (a protein within the thyroid gland) in patients with thyroiditis (inflammation of the thyroid gland).

Almost simultaneously, Noel Rose and Ernest Witebsky, researchers working in the United States, were able to induce thyroiditis in rabbits by mixing a portion of a rabbit's thyroid with bacteria and reinjecting this material into the rabbit's foot. After observing the rabbits' inflamed thyroids and antibodies to the thyroglobulin, Rose looked at the results "with a mixture of awe and fear" because he realized that it might be difficult to convince other researchers of this startling find. For many years, autoimmune diseases were thought not to exist, even though, as far back as 1904, Julius Donath and Karl Landsteiner showed that paroxysmal cold hemoglobinuria (a disease in which red blood cells are destroyed) had an autoimmune component.

Autoimmune diseases often exhibit a genetic predisposition and are among the leading causes of illness in the United States, with about 75 percent of autoimmune cases involving women. The hundreds of autoimmune diseases and autoimmune-related diseases include rheumatoid arthritis (inflammation and erosion of joints), systemic lupus erythematosus (which causes inflammation and can damage many organ systems), and multiple sclerosis (which damages the sheath around nerve fibers). Treatments for these kinds of diseases include such medicines as corticosteroids (hormones to control inflammation) and other immunosuppressants. In some cases, human autoimmune diseases may be triggered by an infection that stimulates the immune system in such a way that the body begins to attack some of its own tissues.

SEE ALSO Tissue Grafting (1597), Thyroid Surgery (1872), Phagocytosis Theory (1882), Allergies (1906), Liver Therapy (1926), Cortisone (1948), Structure of Antibodies (1959), Cyclosporine (1972), and Gene Therapy (1990).

X-ray of the hand of a patient with rheumatoid arthritis, which often leads to the destruction of joint cartilage and crookedness of the joints.

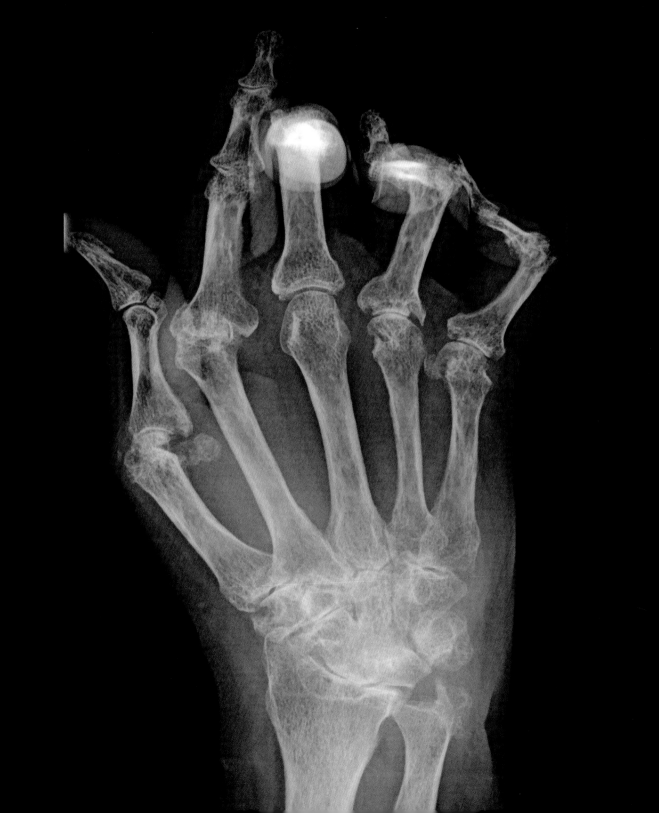

Bone Marrow Transplant

Edward Donnall Thomas (b. 1920)

Various kinds of blood cells develop from "immature cells" called hematopoietic (blood-forming) stem cells (HSCs). Most HSCs reside in the bone marrow, a spongy tissue within bones, but some are also found in the peripheral blood that circulates throughout the body.

A stem cell is a cell that can renew itself through cell division and generate other kinds of specialized cells. Totipotent stem cells (such as fertilized egg cells) can divide and produce all the differentiated cells in an organism. Pluripotent stem cells can give rise to any fetal or adult cell type, but they cannot develop into a fetus or adult because they cannot create extra-embryonic tissue, such as the placenta. Multipotent stem cells (such as HSCs) generally give rise to a limited number of cell types. For example, HSCs can form white blood cells (the cells that fight infection), red blood cells (the cells that carry oxygen), and platelets (the cells that cause clotting for wound healing). Various organs, such as the liver, have dormant stem cells that can be activated when tissue damage occurs and new cells are needed.

A patient with leukemia, a **cancer** of the blood or bone marrow, generally produces an excessive number of abnormal white blood cells. During bone marrow transplants (also called stem cell transplants), physicians often "reset" the bone marrow by first destroying the abnormal marrow with chemotherapy or **radiation** and then injecting healthy donor HSCs into the recipient blood vessels. The injected cells then find their way to the patient's bone marrow. Sometimes, healthy stem cells from the patient can be used, but if healthy stem cells are taken from a separate donor, care must be taken to find a good antigenic match to reduce graft-versus-host disease, in which the donor cells attack the recipient tissues. In 1956, American physician Donnall Thomas carried out the first successful bone marrow transplant, giving a leukemia patient healthy bone marrow from an identical twin. The donated marrow generated healthy blood cells and immune cells, resulting in disease remission.

SEE ALSO Tissue Grafting (1597), Lymphatic System (1652), Radiation Therapy (1903), Corneal Transplant (1905), Kidney Transplant (1954), Thymus (1961), Liver Transplant (1963), Lung Transplant (1963), Hand Transplant (1964), Pancreas Transplant (1966), Heart Transplant (1967), Cyclosporine (1972), Small Bowel Transplant (1987), Face Transplant (2005), and Human Cloning (2008).

Microscopic examination of stained bone marrow cells. Band neutrophils are indicated by the blue-green dots. A large promyelocyte is indicated by the yellow dot. Metamyelocytes are indicated by the orange dots.

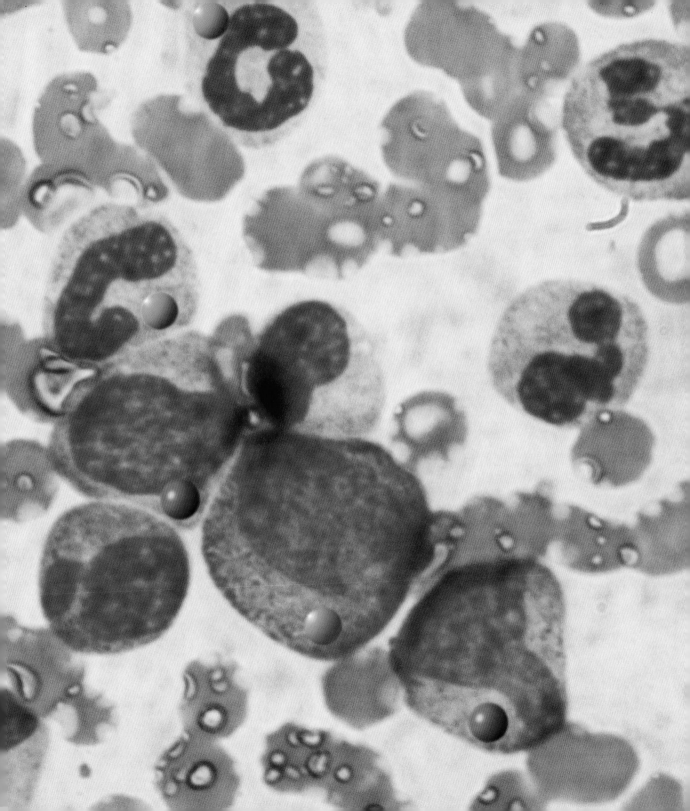

Cardiopulmonary Resuscitation

James Otis Elam (1918–1995), Peter Safar (1924–2003)

Cardiopulmonary resuscitation (CPR) refers to an emergency technique to maintain the life of a person who is usually in cardiac arrest and exhibiting little or no breathing. This technique is often used until additional medical help can arrive at the scene. CPR may involve chest compressions (repeatedly pushing down on the chest to encourage blood circulation), mouth-to-mouth (MM) breathing, or use of a device to push air into the lungs. CPR may also employ the use of electric shocks to encourage a normal heartbeat. Today, a greater emphasis is placed on chest compressions than on artificial breathing in many emergency circumstances, particularly for untrained people.

In 1956, Austrian physician Peter Safar began human experiments to determine if MM resuscitation provides sufficient oxygen to keep the victim alive. In particular, he administered curare (a poison) to 31 volunteers to paralyze their breathing muscles. By monitoring levels of blood oxygen and carbon dioxide for several hours while inflating the lungs with exhaled air, he was able to demonstrate that the exhaled air had sufficient oxygen to validate the practice of MM resuscitation. Based on his research and the research of physicians such as James Elam, Safar encouraged a Norwegian doll maker to manufacture Resusci Anne, a mannequin for CPR training. In his 1957 book *ABC of Resuscitation*, Safar also suggested a combined approach in which a rescuer checked the airway of a victim, facilitated breathing, and performed chest compressions. The book provided a basis for worldwide training of CPR.

The Bible mentions the prophet Elisha putting his mouth upon a child and resuscitating him (2 Kings 4:34). In 1767, the Dutch Humane Society published guidelines suggesting that rescuers keep drowning victims warm, provide MM ventilation, and blow the "smoke of burning tobacco into the rectum." Other methods evolved that were occasionally useful, including lying the victim face down over a barrel and rolling him back and forth. Alternatively, the victim was placed face down on a trotting horse.

SEE ALSO Circulatory System (1628), Ambulance (1792), Defibrillator (1899), Artificial Pacemaker for Heart (1958), and Do Not Resuscitate (1991).

An illustration from U.S. Patent 5,580,255, issued in 1996, describing a mannequin for use when practicing the breathing portion of CPR. The device has an inflatable simulated human chest that rises and falls.

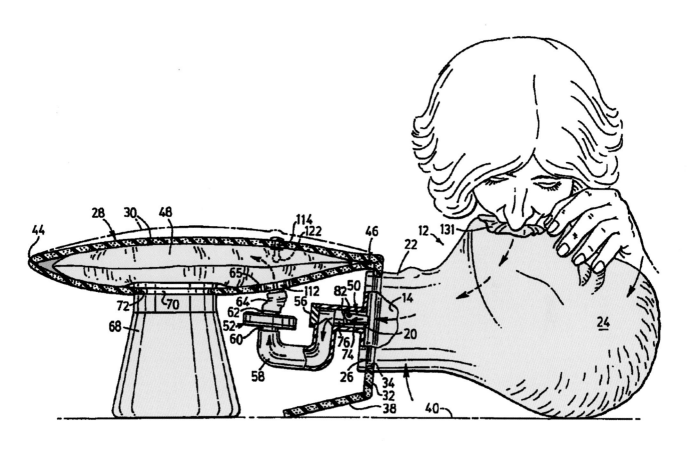

Levodopa for Parkinson's Disease

James Parkinson (1755–1824), **Walther Birkmayer** (1910–1996), **Arvid Carlsson** (b. 1923), **Oleh Hornykiewicz** (b. 1926), **Oliver Wolf Sacks** (b. 1933)

In 1961, Austrian researchers Oleh Hornykiewicz and Walther Birkmayer reported on a seemingly miraculous treatment for Parkinson's, a disease of the central nervous system that impairs movement control and other brain functions. "Bedridden patients who were unable to sit up, patients who could not stand up from a sitting position, and patients who, when standing, could not start walking, performed all these activities after L-dopa [injection] with ease. . . . They could even run and jump. The voiceless speech . . . became forceful and clear."

People afflicted with Parkinson's disease (PD) experience muscle tremors, rigidity, and a slowing down of movement. PD is caused by an insufficient production of the **neurotransmitter** dopamine, normally produced by certain **neurons** in the midbrain. The English apothecary James Parkinson provided a detailed description of PD in an 1817 essay on "shaking palsy." In 1957, Swedish scientist Arvid Carlsson found dopamine in a brain region that is important for the control of movement. He also showed how it was possible to reduce the level of dopamine in animals to cause PD symptoms and reverse the symptoms when giving levodopa (a psychoactive drug, also called L-dopa) to the animals.

Levodopa is able to traverse the blood-brain barrier and enter the brain, where it is transformed into dopamine by certain neurons. Because levodopa produces side effects such as nausea and jerky motions when metabolized outside the brain, other drugs can be given to suppress such metabolism. Deep-brain stimulation with electrical impulses may be used as treatment when drug therapy is no longer effective, and researchers continue to study stem cell transplants in brains as a possible treatment. The neurologist Oliver Sacks used levodopa to treat patients with encephalitis lethargica who had not moved or spoken for years.

PD is also associated with the abnormal accumulation of the alpha-synuclein protein in the brain in the form of Lewy bodies (protein aggregates), which can lead to brain-cell death. A number of genetic mutations are known to cause PD.

SEE ALSO Neuron Doctrine (1891), Alzheimer's Disease (1906), Neurotransmitters (1914), Bone Marrow Transplant (1956), Mitochondrial Diseases (1962), Gene Therapy (1990), and Human Cloning (2008).

A famous illustration of a patient afflicted with Parkinson's disease, from British neurologist William Richard Gowers's A Manual of Diseases of the Nervous System *(1886).*

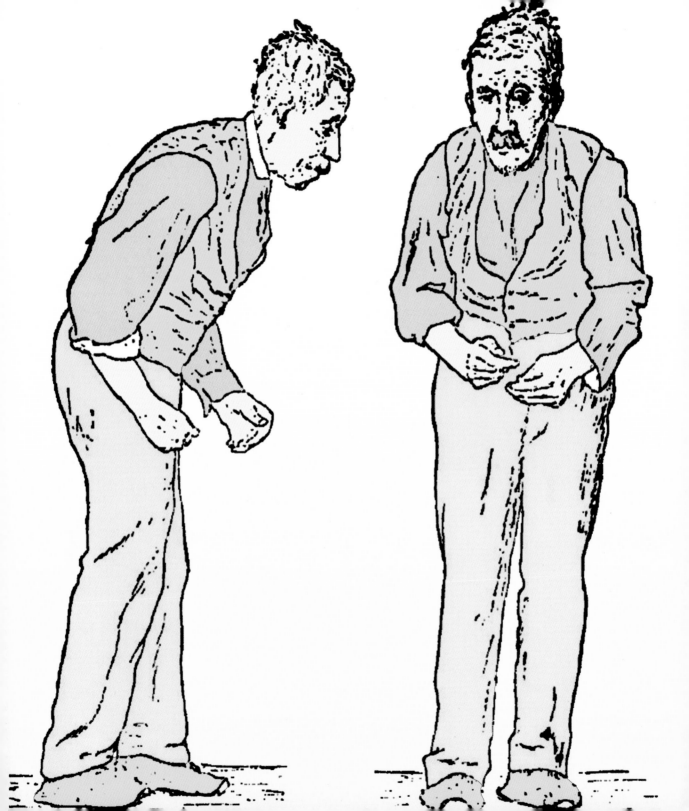

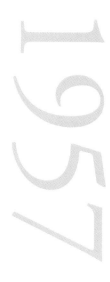

Fetal Monitoring

Orvan Walter Hess (1906–2002), Edward Hon (1917–2001)

The process of birth is among the most stressful situations a human being can endure—yet newborns are wonderfully adapted for surviving this great challenge. Nevertheless, problems can arise that require health professionals to pay careful attention to signs of fetal stress. Before the invention of electronic fetal monitoring, physicians had difficulty in determining a fetus's health, other than by listening to the fetal heart with a special **stethoscope** on the mother's abdomen. However, during the mother's uterine contractions, when fetal stress can arise, the fetal heart may be impossible to hear.

In 1957, American physician Orvan Hess and colleague Edward Hon invented a fetal heart monitor—a machine 6.5 feet (2 meters) in height that could *continuously* monitor electrical cardiac signals from a fetus. Today, cardiotocography (CTG) refers to the simultaneous recording of the fetal heartbeat and uterine contractions during pregnancy. External measurements make use of an **ultrasound** sensor to detect motions of the fetal heart. A pressure-sensitive device simultaneously measures tension on the abdomen, an indirect indicator of pressure within the uterus.

Internal measurements involve inserting an electrode through the mother's cervix and (usually) attaching it to the fetal head to obtain detailed electrical measurements of fetal heart activity. Additionally, a uterine pressure sensor can be inserted into the cavity of the uterus.

With CTG, frequency, duration, and intensity of uterine contractions are continuously monitored. Normal fetal heartbeats are between 110 and 160 beats per minute. Fetal well-being depends on receiving adequate oxygen and waste removal though the umbilical cord and placenta. If the mother smokes cigarettes or has abnormal placenta placement, asthma, diabetes, pneumonia, abnormal blood pressure, or anemia, then fetal needs may be compromised. Fetal monitoring can be used to predict impending fetal hypoxia (low oxygen) so that physicians can prevent injury to the newborn by taking steps to improve uterine-placental blood circulation, for example.

Physicians continue to debate under what circumstances sophisticated fetal monitoring provides the most value, and false indications of fetal distress may result in unnecessary **cesarean sections** and medical costs.

SEE ALSO Stethoscope (1816), Cesarean Section (1882), Amniocentesis (1952), Medical Ultrasound (1957), and Fetal Surgery (1981).

CTG may allow women with high-risk pregnancies to continue pregnancies to greater maturity, and it can also be used to diagnose umbilical cord compression.

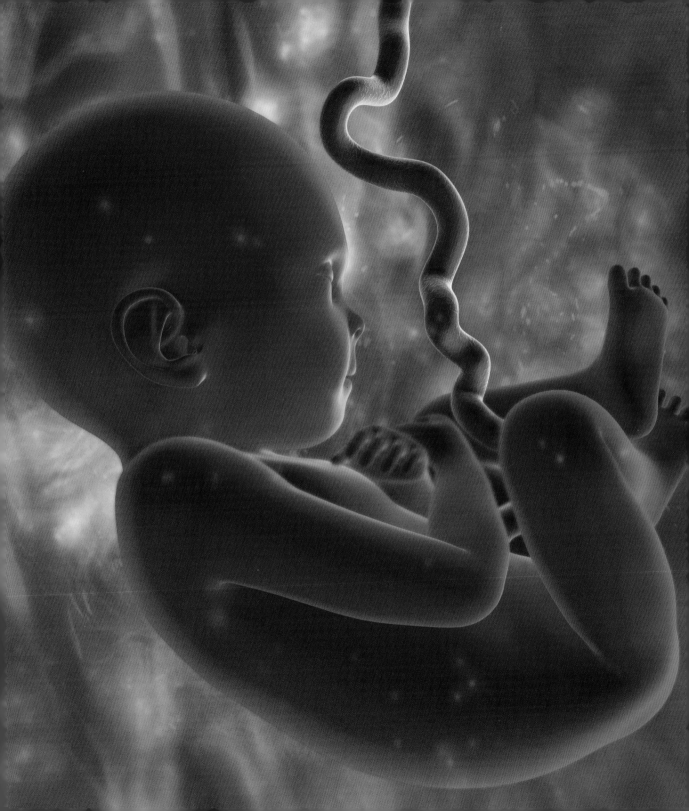

Medical Ultrasound

Paul Langevin (1872–1946), Ian Donald (1910–1987)

The physician Ashok Khurana writes, "Ultrasound is today an integral part of the obstetrician's armamentarium—almost an extension of the examining finger. However, that was never the expectation when it was developed by Professor [Paul] Langevin for the French and British Admiralties during the First World War to combat the growing menace of submarines."

Ultrasound refers to sound waves with frequencies that are so high that humans cannot hear the sounds. Using appropriate signal-producing and detection equipment, trained personnel may use the reflection of such sounds from hidden objects in order to obtain information. For example, an ultrasound probe may transmit pulses of high-pitched sound, with some vibrations reflecting from organs, like an echo from a canyon wall. Scottish physician Ian Donald speculated that the fetus in the womb might be scanned just as warships scanned for enemy submarines in the sea or determined the shape of the seabed. In 1957, he used ultrasound to examine a woman suspected of having a tumor that was too advanced for surgery. He determined she had an ovarian cyst that was easy to remove, and probably saved the woman's life. In 1959, Donald was the first to observe that the head of a fetus produced a clear ultrasound reading, and physicians began to realize the value of ultrasound for determining if a fetus is developing normally, as well as how many fetuses are in the womb. Fetal age, heart defects, and positioning for delivery can also be determined by ultrasound, which is regarded as a safe alternative to **X-rays**.

Ultrasound scanners became commercially available in the mid-1960s, and in the mid-1970s, computer technology became important in producing images. Today ultrasound can also be used to visualize muscles, tendons, organs, and tumors and to create three-dimensional representations. Ultrasound can also be used to produce echocardiograms of the heart structure. Doppler ultrasound is used for studying blood flow in blood vessels. Strong pulses of ultrasound can be used to shatter gallstones and kidney stones during the process of lithotripsy.

SEE ALSO X-rays (1895), Mammography (1949), Amniocentesis (1952), Endoscope (1954), Fetal Monitoring (1957), Thalidomide Disaster (1962), CAT Scans (1967), and Fetal Surgery (1981).

Three-dimensional ultrasound can be used to provide vivid images of the fetus in the womb.

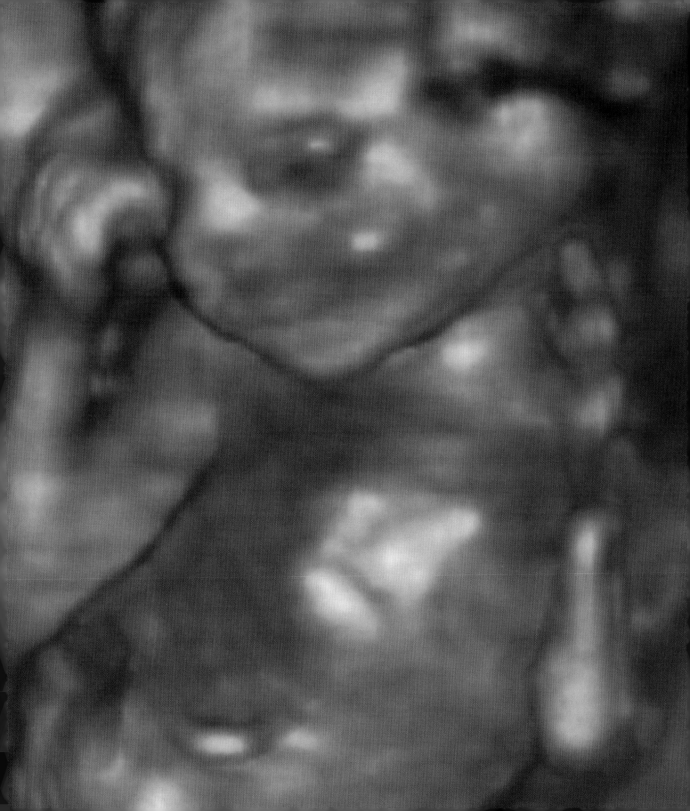

Artificial Pacemaker for Heart

Rune Elmqvist (1906–1996), **Paul Maurice Zoll** (1911–1999), **Wilson Greatbatch** (1919–2011)

The artificial pacemaker for the heart is a device that uses electrical pulses to facilitate the normal beating of the heart. The healthy heart has its own electrical system to control heart rhythms: with each heartbeat, an electric signal spreads from the top of the heart to the bottom, causing the heart to contract and pump blood. The electrical signal begins in a group of cells called the sinoatrial node, located in the right atrium (upper chamber) of the heart. Defects in this electrical signaling system can lead to arrhythmias, in which the heart beats too fast (tachycardia), too slow (bradycardia), or in an irregular fashion.

Numerous individuals have contributed to the artificial pacemaker's evolution from a large and unwieldy machine to a small, modern device implanted in the body and powered by small, long-lasting batteries. For example, in 1952 American cardiologist Paul Zoll built an external pacemaker that applied painful electrical impulses to the chest surfaces. Around 1958, inventors like American Wilson Greatbatch and Swede Rune Elmqvist developed implantable pacemakers that used transistors. Once physicians began to sew electrodes into the heart walls, lower-voltage and battery-powered units became possible. In the mid-1960s, electrode systems could be passed to the heart via blood vessels and then positioned in a heart chamber. In the 1970s, lithium batteries and the use of low-power circuits led to units that could have lifetimes of many years.

Today, pacemakers can provide pulses only when they sense that a pulse is needed to establish proper beating. In a dual-chamber pacemaker, one pacing lead (wire) controls the atrium and another controls the ventricle (lower chamber). In dynamic pacemakers, the pulse-frequency pace can automatically change in response to body needs (e.g., if the pacemaker detects significant body motion, or changes in body temperature or dissolved oxygen levels). Pacemakers may also monitor and store information related to the heart action, which can be accessed by physicians during an examination.

SEE ALSO Digitalis (1785), Defibrillator (1899), Electrocardiograph (1903), and Beta-Blockers (1964).

X-ray image of installed pacemaker, showing some of the wire routing.

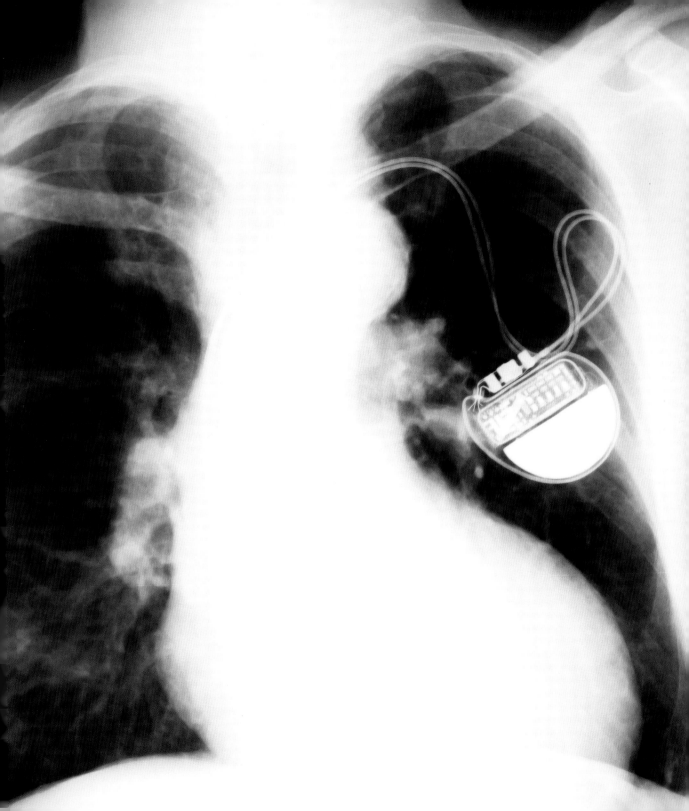

Hip Replacement

Sir John Charnley (1911–1982)

According to medical historian Francis Neary, "The total hip replacement operation has been seen as a landmark in twentieth-century surgery, and is now one of the most performed elective surgical procedures in the world. Since the early 1960s it has played an important role in alleviating pain and restoring mobility to millions of arthritis sufferers. . . . Its development was associated with innovation in materials, instruments and operative procedures—many of which have since been adapted to treat other joints and applied across a range of surgical specialties."

A total hip replacement (or total hip arthroplasty) involves removal of the acetabulum, which refers to the cup-shaped hip socket of the pelvis. In addition, the head of the thigh bone (femur) is also removed. Both are replaced by artificial materials to create a new ball-and-socket joint. In 1958, British orthopedic surgeon John Charnley helped to create a modern artificial hip joint by using a stainless-steel femoral stem with ball-shaped head and a Teflon acetabular cup, both of which were affixed to the bone using acrylic bone cement. In 1962, he replaced the Teflon with more durable polyethylene plastic. Interestingly, Charnley asked his patients if he could have their hips and surrounding tissues after they died to see how well the joint had endured. Most patients were happy to comply.

Today, cement is not always used, because porous coatings on the artificial parts can be employed to form a tight "friction fit" that becomes tighter as bone grows onto or into the porous coatings. Around the normal hip joint, strong ligaments hold the head of the femur within the acetabulum. Computer-assisted orthopedic surgery is currently undergoing increasing refinement to help some surgeons better navigate the surgical process.

Before the development of hip replacement surgery, little could be done for those who fractured their hips, and many people over the age of 60 died as a result of various complications of such fractures.

SEE ALSO Plaster of Paris Casts (1851), Artificial Heart Valves (1952), Bone Marrow Transplant (1956), and Cochlear Implants (1977).

X-ray image of a total hip replacement, involving removal of the natural acetabulum (cup-shaped hip socket of the pelvis) and head of the femur (thigh bone). Both are replaced by artificial materials to create a new ball-and-socket joint.

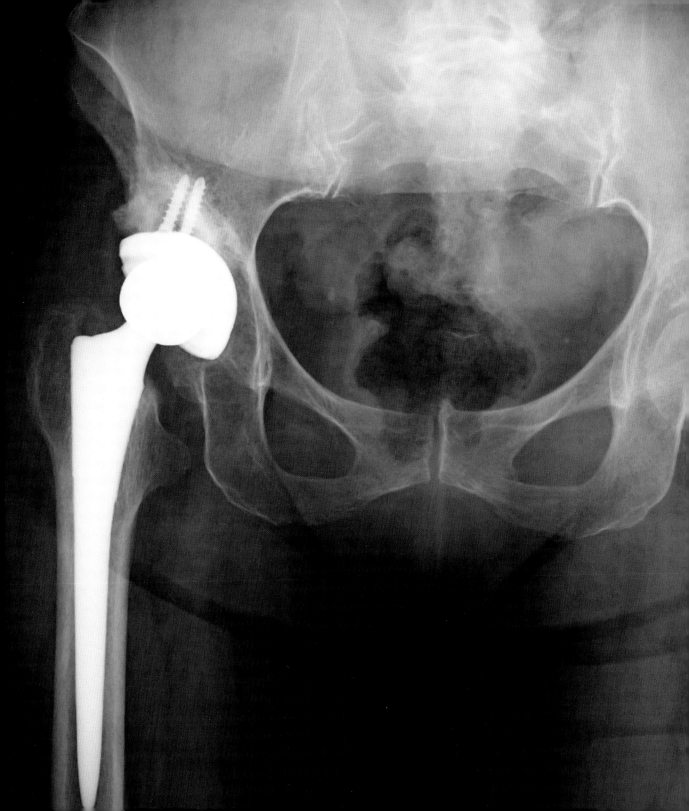

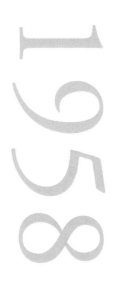

Pineal Body

René Descartes (1596–1650), **Johann Otto Leonhard Heubner** (1843–1926), **Nils Frithiof Holmgren** (1877–1954), **Aaron Bunsen Lerner** (1920–2007), **Rick Strassman** (b. 1952)

For centuries, the function of the pineal body has been shrouded in mystery. In 1640, the French philosopher René Descartes speculated that this small gland was the seat of the soul and the mediator between mind and body. Descartes noted that, unlike many brain features that have two obvious, separate, and symmetrical lobes, the pineal body appeared to be unitary. Its central location nestled between the two human brain hemispheres also suggested to him a special importance.

It wasn't until 1898 that scientific evidence suggested that the pineal body secretes a hormone. During this year, German pediatrician Otto Heubner showed that a pineal tumor caused a boy to enter early puberty. In 1918, Swedish anatomist Nils Holmgren showed that pineal bodies in frogs and dogfish sharks had cells that resembled color-sensitive photoreceptor cells of the eye's retina, and that the pineal body might function like a "third eye." (No such cells reside in the mammalian pineal body.) In 1958, American physician Aaron Lerner and colleagues extracted the hormone melatonin from the pineal glands of cows.

Today, we know that the human pineal gland, the size of a rice grain, produces melatonin, known as the hormone of darkness because darkness stimulates melatonin secretion, while light inhibits secretion. In particular, light entering the eye stimulates the group of nerve cells called the suprachiasmatic nucleus (SCN), located in the brain over the optic nerves. The SCN then inhibits the production of melatonin in the pineal gland.

The pineal gland facilitates the entrainment of circadian (daily) rhythms such as sleep and wakefulness. Melatonin is produced in higher quantities in children than adults and may also play a role in regulating sexual development and immune-system functioning. In 2001, American physician Rick Strassman creatively speculated that the pineal body secreted small amounts of the psychedelic DMT (dimethyltryptamine) and, thus, may mediate "deep meditation, psychosis, and near-death experiences. As we die, the life-force leaves the body through the pineal gland, releasing another flood of this psychedelic spirit molecule."

SEE ALSO Cerebral Localization (1861), Discovery of Adrenaline (1893), Searches for the Soul (1907), Human Growth Hormone (1921), and Near-Death Experiences (1975).

René Descartes's diagram showing the pineal gland (teardrop shape). He wrote, "My view is that this gland is the principal seat of the soul, and the place in which all our thoughts are formed."

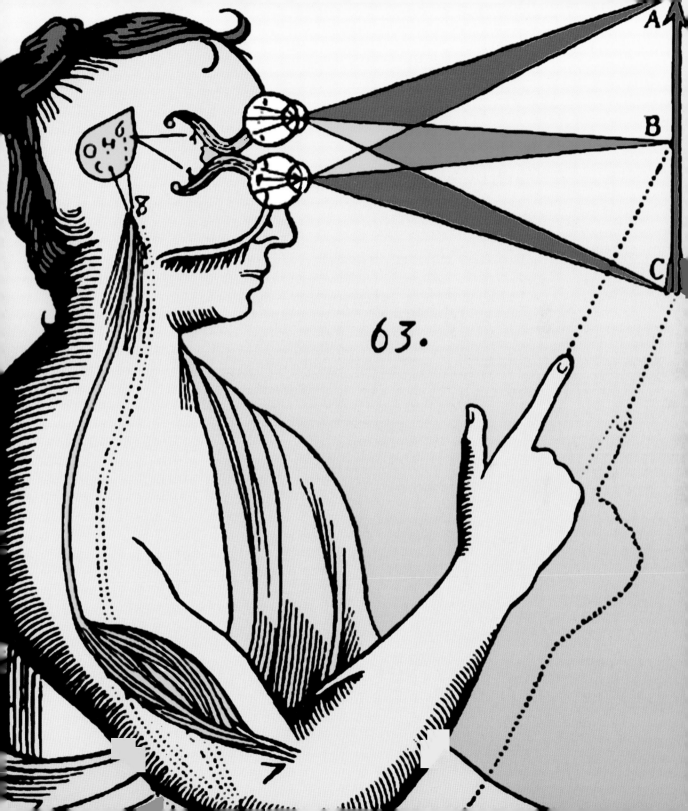

Nanomedicine

Richard Phillips Feynman (1918–1988), **John S. Kanzius** (1944–2009), **Kim Eric Drexler** (b. 1955)

Throughout the history of medicine, researchers have developed increasingly refined tools to investigate and manipulate the human body in greater detail. For example, the ancient Egyptians used linen and animal sinew to close wounds, and today wound closure is assisted with adhesive liquids or **suture** threads smaller than the diameter of a human hair. Following this trend much farther, nanotechnology concerns the manipulation of structures with sizes from 1 to 100 nanometers (nm). For perspective, consider that a human hair is about 10,000 nm in width and that the diameter of a **DNA** double-helix strand is around 2 nm.

The nanotechnology concept was inspired by American physicist Richard Feynman, who in 1959 gave a talk called "There's Plenty of Room at the Bottom," which provided a vision in which tools for manipulating atoms and molecules became a reality. American engineer Eric Drexler also called attention to the vast potential of nanotechnology in *Engines of Creation* (1986).

Nanomedicine—the medical application of nanotechnology—is still in its infancy. One active area of research includes drug delivery, in which nanoscale particles can be used to carry drugs inside particular cells. Nanoparticles are also used to produce high-contrast images and make tumors glow. With Kanzius RF (radio-frequency) therapy, created by American inventor John Kanzius and tested in 2005 at the University of Pittsburgh Medical Center, metallic nanoparticles are attached to **cancer** cells. Radio waves heat the particles, destroying the cancer cells. American bioengineer Jennifer West and colleagues researched gold-coated "nanoshells" with attached antibodies to target cancer cells. Infrared **lasers** heat the gold to kill the cells. Gold nanoshells are also being considered to "weld" delicate tissues together during surgery. American physician James Baker experimented with dendrimers (branching molecular structures with hundreds of hooks) that are absorbed into cancer cells and carry anticancer drugs. Such dendrimers use folic-acid vitamins attached to some hooks as "bait" so that cancer cells with vitamin receptors pull in the dendrimers. Research also continues in producing molecular scaffolding for nerve regeneration.

SEE ALSO Sutures (3000 B.C.), DNA Structure (1953), Structure of Antibodies (1959), Cryonics (1962), Gene Therapy (1990), RNA Interference (1998), and Growing New Organs (2006).

In the future, small molecular "machines" may be used to repair tissues and fight disease. Shown here is an artistic depiction of a nanobot repairing blood cells.

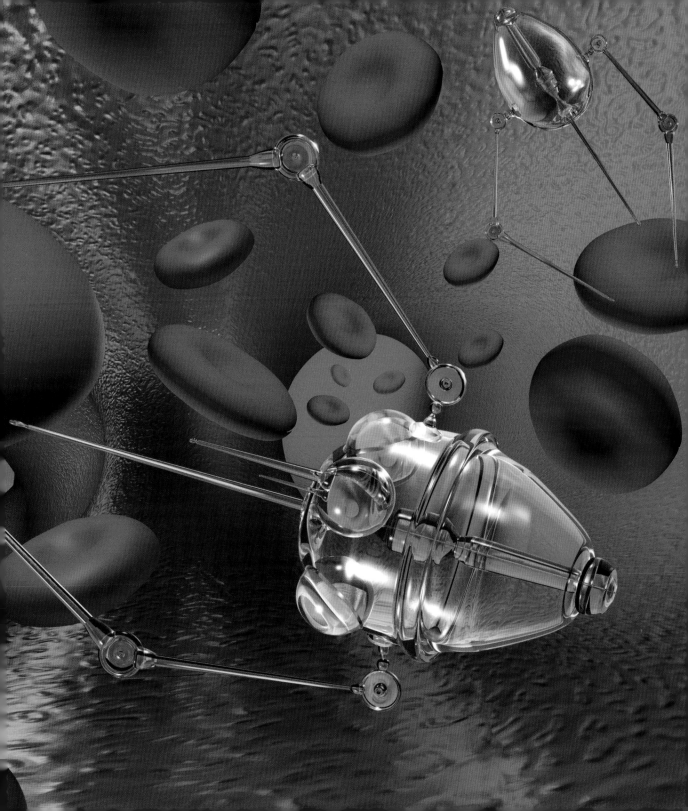

Radioimmunoassay

Solomon Aaron Berson (1918–1972), **Rosalyn Sussman Yalow** (1921–2011)

The invention of the radioimmunoassay (RIA) by American medical physicist Rosalyn Yalow "brought a revolution in biological and medical research," according to the 1977 Nobel Prize committee, a revolution that was "more important than the discovery of **X-rays**." Scientists likened its extreme sensitivity for detecting trace quantities of a substance to detecting a half a lump of sugar in a lake "62 miles long, 62 miles wide, and 30 feet deep."

First discovered by Yalow and her colleague American physician Solomon Berson, RIA has been used to measure minuscule amounts of insulin and other hormones, toxins, viruses, **neurotransmitters**, some **cancers**, and illicit drugs. Several companies have made use of RIA to screen for the hepatitis B virus in donated blood.

To use RIA, the scientist must work with a substance that is an antigen—a molecule recognized by the immune system. A known quantity of the antigen is made radioactive and then mixed in a test tube with a set amount of antibodies. The antigens and antibodies bind to one another. Next, a nonradioactive test substance that contains a tiny amount of the antigen is added to the solution, and some of the test antigens displace the radioactive substances that were joined to the antibodies. Scientists then measure the amount of freed radioactive antigens to determine the small amount of antigens in the sample under study.

Today, related antibody-binding methods such as ELISA (enzyme-linked immunosorbent assay) are also used to detect trace amounts of a substance through the use of observable color changes. These approaches do not require radioactive elements.

Considering the barriers to women in science (and frequent prejudice against Jews), Yalow's receiving her PhD in nuclear physics in 1945 is particularly inspiring. She was the second woman to receive a Nobel Prize in Physiology or Medicine—the first was American biochemist Gerty Theresa Cori, also a Jew. Both Yalow and Berson declined to patent RIA, even though it could have made them rich, because they wanted humankind to easily benefit from the technique.

SEE ALSO Discovery of Viruses (1892), Neurotransmitters (1914), Commercialization of Insulin (1922), Structure of Antibodies (1959), and Positron Emission Tomography (PET) (1973).

Dust mites crawling on pillowcase fabric. A RAST test (short for radioallergosorbent test) is a blood test that uses a radioimmunoassay to detect antibodies to potential allergens, such as mite proteins.

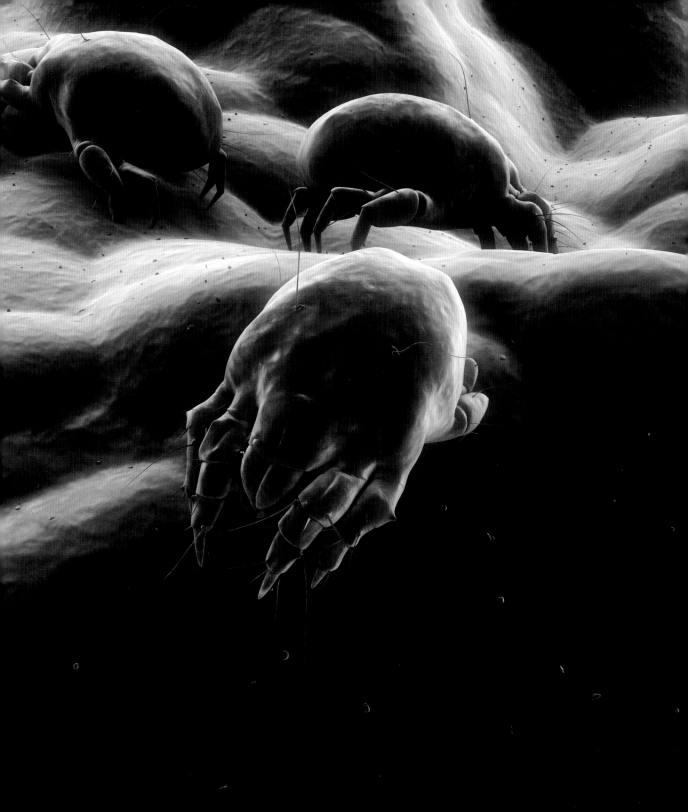

Structure of Antibodies

Paul Ehrlich (1854–1915), **Rodney Robert Porter** (1917–1985), **Gerald Maurice Edelman** (b. 1929)

The **germ theory of disease**, proposed in the mid-1800s, suggested that microorganisms cause many diseases, and people wondered how the body attempted to defend itself against such foreign invaders. Today, we know that antibodies (also called immunoglobulins) are the protective proteins that circulate in our bodies and identify and neutralize foreign substances, called antigens, which include bacteria, viruses, parasites, transplanted foreign tissues, and venoms. Antibodies are produced by plasma B cells (a kind of white blood cell). Each antibody consists of two heavy chains and two light chains made of amino acids. These four chains are bound together to form a molecule shaped like the letter Y. Variable regions at the two upper tips of the Y bind to antigens, thereby marking them for other parts of the immune system to destroy. Many millions of different antibodies can exist with slightly different tip structures. Antibodies can also neutralize antigens directly by binding to them and, for example, preventing the pathogens from entering or damaging cells.

Antibodies circulating in the blood play a role in the humoral immune system. Additional immune players—**phagocytes**—function like single-celled creatures that engulf and destroy smaller particles. The binding of antibodies to an invader can mark the invader for ingestion by phagocytes.

Tests used to detect particular antibodies may lead a physician to suspect, or rule out, certain diseases such as Lyme disease. Autoimmune disorders may be triggered by antibodies binding to the body's own healthy cells. Antiserums can sometimes be made by injecting animals with an antigen and then isolating the antibodies in the serum for use in humans.

Paul Ehrlich coined the word *antibody* (*Antikörper* in German) around 1891, and he proposed a mechanism in which the receptors on cells attached to toxins in a tight lock-and-key fit to trigger antibody production. English biochemist Rodney Porter and American biologist Gerald Edelman won the 1972 Nobel Prize for their independent research, which started around 1959 and elucidated the antibody's Y-like structure, as well as identifying heavy and light chains.

SEE ALSO Lymphatic System (1652), Smallpox Vaccination (1798), Germ Theory of Disease (1862), Phagocytosis Theory (1882), Antitoxins (1890), Allergies (1906), Autoimmune Diseases (1956), Nanomedicine (1959), Radioimmunoassay (1959), and Thymus (1961).

Artist's concept of Y-shaped antibodies circulating through the bloodstream.

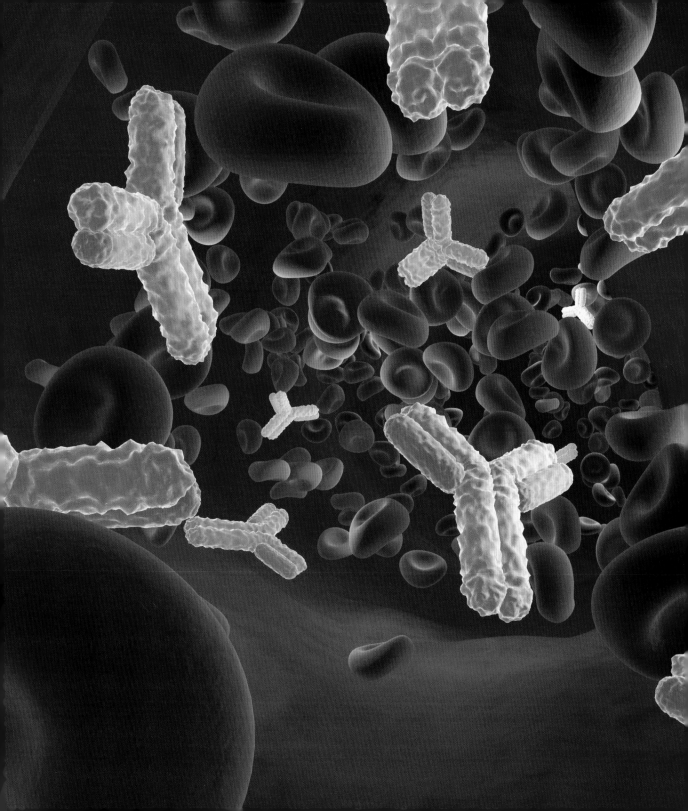

Laser

Albert Einstein (1879–1955), **Leon Goldman** (1905–1997), **Charles Hard Townes** (b. 1915), **Theodore Harold "Ted" Maiman** (1927–2007)

"Laser technology has become important in a wide range of practical applications," writes laser expert Jeff Hecht, "ranging from medicine and consumer electronics to telecommunications and military technology. . . . 18 recipients of the Nobel Prize received the award for laser-related research."

The word *laser* is an acronym for light amplification by stimulated emission of radiation, and lasers make use of a subatomic process known as stimulated emission, first considered by Albert Einstein in 1917. In stimulated emission, a photon (a particle of light) of the appropriate energy causes an electron to drop to a lower energy level, which results in the creation of another photon. This second photon is said to be coherent with the first and has the same phase, frequency, polarization, and direction of travel as the first photon. If the photons are reflected so that they repeatedly traverse the same atoms, an amplification can take place and an intense radiation beam is emitted. Lasers can be created so that they emit electromagnetic radiation of various frequencies.

In 1953, physicist Charles Townes and students produced the first microwave laser (maser), but it was not capable of continuous radiation emission. Theodore Maiman created the first practical working laser in 1960, using pulsed operation. In 1961, dermatologist Leon Goldman was first to use a laser to treat melanoma (a skin **cancer**), and related methods were later used for removing birthmarks and tattoos with minimal scarring. Because of the speed and precision of laser surgery, lasers have since been used in ophthalmology, dentistry, and many other fields. In LASIK eye surgery, a laser beam is used to change the shape of the eye's cornea to correct for nearsightedness and farsightedness. In prostate surgery, a laser may be used to vaporize tumors. Green laser light can be used for coagulation when the light is absorbed by hemoglobin to stop a bleeding blood vessel. The hot beam of a surgical laser can be used to cauterize, or seal off, open blood vessels as the beam moves along tissue.

SEE ALSO Sutures (3000 B.C.), Eye Surgery (600 B.C.), Eyeglasses (1284), Halstedian Surgery (1904), and Corneal Transplant (1905).

An optical engineer studies the interaction of several lasers for potential use aboard a laser-weapons system being developed to defend against ballistic missile attacks. The U.S. Directed Energy Directorate conducts research into beam-control technologies.

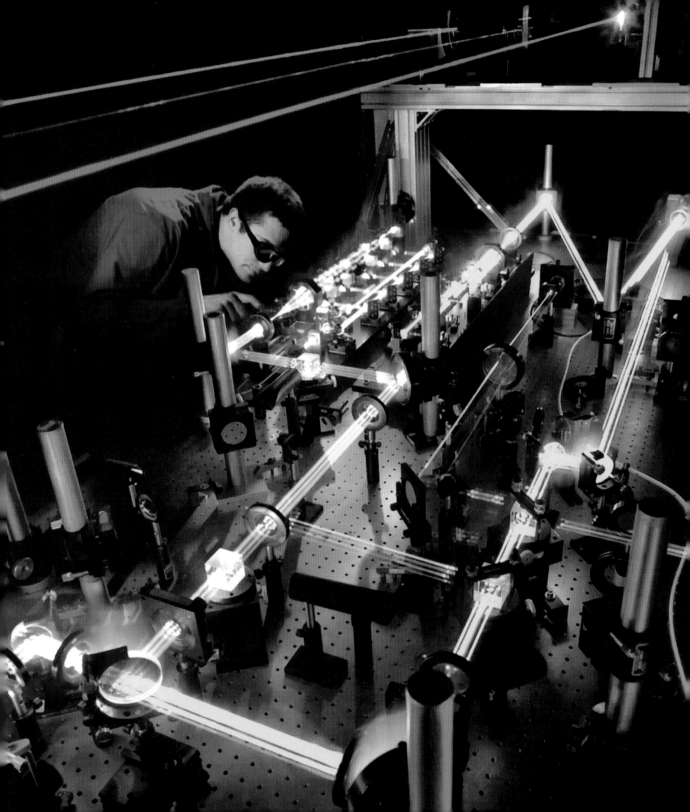

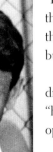

Self-Surgery

Evan O'Neill Kane (1861–1932), **Leonid Ivanovich Rogozov** (1934–2000), **Jerri Lin Nielsen** (née Cahill; 1952–2009), **Inés Ramírez Pérez** (b. 1960)

Several significant milestones in the history of medicine are concerned with acts of self-surgery, in which the patient is also the surgeon performing the operation. Of particular interest are those heroic physicians who performed self-surgery out of necessity in extreme circumstances. For example, on April 30, 1961, Russian general practitioner Leonid Rogozov removed his own infected appendix at the Soviet Novolazarevskaya Research Station in Antarctica. This surgery was probably the first successful self-**appendectomy** undertaken beyond a **hospital** setting, with no possibility of outside assistance, and with no other medical personnel present. Prior to his surgery, Rogozov recorded in his journal: "I did not sleep at all last night. It hurts like the devil! A snowstorm whipping through my soul, wailing like a hundred jackals. . . . I have to think through the only possible way out: to operate on myself. . . . It's almost impossible . . . but I can't just fold my arms and give up."

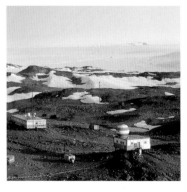

Prior to making the incision, Rogozov injected procaine (a local **anesthetic** drug) near the site, and then he used a mirror to view his operation, which "helps, but also hinders—after all, it's showing things backwards." The operation lasted nearly two hours, and he recovered completely.

Another famous case of self-appendectomy took place on February 15, 1921, when American surgeon Evan O'Neill Kane removed his own appendix, in part to better understand the efficacy of local anesthesia. The operation was completed by his assistants.

In 1999, American physician Jerri Nielsen was forced to biopsy a suspicious breast lump while on duty at the Amundsen-Scott Antarctic research station. The lump was found to be cancerous, and she gave herself chemotherapeutic agents.

In 2000, Inés Ramírez, a Mexican woman with no medical training, performed a successful **cesarean section** on herself using a kitchen knife. After 12 hours of continual pain, she had feared that the fetus was at risk, and her previous pregnancy had ended in fetal death during labor. After surgery, mother and child recovered completely.

SEE ALSO Appendectomy (1848), Cesarean Section (1882), and Medical Self-Experimentation (1929).

LEFT *(upper): Leonid Rogozov, who performed a self-appendectomy.* LEFT *(lower): A portion of Novolazarevskaya Research Station in Antarctica.* RIGHT: *Amundsen-Scott South Pole Station.*

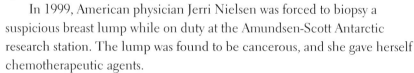

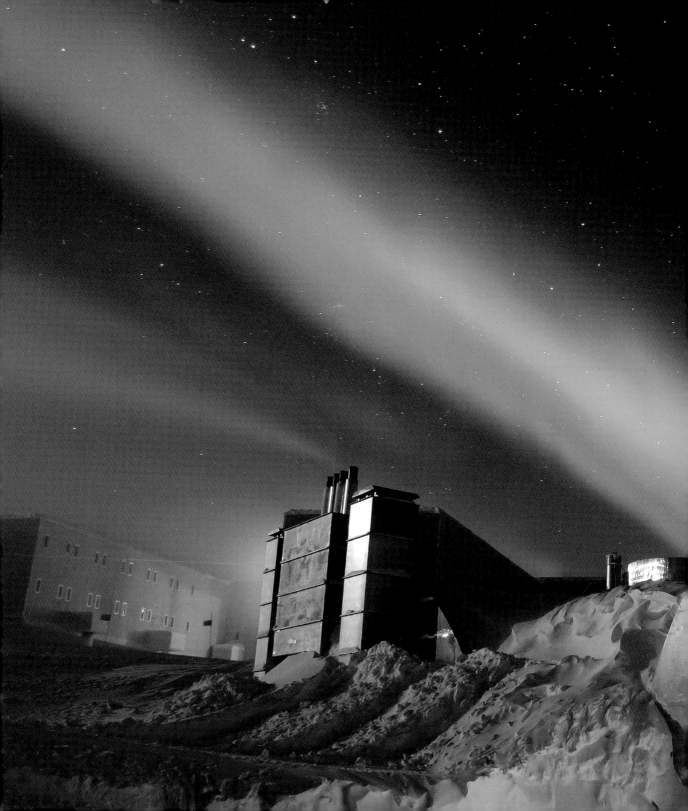

Thymus

Galen of Pergamon (129–199), Jacques Francis Albert Pierre Miller (b. 1931)

Even though Greco-Roman physician Galen noted that the thymus gland, located just behind the breastbone, changed size during a person's adult life, the function of this mysterious gland remained unknown until the 1960s. The riddle of the thymus, however, never stopped people from consuming the cow's thymus (called sweetbread) with great gusto. Gil Marks, author of *The Encyclopedia of Jewish Food*, writes, "Arguably, no community more closely embraced sweetbreads as food than Ashkenazim [German and Eastern European Jews], for whom they followed only liver in popularity among the organs."

In 1961, French scientist Jacques Miller surgically removed the thymus from three-day-old mice and observed the subsequent deficiency of certain lymphocytes (white blood cells), which were later called T cells after the gland from which they originated. Miller also observed that thymectomized mice became highly susceptible to infection and did not reject skin grafts from other mice—rejection that would be expected for mice with properly functioning immune systems.

Today, we know that the thymus has two regions, the outer cortex and the inner medulla. Pre-T cells are produced in bone marrow and circulate to the thymus via the bloodstream. These cells enter the cortex, where a series of molecular events occur that allow the cells to recognize certain antigens—substances that trigger the production of antibodies so that the foreign invaders can be destroyed. During this maturation, cells that *improperly* react to normal tissue components are eliminated. The surviving cells enter the medulla and, eventually, the bloodstream, where they can protect the body from potentially harmful agents. The process of T-cell maturation is controlled by hormones produced by the thymus.

The two-lobed thymus reaches its maximum size at puberty and then begins to dramatically shrink. By the time a person is 75 years old, the thymus becomes hard to distinguish from the surrounding fatty tissue. Loss of a thymus early in life can result in lack of T cells, severe immunodeficiency, and high rates of infection.

SEE ALSO Tissue Grafting (1597), Lymphatic System (1652), Phagocytosis Theory (1882), Autoimmune Diseases (1956), Structure of Antibodies (1959), and Reverse Transcriptase and AIDS (1970).

Artistic rendition of a T cell attacking a cancer cell. A T cell (an infection-fighting white blood cell) can kill some cancer cells and some virus-infected cells. T cells derive their name from the thymus, the main organ responsible for T-cell maturation.

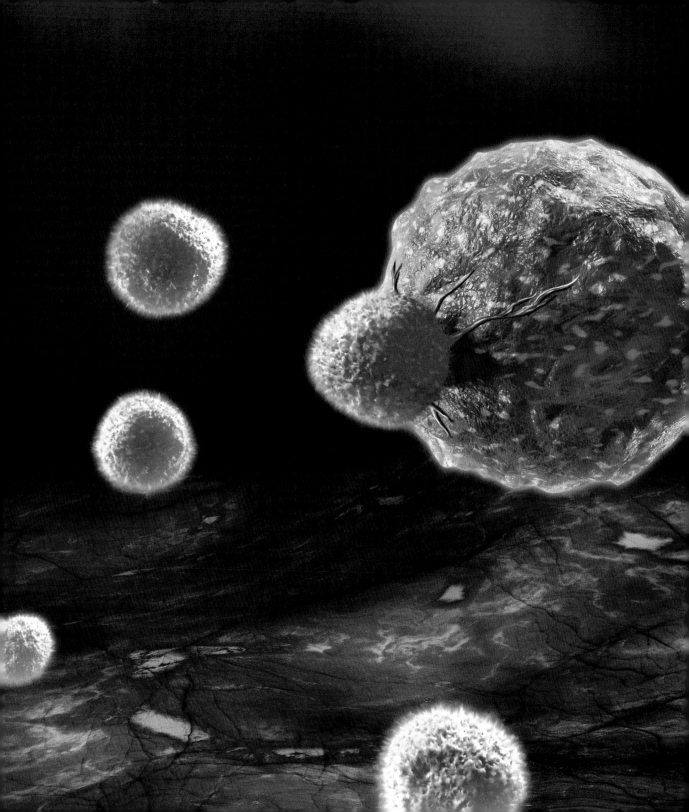

Cryonics

Robert Chester Wilson Ettinger (1918–2011)

In 1773, American statesman Benjamin Franklin regretted that he lived "in a century too little advanced, and too near the infancy of science" that he could not be preserved and revived to satisfy his "very ardent desire to see and observe the state of America a hundred years hence." Perhaps Franklin would have used today's cryonics facilities, in which people are preserved after they are pronounced legally dead by replacing blood with protective fluids and cooling the bodies for long-term storage. These cryoprotectants reduce ice crystal formation that could otherwise damage tissues. Cryonicists hope that technology of the future will be sufficiently advanced to revive such patients and cure whatever diseases they may have suffered from. If our thoughts depend primarily on the brain's structure, then perhaps brains made of other materials or even simulated in software could think.

If cryonic resurrection seems far-fetched, recall that frozen embryos are routinely resurrected to produce healthy children. The modern era of cryonics was stimulated by author Robert Ettinger's book *The Prospect of Immortality*, published in 1962, which discusses the possibility of preserving people. Today, liquid nitrogen is used to store bodies at temperatures of around –320 °F (–196 °C). For religious readers, if scientists were able to freeze *your* disembodied brain and then revive you in a century, would you enter the afterlife during the intervening time of zero brain activity?

In 2006, surgeon Hasan Alam placed pigs into a state of suspended animation—his cold pigs had no pulse, no blood, and no electrical activity in their brains, and the pigs' tissues consumed no oxygen. After a few hours, Alam pumped warm blood into the animals, and the animals jolted back to life. According to Alam, "Once the heart starts beating and the blood starts pumping, voila, you've got another animal that's come back from the other side. . . . Technically I think we can do it in humans."

SEE ALSO Autopsy (1761), Searches for the Soul (1907), Nanomedicine (1959), Hospice (1967), Near-Death Experiences (1975), and First Test-Tube Baby (1978).

This dewar may contain four whole-body patients and six neuropatients (heads only) immersed in liquid nitrogen at –320 °F (–196 °C). This insulated container consumes no electric power. Photo courtesy of Alcor Life Extension Foundation.

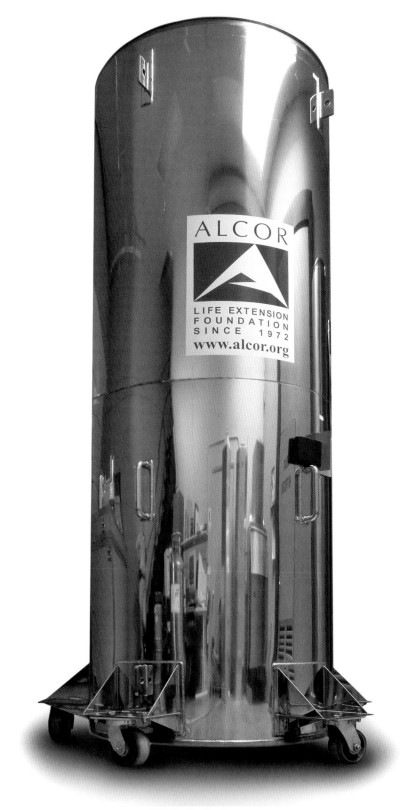

Mitochondrial Diseases

Rolf Luft (1914–2007)

Most of the cells in our bodies harbor the relics of bacteria that more than a billion years ago entered cells and facilitated the emergence of complex life forms like us. These miniature powerhouses of cells, called mitochondria, generate most of the adenosine triphosphate (ATP) needed to supply cellular energy. However, mitochondria are more than mere energy-generation components and affect processes that range from the aging of our bodies to various specialized functions of the different cells in which they reside. They also assist with detoxification and the synthesis of biologically important compounds. A single body cell may have hundreds of mitochondria, each with several copies of its own small, circular, double-stranded **DNA** that contain 37 mitochondrial genes. Mitochondria behave a little like microorganisms and divide separately from the remainder of the host cell.

Mitochondrial diseases (MDs) are caused by malfunctioning mitochondria, which in turn can be caused by mutations in the mitochondria's own DNA (mtDNA) or in the host cell DNA that contributes to mitochondrial structure and function. MDs are extremely varied, but symptoms can include loss of muscle function, visual and hearing problems, mental retardation, blindness, and poor growth. MDs affect the normal process of programmed cell death and "diseases of aging," including dementia, type 2 diabetes, Parkinson's disease, **cancer**, and heart disease. The distribution of abnormal mitochondria may vary from organ to organ and also change through time as mitochondria reproduce within cells. MDs become clinically obvious when the number of defective mitochondria exceeds a certain threshold within cells. Unlike many other human genetic diseases in which father and mother contribute defective genes, mtDNA comes only from the egg cell and, thus, is inherited only from the mother.

In 1962, Swedish endocrinologist Rolf Luft and colleagues elucidated the nature of an MD after studying a woman with improperly functioning mitochondria, which led to energy being wasted as heat. The woman suffered from weight loss and muscular weakness, could not stop sweating, and always felt hot.

SEE ALSO Causes of Cancer (1761), Lavoisier's Respiration (1784), Mendel's Genetics (1865), Chromosomal Theory of Inheritance (1902), Inborn Errors of Metabolism (1902), "Autistic Disturbances" (1943), DNA Structure (1953), and Levodopa for Parkinson's Disease (1957).

Artistic rendition of a mitochondrion, revealing internal compartments, known as cristae, formed by the folds of the mitochondrion's inner membrane (red). The cristae are studded with enzymes (not shown in this rendition) used to make ATP, the energy carrier molecule for cells.

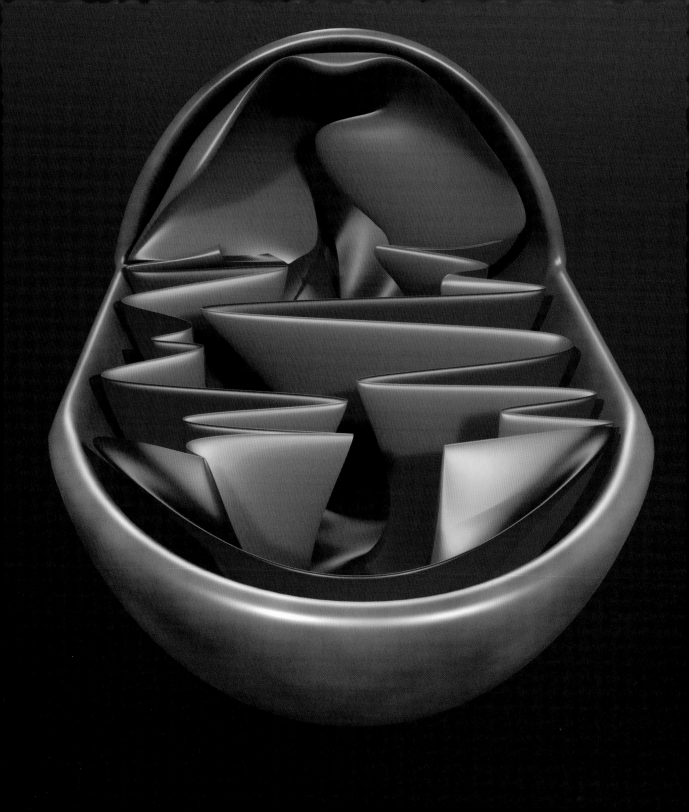

Thalidomide Disaster

Frances Kathleen Oldham Kelsey (b. 1914), **Widukind Lenz** (1919–1995), **William Griffith McBride** (b. 1927)

The August 10, 1962, issue of *TIME* expressed mounting fears as babies continued to be born with phocomelia, or "seal limbs" that looked like flippers. "Appalling reports continued to roll in. So far . . . close to 8,000 babies have been born deformed because their mothers used a sleeping-pill-tranquilizer called thalidomide, [making this] the greatest prescription disaster in medical history." The long bones of the babies' arms failed to develop, and fingers sometimes sprouted from shoulders.

In 1957, thalidomide was promoted by Grünenthal, a German pharmaceutical company, as a tranquilizer, painkiller, sleep aid, and treatment for nausea. Pregnant women used thalidomide to alleviate morning sickness. However, in 1961, the Australian obstetrician William McBride and the German pediatrician Widukind Lenz studied the growing number of babies with seal limbs and warned that thalidomide was the cause.

Although thalidomide was being used around the world, Americans were fortunate because physician Frances Kelsey of the Food and Drug Administration (FDA) rejected several requests to approve thalidomide for use in the United States, believing that it was not adequately tested in pregnant women, nor was it proven to be effective. As a result of the thalidomide disaster, in 1962, the United States enacted laws requiring drugs to be tested for safety during pregnancy before a drug could be approved.

Despite the horrors of thalidomide, researchers began to discover some beneficial uses of the drug in settings totally removed from the drug's intended purpose. When administered to patients with a painful skin inflammation associated with **leprosy**, patients often experienced dramatic pain relief. Also, thalidomide was found to be useful for treating multiple myeloma, a **cancer** of certain white blood cells. In order for women in the United States to be treated with thalidomide today, they must undergo periodic pregnancy tests and take precautions to avoid pregnancy. Because thalidomide has anti-inflammatory effects and also inhibits the growth of new blood vessels (angiogenesis), many possible diseases may benefit from thalidomide treatment.

SEE ALSO Abortion (70), Separation of Conjoined Twins (1689), Cause of Leprosy (1873), Amniocentesis (1952), Fetal Monitoring (1957), Medical Ultrasound (1957), and Fetal Surgery (1981).

FDA inspector Dr. Frances Kelsey receives an award for Distinguished Federal Civilian Service from President John F. Kennedy in 1962 for blocking the sale of thalidomide in the United States. Researchers discovered that thalidomide causes serious birth defects.

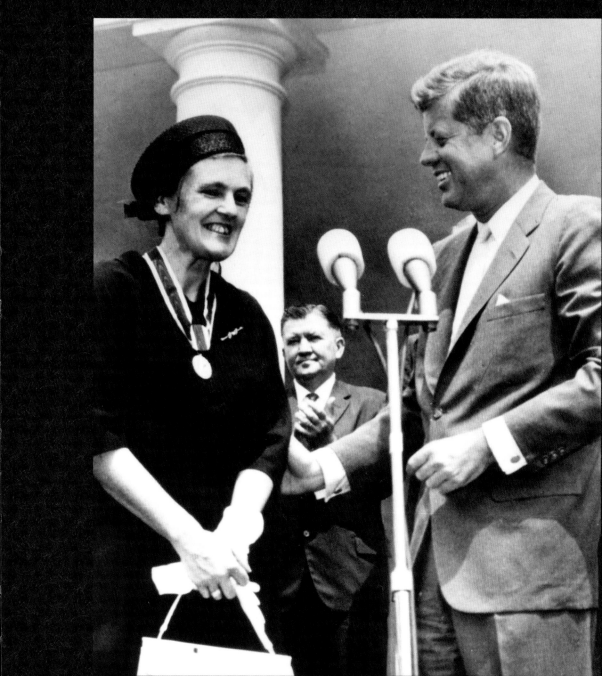

Cognitive Behavioral Therapy

Epictetus (55–135), **Albert Ellis** (1913–2007), **Aaron Temkin Beck** (b. 1921)

Cognitive behavioral therapy (CBT), which emphasizes the role of errors in thinking in producing negative emotions, has ancient roots. The Greek Stoic philosopher Epictetus wrote in the *Enchiridion*, "Men are disturbed not by things, but by the view which they take of them." In CBT, the psychotherapist helps the patient think about situations and circumstances in new ways, in order to change patients' reactions and feelings. If the patient can identify maladaptive or irrational thoughts, the thoughts can be challenged. The resultant improved behaviors serve to educate the patient further and to reinforce the more productive way of thinking. A patient commonly keeps a diary of events and associated feelings and thoughts.

In the 1950s, American psychoanalyst Albert Ellis shaped the development of CBT, partly because of his dislike of the seemingly inefficient and indirect nature of classical psychoanalysis. Ellis wanted the therapist to be heavily involved in helping the client modify unhelpful patterns of thought. In the 1960s, American psychiatrist and psychoanalyst Aaron Beck became the major driving force behind modern CBT.

CBT has often been shown to be helpful in many cases of depression, insomnia, anxiety, obsessive-compulsive disorder, post-traumatic stress disorder, eating disorders, chronic pain, and schizophrenia. When seeing a therapist, a patient is sometimes asked to reframe a thought in terms of a hypothesis that can be tested. In this manner, the patient can "step back" from the belief to allow more objective examination and arrive at a different view. For example, a depressed person may overgeneralize, concluding she will never get a job after a single failed interview. For phobias and compulsions, symptoms are sometimes decreased by gradual exposure to a fearful stimulus. Depressed people may be asked to schedule small pleasurable activities (e.g., meet a friend for coffee). Not only does this modify behavior, but it can be used to test a belief or hypothesis such as "No one enjoys my company." CBT can also be used in conjunction with medications for very serious psychological disorders.

SEE ALSO *De Praestigiis Daemonum* (1563), Psychoanalysis (1899), Jung's Analytical Psychology (1933), Electroconvulsive Therapy (1938), Transorbital Lobotomy (1946), and Antipsychotics (1950).

Using CBT and controlled, gradual exposure to spiders, a therapist can often treat arachnophobia. Functional magnetic resonance imaging studies suggest that CBT can affect the brain in a variety of useful ways.

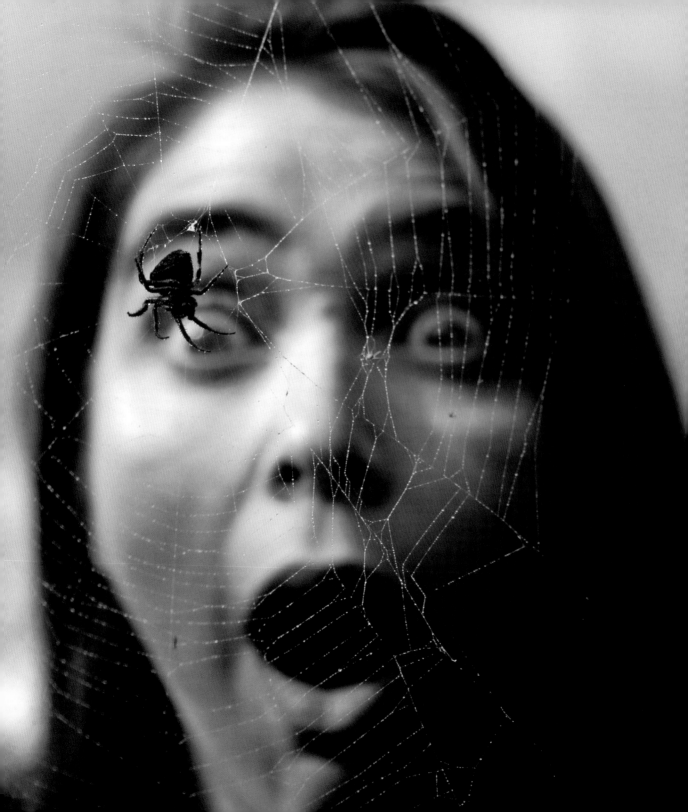

Liver Transplant

Thomas E. Starzl (b. 1926)

In ancient Greek mythology, Prometheus was punished by being bound to a rock while an eagle ate his liver. Each day, the liver regenerated, and the eagle repeated the task. The ancient Babylonians attempted to predict the future by examining the features of animal livers. Today, we know that the liver indeed has remarkable powers of regeneration and can return to its normal size even after more than half of it has been removed.

Individuals may need new livers when their livers are damaged. For example, in adults, chronic hepatitis (inflammation) and cirrhosis (scarring) triggered by viruses or toxins (e.g., alcohol) are common causes of damage. In children, biliary atresia (a blockage of the common bile duct causing liver damage) is the most common reason for transplantation. During liver transplantation, often the recipient's liver is removed and replaced with the cadaver's donor liver. However, transplantations can also be performed using only a portion of a liver from a living donor.

American surgeon Thomas Starzl performed the first human liver transplant in 1963. In the 1980s, the use of immunosuppressant drugs such as **cyclosporine** to reduce foreign-tissue rejection allowed transplants to become more successful and common. During transplants, various vessels need to be reattached, including the inferior vena cava (which receives blood from the liver via hepatic veins), portal vein (which drains nutrient-rich blood from the gastrointestinal tract and spleen into the liver), hepatic artery (which supplies the liver with oxygenated blood), and common bile duct.

The liver serves many functions, including removal of toxins from the bloodstream, protein synthesis and degradation, production of bile used in digestion of foods, production of hormones involved in growth and blood-pressure regulation, metabolization of drugs, and maintenance of blood sugar levels (by converting glucose to glycogen for storing in the liver, and converting glycogen back to glucose when needed). The liver also stores various vitamins, converts ammonia to urea (which is excreted in urine), and creates fibrinogen, needed for blood clotting.

SEE ALSO Tissue Grafting (1597), Vascular Suturing (1902), Corneal Transplant (1905), Kidney Transplant (1954), Bone Marrow Transplant (1956), Lung Transplant (1963), Hand Transplant (1964), Pancreas Transplant (1966), Heart Transplant (1967), Cyclosporine (1972), Small Bowel Transplant (1987), Face Transplant (2005), Growing New Organs (2006), and Human Cloning (2008).

Location of the liver with respect to other major organs. The gallbladder is the teardrop-shaped organ positioned close to the liver.

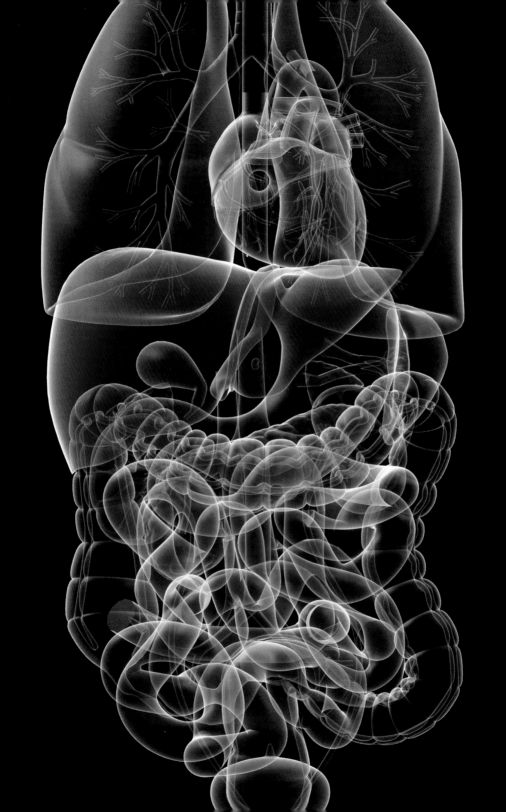

Lung Transplant

James D. Hardy (1918–2003)

The human lungs are a pair of spongy, air-filled organs that facilitate the exchange of oxygen from the atmosphere with carbon dioxide from the bloodstream. Air travels to the lungs through the trachea (windpipe), which leads to the tubular branches called bronchi. The bronchi become divided into increasingly smaller branches (bronchioles), finally becoming microscopic in size. The bronchioles feed microscopic air sacs called alveoli, where the actual gas exchange takes place. Blood containing waste carbon dioxide is sent from the heart to the lungs via the pulmonary arteries. Oxygen-rich blood from the lungs returns to the heart via the pulmonary veins.

Certain kinds of lung damage may be treated by replacing a recipient's diseased lungs with donor lungs. Such damage may be caused by chronic obstructive pulmonary disease (COPD), which includes emphysema (destruction of lung tissue around alveoli, often caused by smoking), cystic fibrosis (a genetic disease that leads to the accumulation of thick, sticky mucus), and pulmonary hypertension (an increase in blood pressure in the lung vasculature).

In 1963, American surgeon James Hardy performed the first human lung transplant, but the patient lived for only 18 days. In 1981, American surgeon Bruce Reitz performed a combined heart-lung transplant by inserting both organs together. American surgeon Joel Cooper performed the first successful *single* lung transplant in 1983 (the patient lived for seven years), followed by the first successful *double* lung transplant in 1986. In 1989, surgeons determined that a bilateral sequential lung transplant, in which each lung is removed and attached separately, gave better outcomes.

Lobe transplants, in which the recipient's diseased lung is replaced with the lobe (section) of a living donor's lung, often require two donors to replace a single recipient lung. In domino transplants, first performed in 1987, the recipient of a new heart and set of lungs offers his or her healthy heart to another recipient. As with other organ transplants, immunosuppressive drugs are required to prevent rejection of the foreign tissue.

SEE ALSO Tissue Grafting (1597), Spirometry (1846), Vascular Suturing (1902), Corneal Transplant (1905), Iron Lung (1928), Kidney Transplant (1954), Liver Transplant (1963), Hand Transplant (1964), Pancreas Transplant (1966), Heart Transplant (1967), Cyclosporine (1972), Small Bowel Transplant (1987), Face Transplant (2005), and Growing New Organs (2006).

Human lungs. The vertical tube is the trachea, or windpipe, which bifurcates at the bottom into the two primary bronchial branches, leading to the lungs.

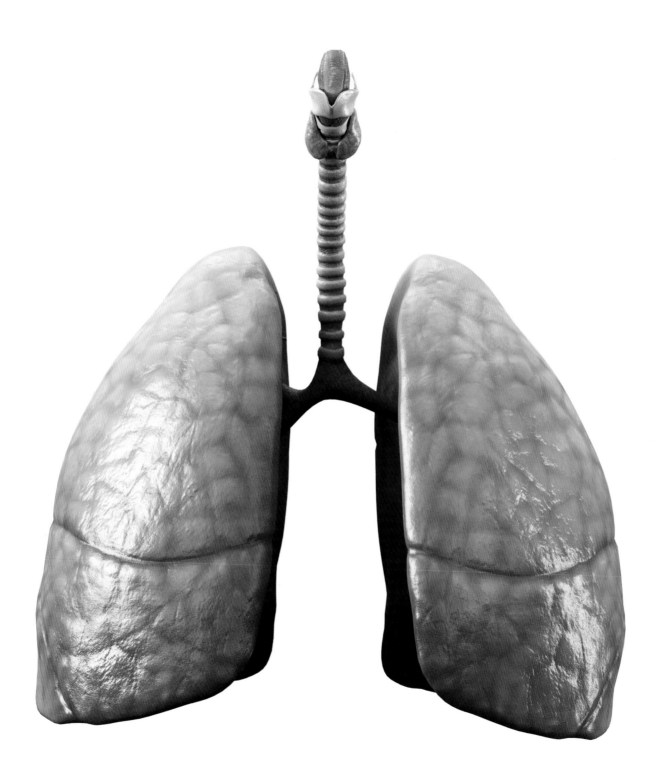

Angioplasty

Charles Theodore Dotter (1920–1985), **Melvin P. Judkins** (1922–1985),
Andreas Roland Grüntzig (1939–1985)

Angioplasty is a medical procedure for widening blood vessels that may be obstructed or narrowed by atherosclerosis, a condition in which an artery wall thickens as the result of an accumulation of fatty materials, such as cholesterol, and calcium. A physician passes an empty balloon on a guide wire into the narrowed vessel and inflates the balloon, a process that crushes some of the fatty deposits and opens the vessel to facilitate blood flow. The balloon is then collapsed and withdrawn. Today, stents (e.g., metal tubes) are often inserted after angioplasty to prevent the vessel from narrowing again. Drug-coated stents can suppress harmful tissue growth and reduce inflammatory response. Patients with stents often take blood-thinner medication to reduce clotting within the stented vessel.

Coronary angioplasty (CA, also known as percutaneous coronary intervention) refers to the widening of coronary arteries, which are the vessels that deliver oxygen-rich blood to the heart muscles. Renal artery angioplasty refers to use in narrow renal arteries, which can lead to high blood pressure and improperly functioning kidneys. Angioplasty is also used for carotid arteries in the neck, cerebral arteries in the brain, and other vessels in the body. Peripheral angioplasty generally refers to widening vessels other than coronary arteries—in the legs, for example.

In 1964, American radiologists Charles Dotter and Melvin Judkins used balloon angioplasty to treat atherosclerotic disease in a leg artery. In 1977, German cardiologist Andreas Grüntzig performed successful balloon angioplasty for coronary arteries. Dotter and colleagues deployed expandable stent structures in coronary arteries in 1986.

Although CA has shown to be helpful for reducing chest pain (angina) and improving quality of life, epidemiological studies continue to be performed to understand the degree to which CA decreases risk of death in various subgroups and in nonacute heart disease. Coronary artery bypass grafting, which bypasses narrowed arteries by connecting other vessels, may actually be more effective than CA for reducing death rates due to heart attacks.

SEE ALSO Circulatory System (1628), Ligation of the Abdominal Aorta (1817), Heart-Lung Machine (1953), Endoscope (1954), Beta-Blockers (1964), and Statins (1973).

A physician passes an empty balloon on a guide wire into the narrowed vessel and inflates the balloon to widen the vessel. Stents (e.g., metal, cagelike cylinders) are often inserted and left inside to prevent the vessel from narrowing again.

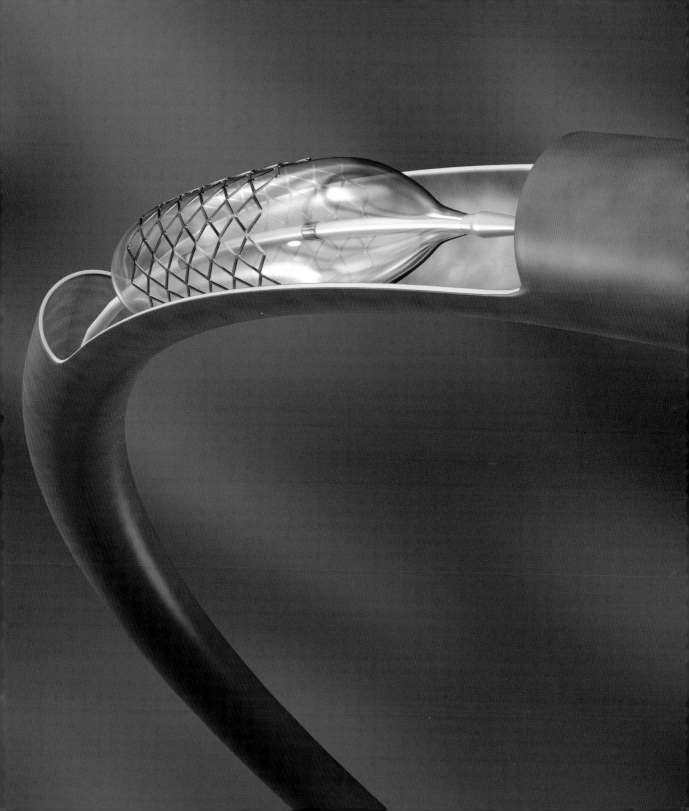

Beta-Blockers

Sir James Whyte Black (1924–2010)

Scottish physician James Black revolutionized the pharmaceutical industry and saved millions of lives with his rational and targeted drug design, an approach he used to create the world's first drugs that generated billions of dollars.

Black had been aware that the hormone **adrenaline**, also referred to as epinephrine, is secreted in larger quantities during times of stress, increasing heart rate and contraction force, which requires that the heart be supplied with more oxygen. He reasoned that if he could reduce such stress, this could be beneficial for those with weakened hearts.

Black turned his attention to the beta-receptors—sites on the heart muscles to which adrenaline binds to make the heart work harder. Black believed that if he could design a drug that structurally resembled adrenaline, this molecule might bind to the receptor and block the action of adrenaline, like sticking a wad of gum into a lock to prevent a key from opening the door. Black and his colleagues used a rational design process (i.e., based on their understanding of molecular and physiological processes and biological targets), which was counter to the common method of starting with a chemical found in nature and then looking for possible uses.

In the early 1960s, Black discovered the first clinically important beta-blocker drug, propranolol. Beta-blockers have since played significant roles in the protection of the heart after a heart attack and in the treatment of angina pectoris (pain caused by lack of blood and oxygen to the heart), high blood pressure, cardiac arrhythmias, migraines, performance anxiety (e.g., for musicians and public speakers), and glaucoma (often associated with increased pressure in the eye). Beta-blockers have been used by surgeons, marksmen, and archers to reduce tremors and enhance performance, although such drugs are banned by the International Olympic Committee.

Black was awarded the Nobel Prize in 1988 for his drug design work, which included the creation of cimetidine (brand name Tagamet) used to treat stomach ulcers. When informed that he had won the prize, Black quipped, "I wished I had my beta-blockers handy."

SEE ALSO Discovery of Adrenaline (1893), Artificial Pacemaker for Heart (1958), Angioplasty (1964), and Statins (1973).

The famous cellist Pablo Casals often experienced classic signs of performance anxiety: a thumping heart, shortness of breath, and tremors prior to and during his performances. Today, musicians sometimes use beta-blockers to enhance their performances.

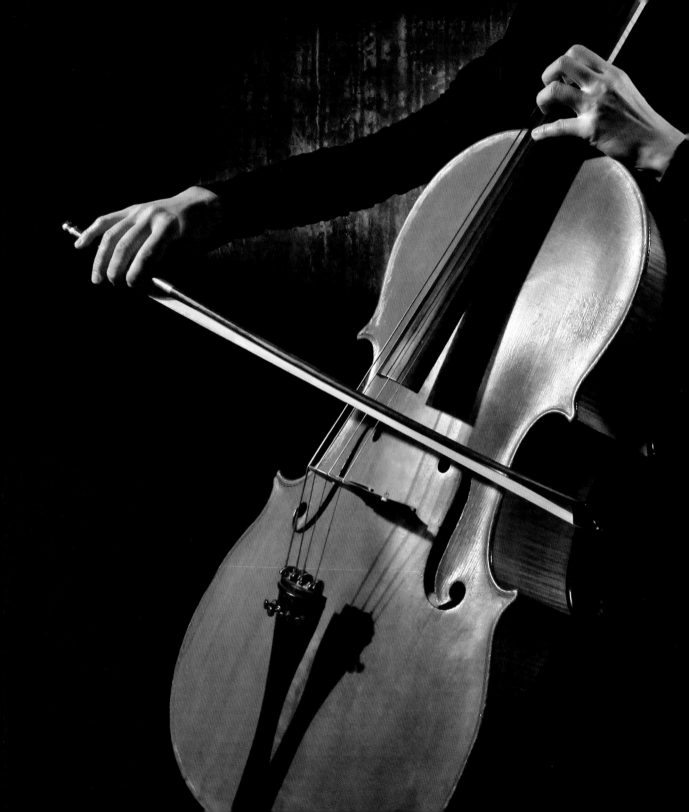

Hand Transplant

Roberto Gilbert Elizalde (1917–1999), Jean-Michel Dubernerd (b. 1941)

In 1833, Scottish anatomist Charles Bell wrote of his admiration for the human hand: "We have seen that the system of bones, muscles, and nerves of this extremity is suited to every form and condition . . . and we must confess that it is in the human hand that we have the consummation of all perfection as an instrument." In 1803, English physician Erasmus Darwin called the human hand the "first gift of Heaven."

Sadly, sometimes hands are lost due to accidents, thus motivating the need for hand transplants. In 1964, Ecuadoran surgeon Roberto Elizalde performed a hand transplant on a sailor with a blast injury, but the patient's body rejected the foreign tissue after only two weeks because only primitive immunosuppressant drugs were available at that time. In 1998, Australian surgeon Earl Owen and French surgeon Jean-Michel Dubernerd performed a successful hand transplant for Clint Hallam, who had lost his hand in a circular-saw accident. During the surgery, the surgeons first joined the two bones of the donor's forearm to Hallam's bones. Tendons, arteries, nerves, and veins also had to be connected. Finally, the skin was sewed together.

After a successful period of two years, during which Hallam learned to move his new fingers, Hallam decided to stop taking the immunosuppressive drugs that kept his hand from being rejected. He felt as if the donor hand did not belong to his body. Slowly, his hand rotted away, and he lost all sensation. He begged surgeons to remove the hand, and they complied in 2001. The Hallam case reinforces the need to ensure that transplant recipients are psychologically motivated to continue taking their medications well after a transplant is undertaken.

In 2009, Jeff Kepner underwent the first double hand transplant in the United States. In 2010, a male Polish soldier received two new hands from a female donor after losing his hands in a bomb explosion.

SEE ALSO Tissue Grafting (1597), Vascular Suturing (1902), Corneal Transplant (1905), Kidney Transplant (1954), Bone Marrow Transplant (1956), Liver Transplant (1963), Lung Transplant (1963), Pancreas Transplant (1966), Heart Transplant (1967), Cyclosporine (1972), Small Bowel Transplant (1987), Face Transplant (2005), Growing New Organs (2006), and Human Cloning (2008).

Muscles and tendons of the hand and forearm.

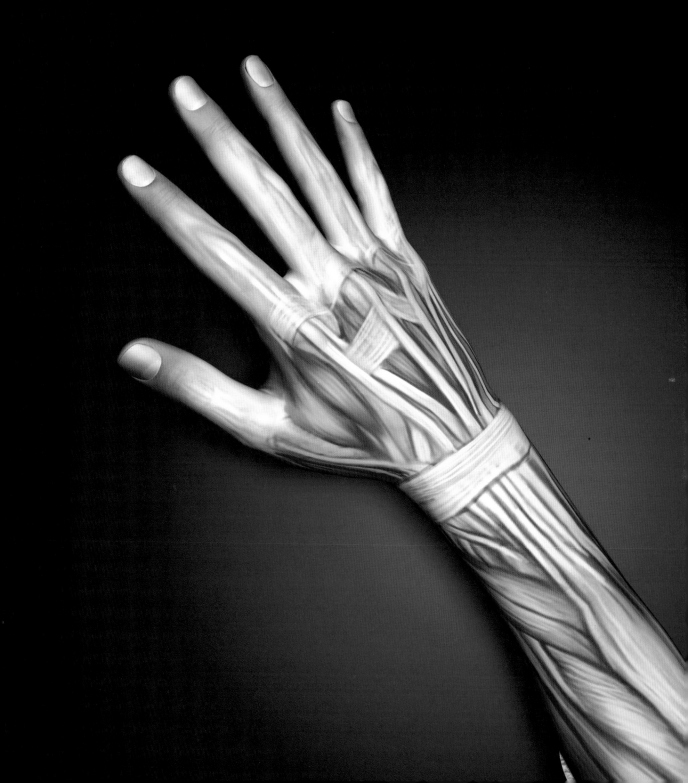

Pancreas Transplant

Herophilus of Chalcedon (335 B.C.–280 B.C.), **Richard C. Lillehei** (1927–1981)

The pancreas is an elongated, light-colored organ, about 7 inches (17.8 cm) long and 1.5 inches (3.8 cm) wide, that lies beneath the stomach and connects to the small intestine at the duodenum. The pancreas was first described in Western civilization by Greek anatomist Herophilus of Chalcedon around 300 B.C., but it wasn't until the 1890s that scientists demonstrated that removal of the pancreas in dogs led to diabetes. Today, we know that the pancreas is both an endocrine gland (which secretes hormones directly into the blood) and an exocrine gland (which secretes substances into ducts). In particular, the pancreas secretes digestive enzymes that pass into the small intestine to break down foods. Among the several hormones produced by the islets of Langerhans in the pancreas is insulin, which decreases glucose in the blood. Individuals afflicted with type 1 diabetes mellitus (DM1) have an immune system that destroys the insulin-secreting cells. Thus, these patients require insulin, often in the form of injections. Even though patients can attempt to stabilize blood sugar levels using insulin injections, the results are not as good as having a functioning pancreas, and DM1 may also cause a variety of secondary problems, such as kidney disease, cardiovascular disease, and damage to the retina.

Pancreas transplants can be performed when an individual is not responding favorably to insulin injections. During such a transplant, the recipient's current pancreas is left in place, where it can continue to help with food digestion, and the donor pancreas (with good insulin-producing cells) is attached to blood vessels in the right lower abdomen.

Pancreatic transplants are not yet considered effective options for individuals with pancreatic **cancer**. The most common form of pancreas transplant involves a simultaneous pancreas-kidney transplant, particularly when the patient is already suffering from diabetes-induced kidney damage. In 1966, the first pancreas transplant was performed by American surgeons Richard Lillehei, William Kelly, and colleagues.

SEE ALSO Tissue Grafting (1597), Murder and Wirsung's Duct (1642), Corneal Transplant (1905), Commercialization of Insulin (1922), Kidney Transplant (1954), Bone Marrow Transplant (1956), Liver Transplant (1963), Lung Transplant (1963), Hand Transplant (1964), Heart Transplant (1967), Cyclosporine (1972), Small Bowel Transplant (1987), Face Transplant (2005), Growing New Organs (2006), and Human Cloning (2008).

Illustration showing the shape and position of the pancreas relative to other organs.

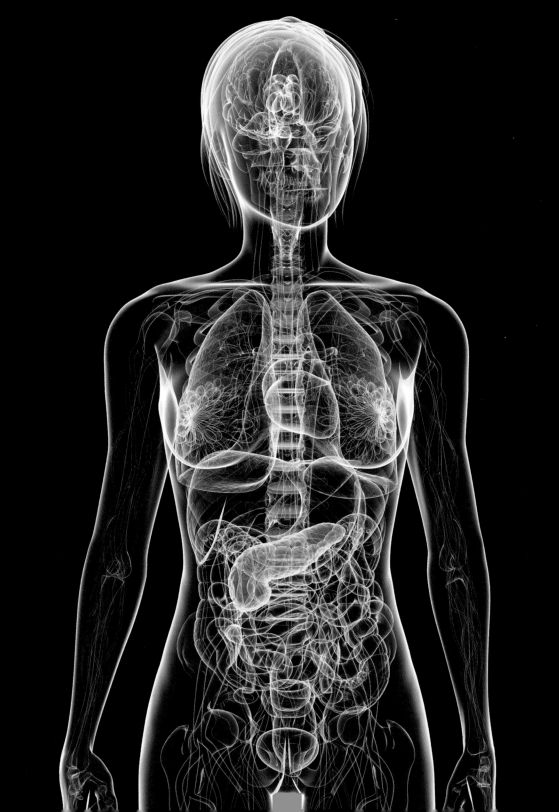

CAT Scans

Sir Godfrey Newbold Hounsfield (1919–2004), **Allan MacLeod Cormack** (1924–1998)

Not long after the 1895 discovery of **X-rays** by physicist Wilhelm Röntgen, X-ray devices were built to examine the interior of the human body. As important as this development was, X-ray images are limited because the body has important anatomical features and tissues, with only slightly different densities, that cannot be distinguished in X-ray images. Also, the traditional X-ray image penetrates through the body, producing images of organs that fall atop one another and cannot be distinguished. Many of these shortcomings were overcome with the invention of the CAT scan (computerized axial tomography—from the Greek word *tomos*, meaning "slice" or "section"—also referred to as the CT scan). For example, a conventional X-ray of a head shows the skull, but a CT scan shows the skull and brain in great detail.

Using a computer, the CT device combines many X-ray images to generate cross-sectional views of the human body. Additionally, the views can be combined to create three-dimensional reconstructions of organs and other structures. The CT hardware includes a doughnut-shaped portion that shoots X-rays—from many different angles—through the body into detectors. CT scans represent one of the first major uses of information-processing technology in medicine.

English electrical engineer Godfrey Hounsfield shared the Nobel Prize with South African physicist Allan Cormack for their work on CT methods and theory. In 1967, Hounsfield began developing the first commercially viable CT scanner while working for the British music and entertainment company EMI. In 1971, a prototype EMI scanner was first used to detect a brain tumor in a patient.

Today, CT scans are useful in detecting tumors, ruling out coronary artery disease, and elucidating bowel obstructions, complex fractures, and damage to intervertebral discs. The CT scan helps surgeons plan reconstructive surgery and design replacement parts, such as hip replacements. With CT pulmonary angiography, CT scans are used with contrast-enhancing dyes to visualize pulmonary embolisms (blockages of arteries of the lung). Helical, or spiral, CT machines continuously slide the patient through the device's X-ray circle.

SEE ALSO X-rays (1895), Radiation Therapy (1903), Mammography (1949), Medical Ultrasound (1957), and Magnetic Resonance Imaging (MRI) (1977).

A CAT scan "slice" through the head and brain. A cross section of the right eye is visible at the upper right.

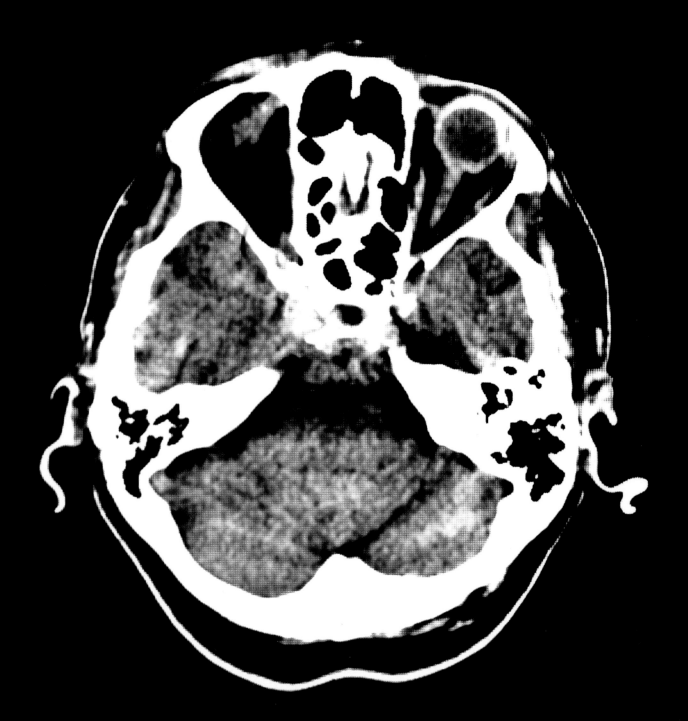

Heart Transplant

James D. Hardy (1918–2003), Christiaan Neethling Barnard (1922–2001), Robert Koffler Jarvik (b. 1946)

Journalist Laura Fitzpatrick writes, "For much of recorded history, many doctors saw the human heart as the inscrutable, throbbing seat of the soul, an agent too delicate to meddle with." However, the possibility of heart transplantation—in which the damaged heart of a recipient is replaced with the healthy heart of a deceased donor—became a possibility after the 1953 invention of the heart-lung machine, a device that could temporarily bypass the heart and lungs during surgery and ensure adequate oxygenation of the blood (see entry "**Heart-Lung Machine**").

In 1964, American surgeon James Hardy performed the first heart transplant when he transplanted the heart of a chimpanzee into the chest of a dying man (no human heart was available). The animal heart beat inside the patient but was too small to keep him alive, and he died after 90 minutes. The world's first successful human-to-human heart transplant took place in 1967, when South African surgeon Christiaan Barnard removed the heart of a young woman who was killed in a car accident. The recipient was Louis Washkansky, a 54-year-old man who suffered from heart disease. A day later, he was awake and talking. He lived for 18 days and then succumbed to pneumonia caused by the immunosuppressive drugs he was taking to combat rejection of the foreign organ tissue.

Organ transplants became much more successful after the 1972 discovery of **cyclosporine**, a compound derived from fungus that suppressed organ rejection while allowing a significant portion of the body's immune system to function normally and fight general infection. The prognosis for heart transplant patients was no longer so bleak. For example, although an extreme case, American Tony Huesman survived for 31 years with a transplanted heart. Today, organs that can be transplanted include the heart, kidneys, liver, lungs, pancreas, and intestines. In 1982, American researcher Robert Jarvik implanted the first permanent artificial heart.

SEE ALSO Tissue Grafting (1597), Vascular Suturing (1902), Artificial Heart Valves (1952), Heart-Lung Machine (1953), Kidney Transplant (1954), Bone Marrow Transplant (1956), Liver Transplant (1963), Lung Transplant (1963), Hand Transplant (1964), Pancreas Transplant (1966), Cyclosporine (1972), Small Bowel Transplant (1987), Face Transplant (2005), and Growing New Organs (2006).

Artwork titled "Transplants, Resurrection, and Modern Medicine." A creative artist depicts the human heart growing from a tree, symbolizing the rejuvenation of life provided to recipients of donor hearts—as well as the "miracle" of modern transplant surgery.

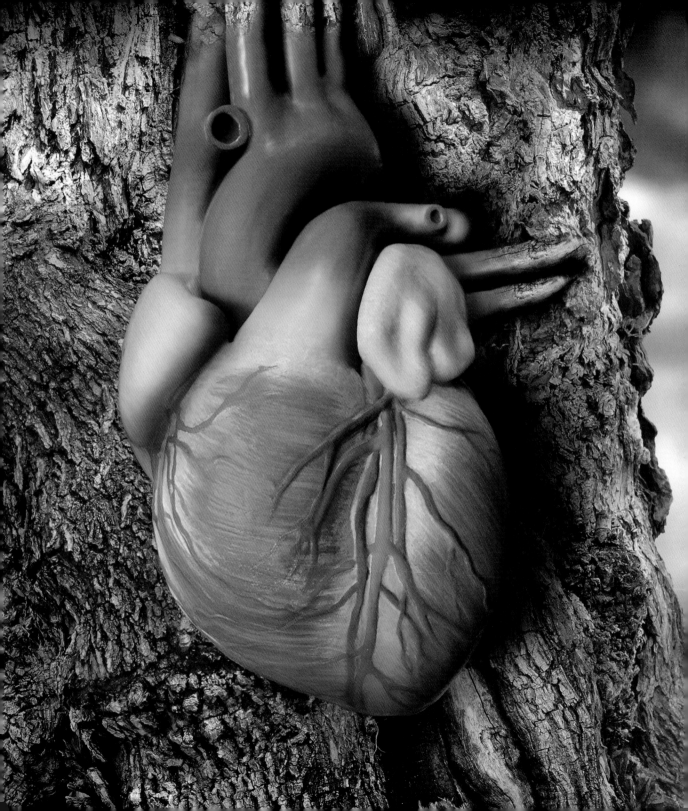

Hospice

Jeanne Garnier (1811–1853), **Cicely Mary Saunders** (1918–2005), **Elisabeth Kübler-Ross** (1926–2004)

Hospice refers to both a philosophy and an approach to caring for the terminally ill, and it often involves reducing pain and addressing the psychological and spiritual needs of the dying. Such care may take place in **hospitals**, nursing homes, and homes of individuals. In the fourteenth century, the Knights Hospitaller of the Order of St. John of Jerusalem (a Christian military order) opened a hospicelike facility on the Greek island of Rhodes to care for the sick and dying. In 1842, widow and bereaved mother Jeanne Garnier helped to found the hospice of L'Association des Dames du Calvaire in Lyon, France.

One of the most important founders of the modern hospice was British **nurse**, physician, and writer Cicely Saunders, who defined the mission of the hospice movement when she said, "We do not have to cure to heal." In 1967, she opened St. Christopher's Hospice in South London.

At about the same time that Saunders was promoting hospice care in the United States and England, along with the notion that dying did not have to be a painful and bleak experience, the Swiss-born psychiatrist Elisabeth Kübler-Ross was also studying how hospitals and society responded to terminal illness. In her 1972 testimony to the U.S. Senate Special Committee on Aging, Kübler-Ross stated, "We live in a very particular death-denying society. We isolate both the dying and the old, and it serves a purpose. They are reminders of our own mortality. We should not institutionalize people. We can give families more help with home care and visiting nurses, giving the families and the patients the spiritual, emotional, and financial help in order to facilitate the final care at home."

As for Saunders, she died at age 87 in the London hospice she founded. Before she died, she wrote, "You matter because you are you. You matter to the last moment of your life, and we will do all we can, not only to help you die peacefully, but also to live until you die."

SEE ALSO Hospitals (1784), Ambulance (1792), Informed Consent (1947), Cryonics (1962), Near-Death Experiences (1975), and Do Not Resuscitate (1991).

Before the Order of the Knights Hospitaller opened the first hospice, the order was first attached to a hospital in Jerusalem, founded around 1023. Shown here is the Siege of Acre (located today in northern Israel), with the Hospitaller Master Mathieu de Clermont defending the walls in 1291. (Painted by D. Papety, 1815–1849.)

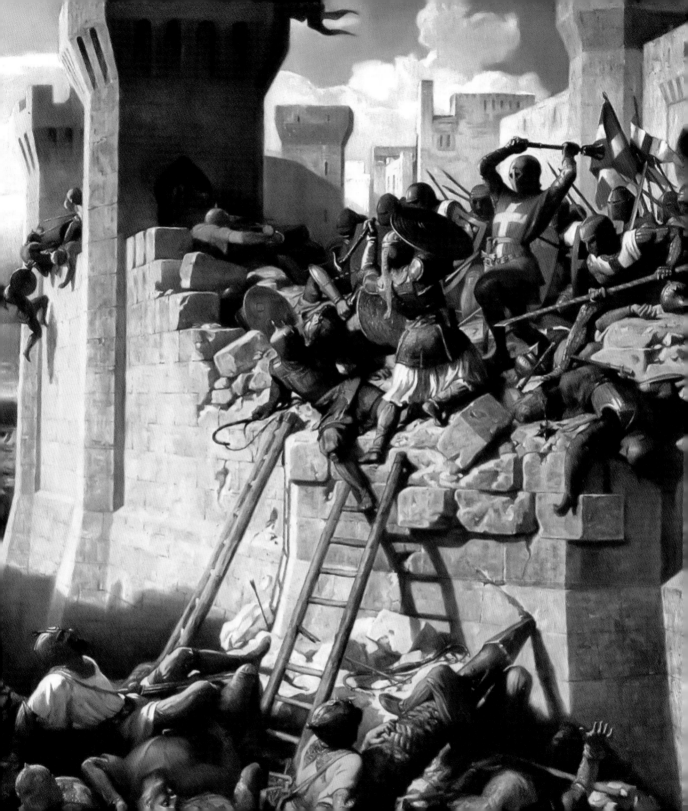

Reverse Transcriptase and AIDS

Howard Martin Temin (1934–1994), **David Baltimore** (b. 1938)

According to one of the central dogmas of biology, information contained in the **DNA** sequences in our cells may be transcribed into RNA molecules, which may be subsequently translated into proteins. However, in 1970 American biologists Howard Temin and David Baltimore independently discovered reverse transcriptase (RT), an enzyme that transcribes single-stranded **RNA** into double-stranded DNA. This discovery led to a more complete understanding of retroviruses such as HIV (human immunodeficiency virus), which causes acquired immunodeficiency syndrome (AIDS), a disease of the human immune system.

A simplified model of a retrovirus consists of a lipid outer membrane (derived from an infected cell's outer membrane) and envelope proteins embedded in this membrane. Within this outer envelope resides a virus protein shell that surrounds two identical single-stranded RNA molecules and molecules of RT. When a retrovirus invades a cell, the virus's envelope protein first binds to a protein receptor on the cell's surface. For example, the envelope protein of HIV subtype-1 binds to a receptor on human T cells (a type of white blood cell). The virus's RT is carried inside the host cell and begins to synthesize DNA copies of the viral RNA. This DNA enters the cell's nucleus, and integrase (an enzyme from the virus) inserts this new DNA into the host's DNA.

These inserts are transcribed by the host's own enzymes into new RNA molecules that are translated by the host into capsid proteins, RT, and envelope proteins. Other copies of these new RNAs are inserted into newly forming virus particles.

In order to combat HIV, drugs have been developed to inhibit RT. Additionally, protease inhibitors can be used to block the action of a virally encoded HIV protease enzyme that the retrovirus needs to mature properly. Fusion inhibitor drugs interfere with the entry of an HIV virion into a human cell, and integrase inhibitors suppress the integrase enzyme. Note that various kinds of retroviruses can cause **cancer** when the newly made viral DNA is inserted in the host DNA, as described in the entry **"Oncogenes."**

SEE ALSO Persecution of Jewish Physicians (1161), Condom (1564), Koch's Tuberculosis Lecture (1882), Discovery of Viruses (1892), Stanley's Crystal Invaders (1935), DNA Structure (1953), Thymus (1961), Oncogenes (1976), and RNA Interference (1998).

Colorized scanning electron micrograph of HIV-1 budding (green) from a cultured lymphocyte. The numerous round bumps on the cell surface represent sites of assembly and budding of virions.

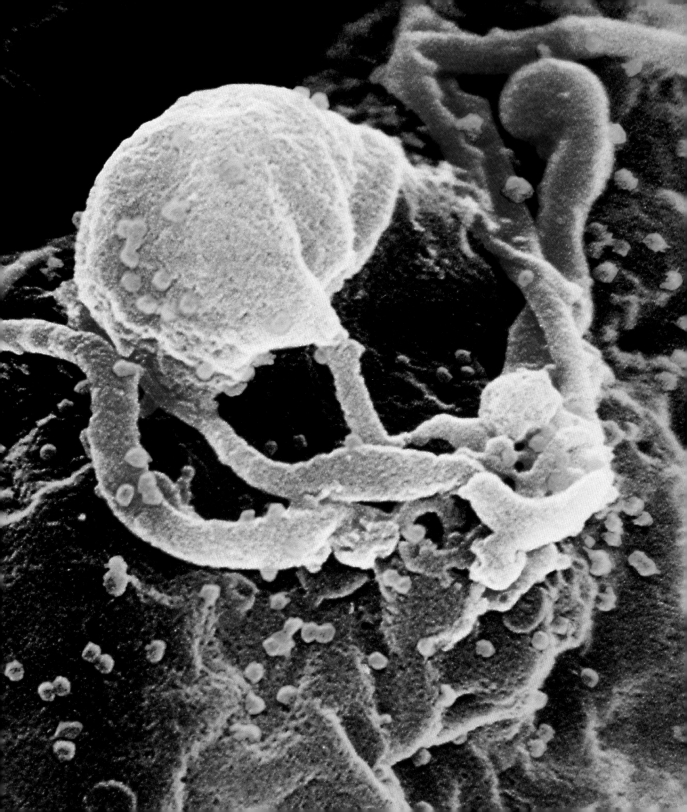

Cyclosporine

Hartmann F. Stähelin (b. 1925), **Thomas E. Starzl** (b. 1926), **Roy Yorke Calne** (b. 1930)

In the 1960s, the odds of surviving organ transplantation (moving an organ from one body to another) were improving, but bodies usually rejected the foreign donor tissue. Journalist Richard Hollingham writes, "Organ transplants were increasingly perceived as the last desperate measure of an increasingly desperate branch of surgery." It was fortuitous that surgeons would soon have a new ally in the quest to save lives.

Immunosuppressive drugs, which inhibit the body's immune system, help to prevent the rejection of transplanted organs. In 1972, researchers at Sandoz, a Swiss pharmaceutical company, implemented a screening test designed by physician Hartmann Stähelin and discovered the immunosuppressive effects of **cyclosporine** (abbreviated Cy and also spelled as cyclosporin and ciclosporin), a compound derived from a fungus. British surgeon Roy Calne and colleagues demonstrated the success of Cy in kidney transplants, and in 1983, the drug was approved for use in the United States for all transplant patients.

American physician Thomas Starzl, who showed that Cy worked most effectively when administered with steroids, demonstrated the success of cyclosporine in decreasing organ rejection in **liver transplants**. Journalist Barry Werth writes, "Cyclosporine made Tom Starzl the most famous and influential transplanter in the world. Transplantation, which had been macabre and dismaying, now gleamed with optimism. . . . There seemed to be no limit to what Starlz could do. In 1984 . . . he replaced both the heart and liver of a six-year-old girl . . . who within two weeks was skipping around the **hospital**."

Cy is notable because it was the first strongly immunosuppressive drug that allowed selective inhibition of T cells (a type of white blood cell) without excessive toxicity, allowing a significant portion of the body's immune system to fight general infection. However, the drug is not perfect, and not all organ rejection can be prevented. Cy must be taken indefinitely by people who have received organ transplants, and the drug may cause kidney damage, in addition to increasing **cancer** risk. Twenty-five years after its discovery, around 200,000 people relied on Cy for transplants.

SEE ALSO Tissue Grafting (1597), Corneal Transplant (1905), Kidney Transplant (1954), Bone Marrow Transplant (1956), Liver Transplant (1963), Lung Transplant (1963), Hand Transplant (1964), Pancreas Transplant (1966), Heart Transplant (1967), Small Bowel Transplant (1987), and Face Transplant (2005).

Molecular ribbon diagram of human cyclophilin A (a protein) in complex with cyclosporine (yellow). The complex inhibits an enzyme, and this inhibition suppresses organ rejection by stopping the production of pro-inflammatory molecules.

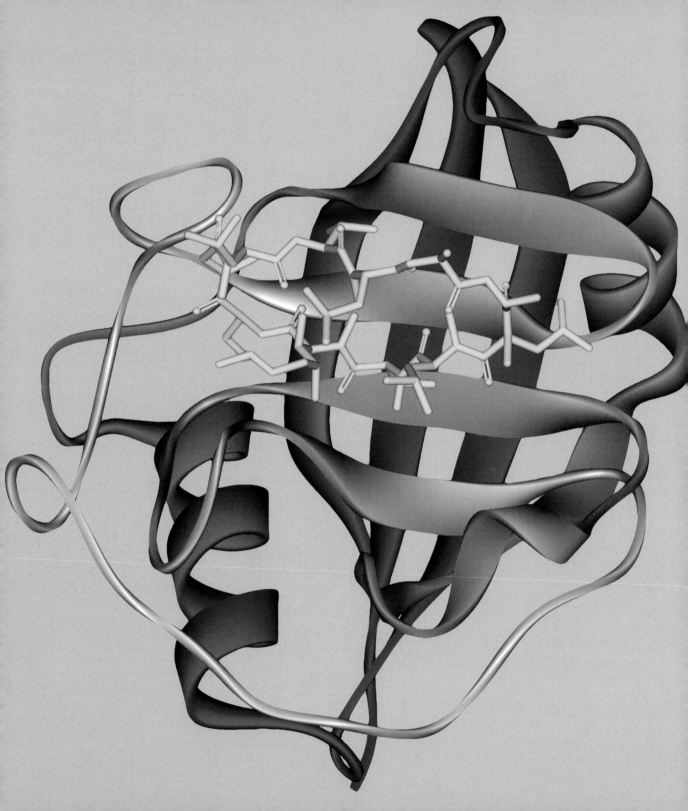

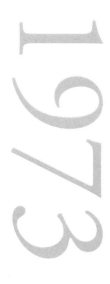

Positron Emission Tomography (PET)

Gordon L. Brownell (1922–2008), **Michael E. Phelps** (b. 1939)

The fictional spaceships in *Star Trek* were powered by antimatter-matter reactions, yet real antimatter-matter reactions have practical applications today in the three-dimensional medical imaging technique called positron emission tomography (PET). Unlike other scanning methods—such as **CAT** or **MRI** scans, which employ **X-rays** and magnetism, respectively—the PET scan provides detailed information on body and tissue *function*.

In preparation for a PET scan, a patient may be injected with a radioactive substance such as the sugar fluorodeoxyglucose (FDG), which contains a radioactive fluorine atom that was made in a cyclotron (particle accelerator). Metabolically active cells, such as **cancer** cells, absorb more FDG than less active cells and tissues. When the fluorine atom decays, it emits a positron—the antimatter form of an electron, with a positive electrical charge. The positron collides with an ordinary electron, creating a burst of energy in the form of gamma rays (high-energy radiation). These gamma rays are then detected by circular detectors that surround the patient and help identify the locations of high FDG concentrations. Today, PET scanners are often integrated with CAT scanners to better show the correspondence between metabolic and anatomical information. Because the radioactive fluorine is short-lived, the patient radiation dose can be low.

Many technologists contributed to the development of PET. For example, in 1953, American physicist Gordon Brownell conducted early research in using positrons for medical imaging of the brain. In 1973, American biophysicist Michael E. Phelps invented a PET device and later worked on other generations of PET scanners that served as prototypes for today's systems.

Although PET scans are not as sharp as CAT and MRI scans, PET scans can be useful in detecting tumors and the spread of cancer, determining the effectiveness of a cancer treatment, studying blood flow in heart muscle, evaluating seizures and **epilepsy**, and predicting the onset of **Alzheimer's disease**, as well as differentiating this disease from other disorders such as Parkinson's disease, Huntington's chorea, and vascular dementia.

SEE ALSO X-rays (1895), Radiation Therapy (1903), Mammography (1949), Medical Ultrasound (1957), Radioimmunoassay (1959), CAT Scans (1967), and Magnetic Resonance Imaging (MRI) (1977).

PET-scan "slice" of a brain, after the patient was injected with the tracer substance FDG. Red areas show high concentrations of accumulated FDG. Blue areas are regions where little tracer has accumulated.

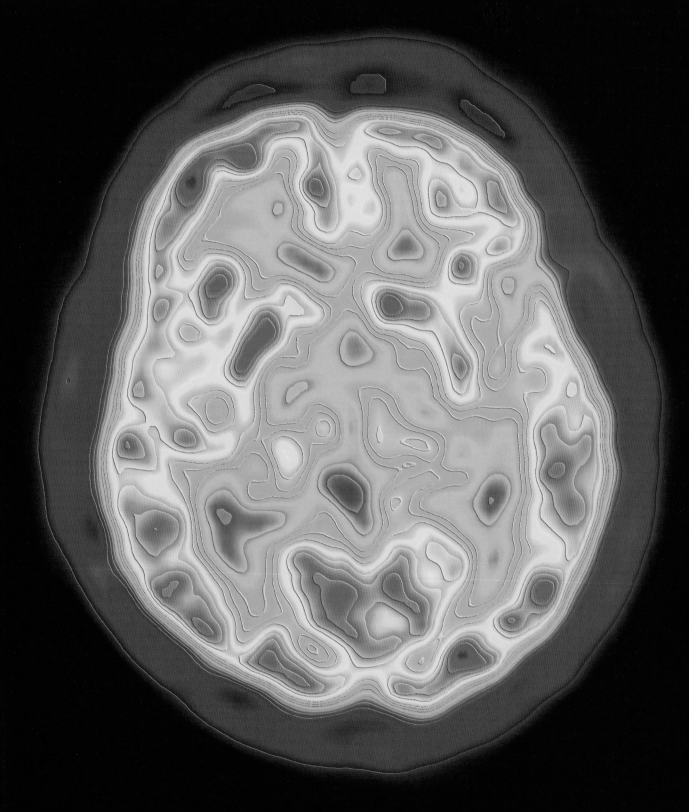

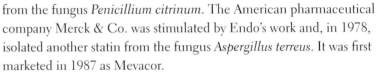

Statins

Akira Endo (b. 1933)

Reporter Peter Landers writes, "It took two years and thousands of moldy broths for Akira Endo to find something that reduces cholesterol. His breakthrough, drawn from a mold like one that grows on oranges, turned out to be the first in a class of medicines that [in 2006] brings $25 billion a year to pharmaceutical companies."

Cholesterol is important to the functioning of every cell in our bodies, but it also contributes to atherosclerosis, in which cholesterol-containing deposits accumulate on the inside of artery walls. These deposits, or plaques, can rupture, leading to the formation of a blood clot. The plaques or clots can reduce the flow of blood and result in angina (chest pain) or heart attack if coronary arteries become blocked. Atherosclerosis is also associated with inflammation of artery walls.

Statins are a class of drugs used to lower cholesterol levels by inhibiting the enzyme HMG-CoA reductase, which the liver uses to produce cholesterol. In 1973, Japanese biochemist Akira Endo discovered the first anticholesterol statin—mevastatin—isolated

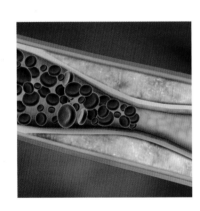

from the fungus *Penicillium citrinum*. The American pharmaceutical company Merck & Co. was stimulated by Endo's work and, in 1978, isolated another statin from the fungus *Aspergillus terreus*. It was first marketed in 1987 as Mevacor.

Statins appear to function in multiple beneficial ways. For example, they reduce LDL (low-density lipoprotein) cholesterol (the "bad" form of cholesterol that contributes to the formation of plaques in the arteries) and inflammation, while maintaining plaque stability. In addition, they increase LDL uptake when liver cells detect reduced levels of liver cholesterol due to statins and compensate by creating LDL *receptors* that draw cholesterol out of the general circulation. Statins are generally accepted as useful in decreasing mortality in people with preexisting cardiovascular disease— and those at high risk—but possible adverse side effects include abnormally elevated liver enzymes and the breakdown of skeletal muscles, which releases products into the bloodstream that are harmful to kidneys and can lead to kidney failure.

SEE ALSO Pulse Watch (1707), Ligation of the Abdominal Aorta (1817), Cortisone (1948), Angioplasty (1964), and Beta-Blockers (1964).

LEFT: *Plaque in artery restricting blood flow.* RIGHT: *The oyster mushroom* (Pleurotus ostreatus, *a culinary mushroom*) *contains the statin lovastatin.*

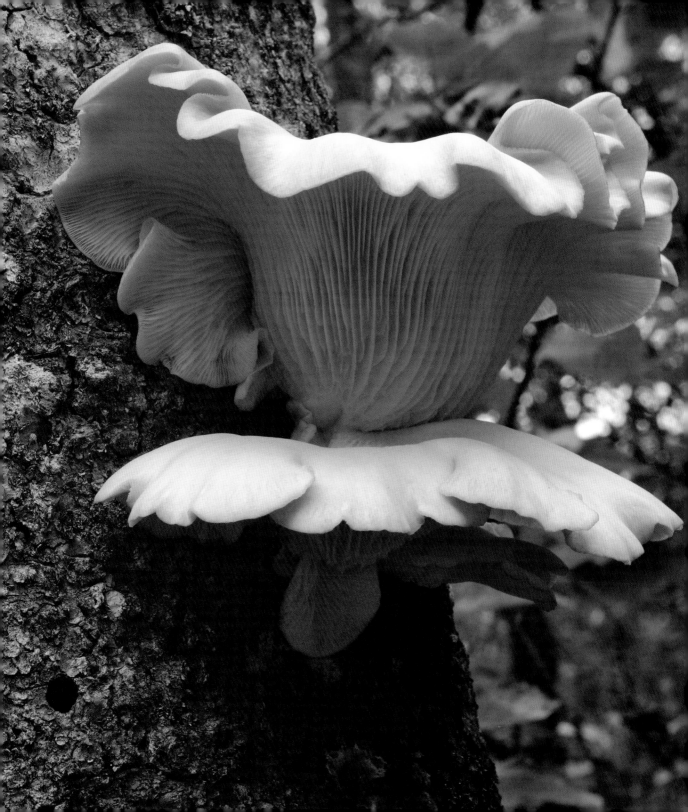

Near-Death Experiences

Plato (428 B.C.–348 B.C.), **Hieronymus Bosch** (1450–1516), **Raymond Moody** (b. 1944)

The Bengali poet Rabindranath Tagore once wrote, "Death is not extinguishing the light; it is putting out the lamp because the dawn has come." Scientists and mystics have long pondered the physical and mental transitions that occur at the threshold of death. In 1975, physician Raymond Moody published his best-selling book *Life After Life*, which provided case studies of people who were without vital signs—including some who were pronounced dead by their physicians—and later revived. Some of the people had NDEs, or near-death experiences (a term Moody coined), in which they felt that they were leaving their bodies and floating up to the ceiling. During an NDE, many saw light at the end of a tunnel and felt serenity or fear, sometimes followed by a loss of fear of death. Some reported seeing the doctors performing medical resuscitation efforts.

While some researchers have suggested that NDEs provide evidence of life after death, or perhaps a movement of consciousness away from the body, others explain such phenomena in purely biological terms, suggesting that the experiences are hallucinations caused by a brain deprived of oxygen (hypoxia) or excess carbon dioxide in the blood (hypercarbia). Some have theorized that endorphins (brain chemicals) may create the euphoric sensations of NDEs. Researchers have also experimented with the hallucinogen ketamine, which can produce an altered state of consciousness resembling an NDE. However, even if the NDEs are hallucinations, physicians study them to better understand the mechanism of NDEs, which often have a profound, lasting psychological effect on the person with the experience.

Of course, the idea of NDEs is not new. In *Republic*, Plato tells the story of Er, a soldier who is killed and journeys toward "a straight light like a pillar, most nearly resembling a rainbow, but brighter and purer." Er later returns to life to spread the news about another world. Hieronymus Bosch produced the startling painting *Ascent into the Empyrean*, showing souls passing through a tunnel toward a light.

SEE ALSO Defibrillator (1899), Searches for the Soul (1907), Jung's Analytical Psychology (1933), Pineal Body (1958), Cryonics (1962), and Hospice (1967).

Ascent of the Blessed (c. 1500), painted by Dutch artist Hieronymus Bosch (c. 1450–1516).

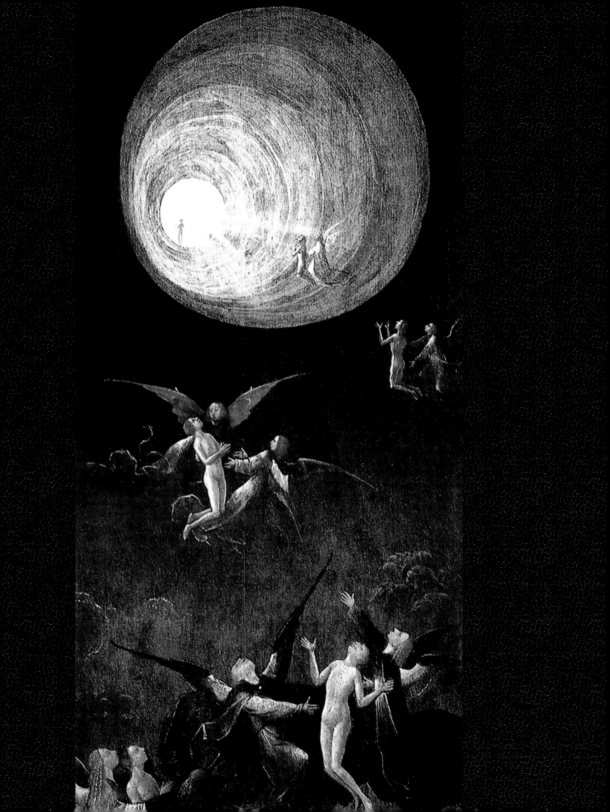

Oncogenes

John Michael Bishop (b. 1936), Harold Elliot Varmus (b. 1939)

The process of cell division relies on a specific sequence of events that involves the proper processing of information contained in our genes. When this process malfunctions, unregulated cell growth, or **cancer**, can occur. Two general mechanisms exist that facilitate the cell's progression to a cancer state. The first involves proto-oncogenes, whose normal activity promotes healthy cell proliferation. In an altered form, such as might occur due to mutation in its genetic sequence, the proto-oncogene becomes an oncogene that, in turn, promotes excessive cell growth. Mutation may be triggered by radiation, chemicals, or other means.

On the other hand, tumor-suppressor (TS) genes *inhibit* events that promote a cancerous state. For example, some useful TS gene products may lead abnormal cells to apoptosis (a normal and beneficial process of cell death). By analogy with a car, oncogenes are accelerator pedals that are stuck, as if pressed down to the floor, and TS genes are the brakes. If either the pedal or the brakes malfunction, the car may careen wildly out of control.

In 1976, American biologists J. Michael Bishop and Harold E. Varmus showed that oncogenes were defective proto-oncogenes found in many organisms, including humans. Bishop once likened proto-oncogenes to the material on which cancer-causing agents can act, the "keyboards on which various carcinogens can play."

Cancer-causing genes were first discovered in viruses and shown to be copies of normal cellular genes. In short, the viral oncogenes were proto-oncogenes that had been incorporated into the viruses in slightly altered form. When the virus invades a host cell, inserting additional viral oncogenic genes, these may dangerously enhance the existing proto-oncogene activity. Cancers caused by these oncoviruses may sometimes be prevented by vaccinations against the virus, and some oncogenic proteins in cancer cells can be targeted by monoclonal antibodies. Additionally, the expression of oncogenes can sometimes be suppressed by small **RNA** molecules called microRNAs. On the other hand, mutations in such microRNAs (oncomirs) can activate oncogenes.

SEE ALSO Causes of Cancer (1761), Cell Division (1855), Mendel's Genetics (1865), Discovery of Viruses (1892), Stanley's Crystal Invaders (1935), Reverse Transcriptase and AIDS (1970), Epigenetics (1983), Gene Therapy (1990), and RNA Interference (1998).

Molecular model of tumor-suppressor protein p53 binding to a strand of DNA. Cancers may be caused by mutations that inactivate this protein, which normally behaves as a "guardian of the genome." Oncogenes are the accelerator pedals, and p53 is a brake.

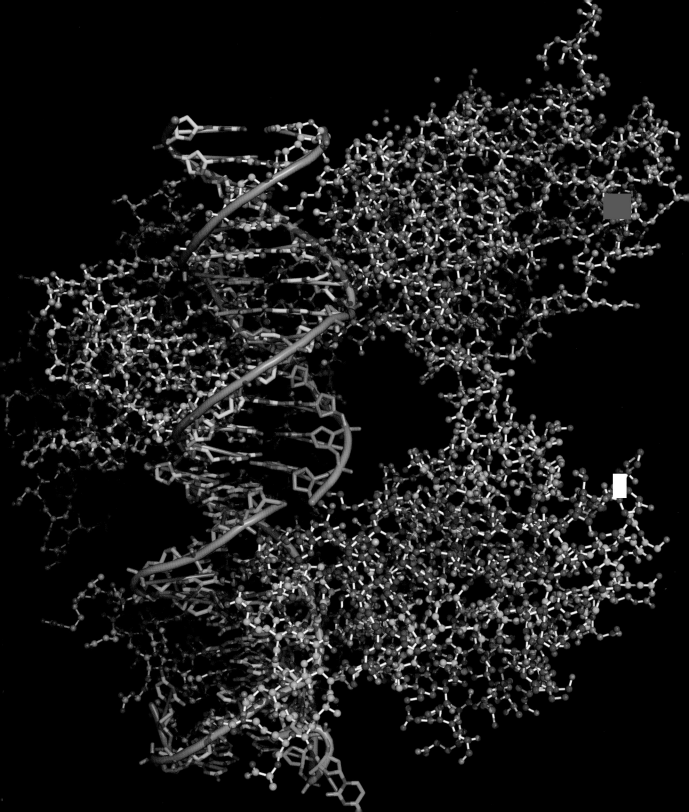

Cochlear Implants

André Djourno (1904–1996), **Charles Eyries** (1908–1996),
Adam M. Kissiah Jr. (b. 1947)

According to the biblical prophet Isaiah, there will come a time when "the eyes of the blind shall be opened, and the ears of the deaf unstopped." Nevertheless, throughout history, the deaf have been mistreated or seen as outcasts. One of the most prejudiced pronouncements is attributed to the Greek polymath Aristotle: "Those who are born deaf all become senseless and incapable of reason."

In humans, sound travels to the cochlea, a spiral, fluid-filled organ of the inner ear. Microscopic hairs project into the fluid, vibrate in response to sound waves, and convert the sounds into nerve impulses that travel along the auditory nerve to the brain. Missing or abnormal hair cells may result in a sensorineural hearing impairment, which results from developmental abnormalities, trauma, or disease.

A cochlear implant (CI) is an electronic device that provides a sense of sound to the deaf. The external portion makes use of a microphone, a speech processor that divides the sounds into several frequency channels, and a transmitter that sends the processed sound (through electromagnetic induction) to a receiver beneath the skin. The signals are then sent to an array of electrodes that wind through the cochlea. CIs are usually most effective for the newly deaf or when implanted in deaf children at a very early age (younger than two). For an older person who has been deaf for a long period of time or has never heard, the brain may have great difficulty adapting to this new sensory input.

Early research in CIs included the 1957 work of French-Algerian surgeons André Djourno and Charles Eyries, who placed a wire on an auditory nerve exposed during an operation. The deaf patient heard sounds like "a roulette wheel" and "a cricket" when a current was applied. Early devices could not be used to understand speech but helped with lip-reading. In 1977, American engineer Adam Kissiah received a foundational U.S. patent for digital-electronics stimulation of the acoustic nerve in humans.

SEE ALSO Eyeglasses (1284), Cranial Nerves Classified (1664), Exploring the Labyrinth (1772), Stethoscope (1816), and Hearing Aids (1899).

Illustration of electric acoustic stimulation, a combination of a hearing aid and a cochlear implant in the same ear. A collection of electrodes winds through the spiraling cochlea.

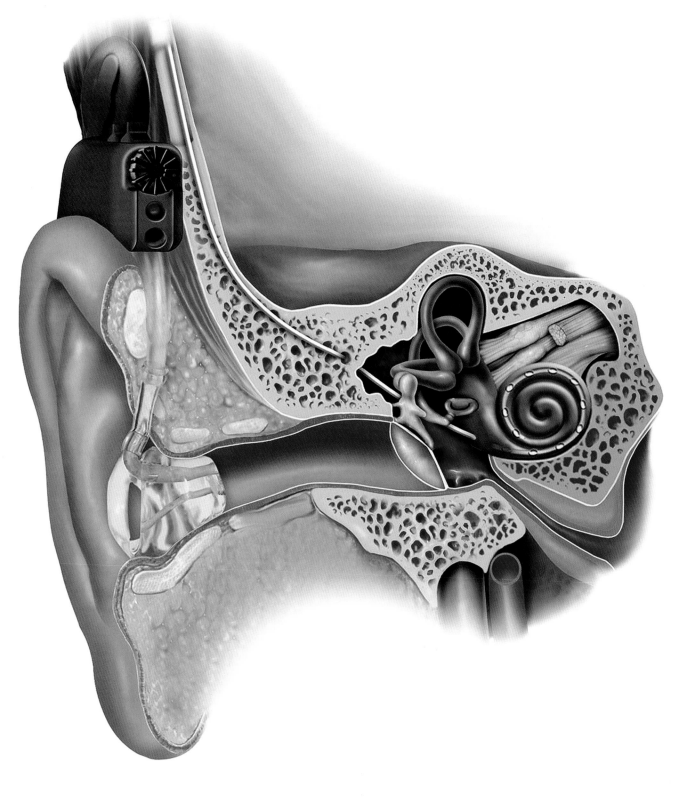

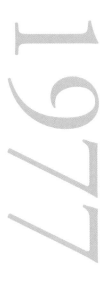

Magnetic Resonance Imaging (MRI)

Paul Christian Lauterbur (1929–2007), **Peter Mansfield** (b. 1933), **Raymond Vahan Damadian** (b. 1936)

MRI (magnetic resonance imaging) uses magnetism, radio waves, and a computer to visualize internal structures of the body—with greater contrast between soft tissues than provided by **X-ray** images or **CAT scans**. During an MRI scan, a patient is typically placed within a large circular tube that creates a strong magnetic field.

If an atomic nucleus has at least one neutron or proton unpaired, the nucleus may act like a tiny magnet. The magnetic field exerts a force that can be visualized as causing the nuclei to precess, or wobble, like a spinning top. The energy difference between nuclear spin states can be made larger by increasing the external magnetic field. After turning on the magnetic field, radio waves induce transitions between spin states, placing some of the spins into their higher-energy states. If the radio wave is turned off, the spins return (or "relax") to the lower state and produce a detectable radio signal at the resonant frequency of the spin flip.

In 1971, American physician Raymond Damadian showed that the hydrogen relaxation rates of water could be different in normal and malignant cells, opening the possibility of using MRI in medical diagnosis. In 1977, he performed a scan of an entire human body. American chemist Paul Lauterbur contributed to the generation of MRI images using gradients in the magnetic field, and British physicist Peter Mansfield created mathematical methods for efficiently producing the images.

MRI is useful for scanning tissues containing many hydrogen nuclei (e.g., water molecules) such as the brain, spinal cord, intervertebral discs, and heart. Unlike X-rays, MRI uses no dangerous ionizing radiation and can provide information on the chemical composition of a tissue. Contrast agents (e.g., solutions containing the metal gadolinium) may be injected to enhance visual contrast. Diffusion MRI can be used to measure the diffusion of water in tissues. Functional MRI enables the study of brain activity in real time.

SEE ALSO X-rays (1895), Radiation Therapy (1903), Mammography (1949), Medical Ultrasound (1957), CAT Scans (1967), and Positron Emission Tomography (1973).

An MRI/MRA (magnetic resonance angiogram) of the brain vasculature (arteries). This kind of MRI study is often used to reveal brain aneurysms.

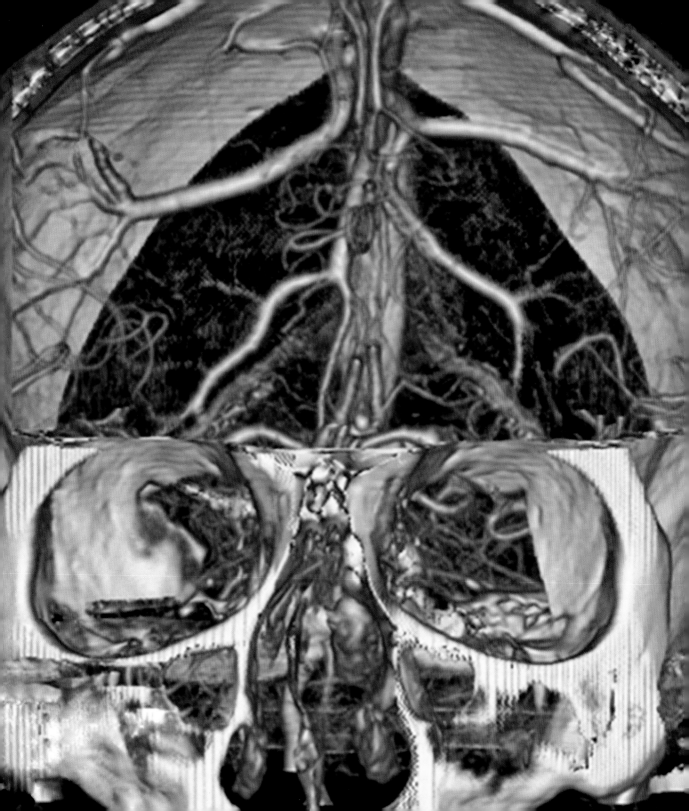

First Test-Tube Baby

Patrick Christopher Steptoe (1913–1988), **Robert Geoffrey Edwards** (b. 1925), **Louise Joy Brown** (b. 1978)

According to a July 1978 issue of *TIME*, "Banner headlines . . . called it OUR MIRACLE and BABY OF THE CENTURY. Some commentators heralded the coming birth as a miracle of modern medicine, comparable to the first **kidney** and **heart transplants**. Theologians [and some] scientists sounded warnings about its disturbing moral, ethical, and social implications."

In vitro fertilization (IVF) refers to a procedure in which egg cells are fertilized by **sperm** outside the body. A woman is given hormones to stimulate her ovaries to produce several eggs, and a physician subsequently inserts a needle through the vagina and into the woman's ovaries to remove eggs. Sperm and eggs are combined in a laboratory dish that contains a supportive medium to nourish the eggs. After a period of time (two or three days), the doctor transfers the very early embryos (e.g., consisting of eight cells) into the woman's uterus, and she is given hormones (e.g., progesterone) for a period of time to sustain the uterine lining and facilitate embryo survival. The resulting babies have been informally referred to as test-tube babies.

Couples who are infertile—for example, because the woman has damaged fallopian tubes that prevent eggs from entering the uterus from the ovaries—may chose IVF as a means to facilitate pregnancy. Intracytoplasmic sperm injection (ICSI) may be used to directly inject a sperm cell into an egg in some cases of male infertility.

More than one embryo is typically transferred to the uterus to increase the likelihood that at least one embryo will develop. Preimplantation genetic diagnosis (PGD) can be used to screen embryos for chromosomal abnormalities before they are implanted in the uterus. Embryos may also be frozen and stored for later use.

On July 25, 1978, Louise Brown, the first test-tube baby, was born as a result of the pioneering IVF methods of British physician Patrick Steptoe and physiologist Robert Edwards. More than a million babies have since been born using IVF methods. Citing the dissociation of the sexual act and the procreative act, the Roman Catholic Church opposes the practice of IVF.

SEE ALSO Abortion (70), Discovery of Sperm (1678), Separation of Conjoined Twins (1689), Salpingectomy (1883), Amniocentesis (1952), Cryonics (1962), and Human Cloning (2008).

Although actual "test-tube babies" are created when a physician transfers very early embryos into the woman's uterus, in the early days of IVF, some people thought it meant that the baby was raised outside the womb, creatively illustrated here.

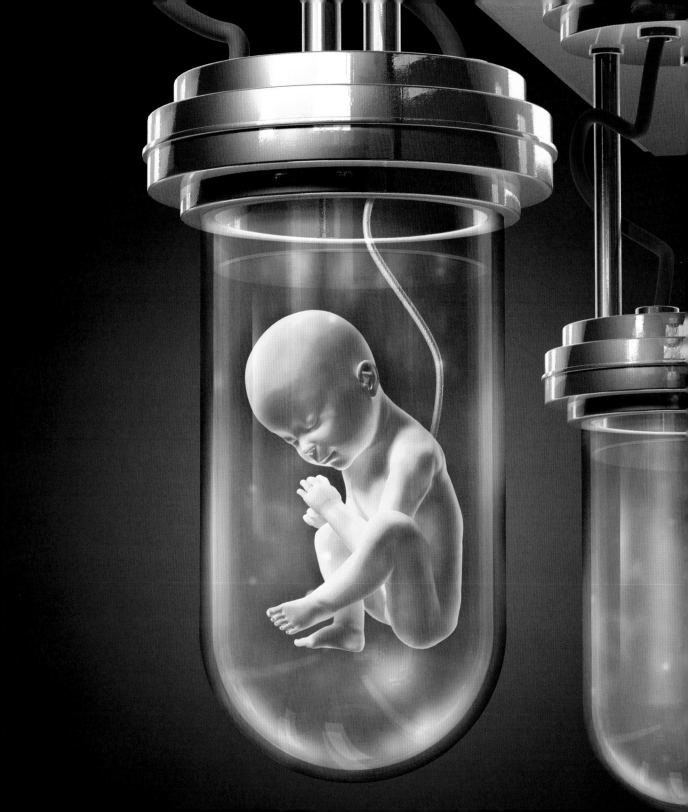

Fetal Surgery

Michael R. Harrison (b. 1943)

Physician Pamela Camosy writes, "Treatment of the *unborn* patient is an exciting endeavor that is itself in its infancy. The heretofore hidden world of the fetus is coming under closer scrutiny, and the scope of medicine, both its science and its humanity, has been forever broadened." Fetal surgery refers to operations performed on the fetus before birth, while it is still in the womb. Usually performed when the life of the fetus is in jeopardy, fetal surgery comes in several forms. In open fetal surgery, a surgeon cuts into the mother's abdomen and uterus in order to operate on the fetus, which still remains connected to the mother via the umbilical cord and placenta. The fetus is returned to the uterus, and the uterine and abdominal walls are closed. A second surgery (a **cesarean section**) is performed when the baby is finally delivered. One challenge of this surgery is to prevent the mother from going into labor prematurely as a result of the surgeon's damaging the uterus. Minimally invasive fetoscopic surgery, also called Fetendo (because of its similarity to playing a Nintendo video game), uses real-time video and a tubelike fetoscope (see entry "**Endoscope**") to guide small surgical instruments to the site of the surgery.

In 1981, pediatric surgeon Michael Harrison performed the first human open fetal surgery at the University of California, San Francisco, in order to save a fetus whose bladder was dangerously enlarged due to a blockage in its urinary tract. Harrison inserted a catheter (tube) to allow the urine to drain, and the baby survived.

Ultrasound may reveal a variety of malformations of the fetus, and fetal surgery may be performed to open fetal heart valves, repair hernias of the diaphragm, remove life-threatening tumors attached to the fetus's tailbone (sacrococcygeal teratomas), and repair incomplete closures of the embryonic neural tube associated with the spina bifida birth defect. Selective **laser** photocoagulation is used to seal off blood vessels that can allow certain improper and dangerous flow of blood between twin fetuses.

SEE ALSO Separation of Conjoined Twins (1689), Cesarean Section (1882), Amniocentesis (1952), Endoscope (1954), Fetal Monitoring (1957), Medical Ultrasound (1957), and Thalidomide Disaster (1962).

LEFT: *Minimally invasive fetal surgery can be used to treat twin-to-twin transfusion syndrome (TTTS) in which one twin receives a disproportionate blood supply.* RIGHT: *De Wikkellkinderen (1617), by an unknown artist, with one pale twin, may represent a TTTS outcome.*

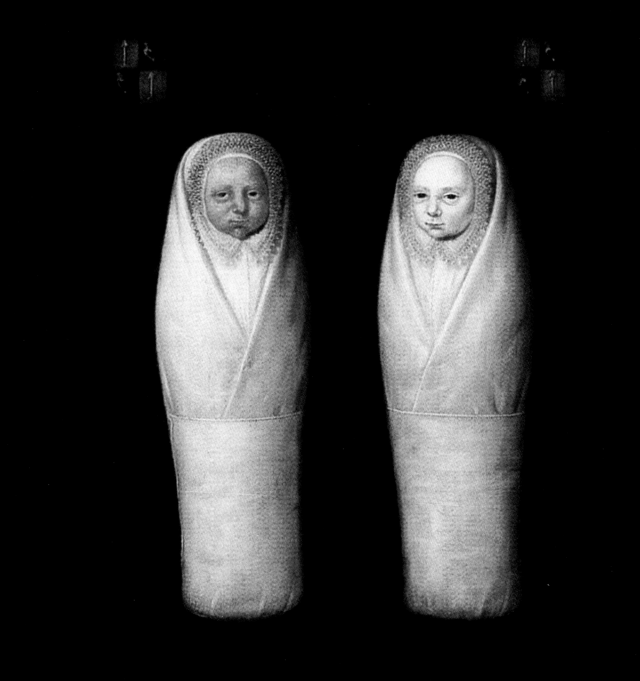

Laparoscopic Surgery

Georg Kelling (1866–1945), **Hans Christian Jacobaeus** (1879–1937), **Kurt Karl Stephan Semm** (1927–2003), **Philippe Mouret** (1938–2008), **Erich Mühe** (1938–2005)

Laparoscopic surgery, also referred to as keyhole surgery or minimally invasive surgery, is performed through small incisions. An **endoscope** is a tubelike device used by physicians to peer within the body, often through an existing orifice such as the mouth. In abdominal or pelvic surgery, a laparoscope is often used, which includes digital electronics such as a charge-coupled device placed at the end of the laparoscope to capture video images. Additionally, a fiber-optic system provides illumination within the body. In endoscopic procedures, instruments are usually passed through small channels in the endoscope itself, but laparoscopic surgery usually involves instruments that are introduced through trocars (sharp-pointed surgical shafts used as entry ports to the body), which provide different channels for manipulation of surgical instruments. Laparoscopic surgery has several potential advantages over traditional surgery, including reduced bleeding, quicker patient recovery with less pain and less scarring, and reduced infections.

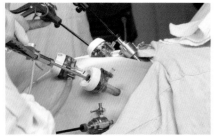

Some of the forerunners of laparoscopic procedures were performed by Swedish physician Hans Jacobaeus, starting around 1910. In 1981, German surgeon Kurt Semm performed the first laparoscopic **appendectomy**. German surgeon Erich Mühe (in 1985) and French surgeon Philippe Mouret (in 1987) performed the earliest laparoscopic cholecystectomies (gallbladder removals). It wasn't until around 1986, however, that laparoscopic surgical methods became an integral part of general surgery, following the development of a video computer chip that allowed the magnification and projection of images onto television screens.

Physicians Shelly Spaner and Garth Warnock write, "The rapid acceptance of the technique of laparoscopic surgery by the general population is unparalleled in surgical history. It has changed the field of general surgery more drastically and more rapidly than any other surgical milestone."

SEE ALSO Sutures (3000 B.C.), Hysterectomy (1813), General Anesthesia (1842), Appendectomy (1848), Salpingectomy (1883), Endoscope (1954), Laser (1960), Robotic Surgery (2000), and Telesurgery (2001).

LEFT: *Preparing for gastric bypass surgery.* RIGHT: *Diagram of a laparoscopic surgical instrument from U.S. Patent 5,480,409. The jaws labeled 215 and 216 can be opened and closed within the body.*

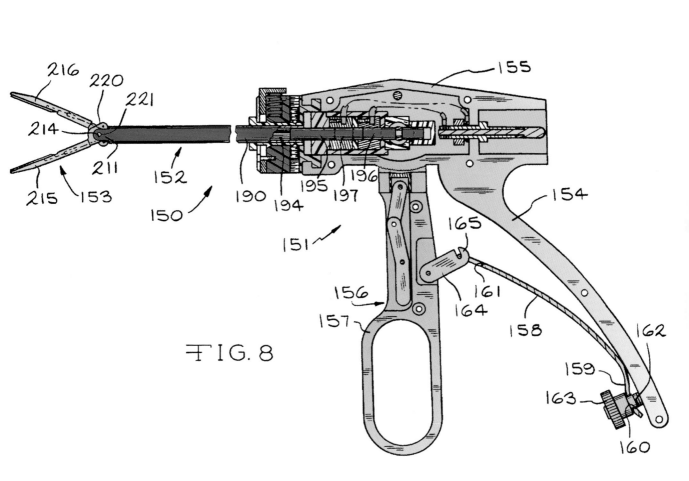

216
220
221
214
211
215
153
152
150
151
190
194
195
197
196
155
154
165
161
164
156
157
158
162
159
163
160

FIG. 8

Prions

Stanley Ben Prusiner (b. 1942), Daniel Carleton Gajdusek (1923–2008)

As in the fictional story of Dr. Jekyll and Mr. Hyde, in which a good personality and an evil personality lurk within the same person, the devastating prion diseases appear to be caused by a protein that has a beneficial and a devastating form. In 1982, American neurologist and biochemist Stanley Prusiner coined the term *prion* when referring to a disease-causing agent he researched that appeared to be solely composed of protein. In contrast, even **viruses** contain genetic information in the form of **DNA** or RNA, in addition to protein.

The small prion protein (PrP) exists in at least two three-dimensional shapes. In the normal cellular form (PrP-C), the protein may serve several useful purposes, such as maintaining the insulation that facilitates electrical signals along nerve fibers. In its deadly shape (PrP-Sc, where the Sc indicates scrapie, a prion disease of sheep), the protein causes destruction of the brain. Some prion diseases that run in families, such as Creutzfeldt-Jakob disease, can be acquired genetically through a mutation of the gene that codes for PrP. However, the same kind of disease can also be acquired by eating beef from cows infected with prions. In cows, the disease is known as bovine spongiform encephalopathy (BSE), or "mad cow" disease. Another example of acquired prion disease is kuru, which American physician Daniel Gajdusek researched in the Fore tribe of Papua New Guinea. Kuru appears to be caused by eating the brains of dead, infected kinsmen.

Researchers are still investigating how the deadly PrP-Sc converts PrP-C into more PrP-Sc. As the abnormal protein accumulates in the brain, it forms clumps and destroys brain cells, producing spongelike holes in the brain, loss of motor control, dementia, and death. Unfortunately, PrP-Sc is very stable and resists destruction by chemicals and physical agents. Also, it does not stimulate inflammation, and the immune system is not triggered to fight the disease. Genetically engineered mice that do not produce any PrP cannot be infected with prion disease.

SEE ALSO Mendel's Genetics (1865), Discovery of Viruses (1892), Alzheimer's Disease (1906), Meat Inspection Act of 1906 (1906), and DNA Structure (1953).

A British outbreak of BSE occurred when cattle were fed infected meat and bonemeal. The disease may infect people who eat food containing parts of infected animals. Today, laws restrict the use of ruminant-derived protein supplements in cattle feed.

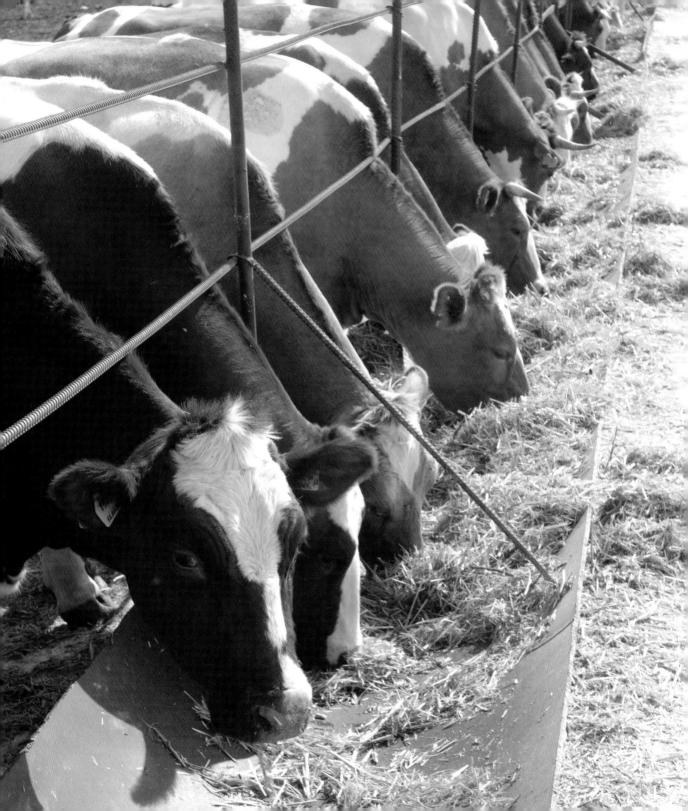

Epigenetics

Bert Vogelstein (b. 1949)

Just as a pianist interprets the notes in a musical score, controlling the volume and tempo, epigenetics affects the interpretation of **DNA genetic** sequences in cells. Epigenetics usually refers to the study of heritable traits that do not involve changes to the underlying DNA sequences of cells.

One way in which DNA expression can be controlled is by the addition of a methyl group (a carbon atom with three attached hydrogen atoms) to one of the DNA bases, making this "marked" area of the DNA less active and potentially suppressing the production of a particular protein. Gene expression can also be modified by the histone proteins that bind to the DNA molecule.

In the 1980s, Swedish researcher Lars Olov Bygren discovered that boys in Norrbotten, Sweden, who had gone from normal eating to vast overeating in a single season produced sons and grandsons who lived much shorter lives. One hypothesis is that inherited epigenetic factors played a role. Other studies suggest that environmental factors such as stress, diet, smoking, and prenatal nutrition make imprints on our genes that are passed through generations. According to this argument, the air your grandparents breathed and the food they ate can affect your health decades later.

In 1983, American medical researchers Bert Vogelstein and Andrew P. Feinberg documented the first example of a human disease with an epigenetic mechanism. In particular, they observed widespread loss of DNA methylation in colorectal **cancers**. Because methylated genes are typically turned off, this loss of methylation can lead to abnormal *activation* of genes in cancer. Additionally, too much methylation can undo the work of protective tumor-suppressor genes. Drugs are currently being developed that affect epigenetic markers that silence bad genes and activate good ones.

The general concept of epigenetics is not new. After all, a brain cell and liver cell have the same DNA sequence, but different genes are activated through epigenetics. Epigenetics may explain why one identical twin develops asthma or bipolar disorder while the other remains healthy.

SEE ALSO Causes of Cancer (1761), Mendel's Genetics (1865), Chromosomal Theory of Inheritance (1902), DNA Structure (1953), Oncogenes (1976), Gene Therapy (1990), RNA Interference (1998), and Human Genome Project (2003).

Loss of DNA methylation (marking) can occur in colorectal cancer, such as in the polyps shown here. Because methylated genes are typically turned off, this loss of methylation can lead to abnormal activation of genes involved in cancer.

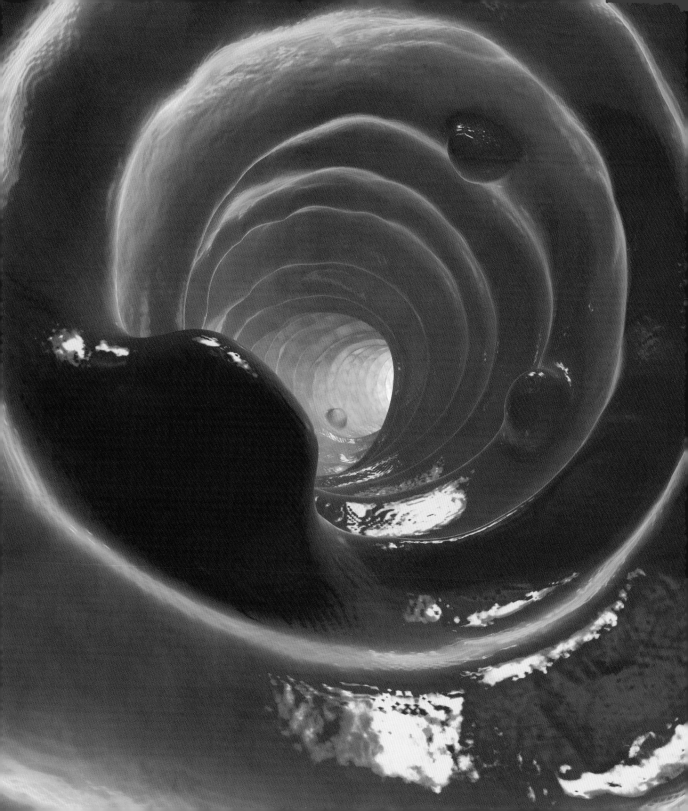

Polymerase Chain Reaction

Kary Banks Mullis (b. 1944)

In 1983, while driving along a California highway, biochemist Kary Mullis had an idea for how to copy a microscopic strand of genetic material billions of times within hours—a process that has since had countless applications in medicine. Although his idea for the polymerase chain reaction (PCR) turned into a billion-dollar industry, he received only a $10,000 bonus from his employer. Perhaps his Nobel Prize ten years later can be viewed as a sufficiently awesome consolation prize.

Scientists usually require a significant amount of a particular **DNA** genetic sequence in order to study it. The groundbreaking PCR technique, however, can start with as little as a single molecule of the DNA in a solution, with the aid of Taq polymerase, an enzyme that copies DNA and that stays intact when the solution is heated. (Taq polymerase was originally isolated from a bacterium that thrived in a hot spring of America's Yellowstone National Park.) Also added to the brew are primers— short segments of DNA that bind to the sample DNA at a position before and after the sequence under study. During repeated cycles of heating and cooling, the polymerase begins to rapidly make more and more copies of the sample DNA between the primers. The thermal cycling allows the DNA strands to repeatedly pull apart and come together as needed for the copying process. PCR can be used for detecting food-borne pathogens, diagnosing genetic diseases, assessing the level of HIV viruses in AIDS patients, determining paternity of babies, finding criminals based on traces of DNA left at a crime scene, and studying DNA in fossils. PCR was important in advancing the **Human Genome Project**.

Medical journalist Tabitha Powlege writes, "PCR is doing for genetic material what the invention of the printing press did for written material—making copying easy, inexpensive, and accessible." The *New York Times* referred to Mullis's invention as "dividing biology into the two epochs of before PCR and after PCR."

SEE ALSO DNA Structure (1953), Reverse Transcriptase and AIDS (1970), and Human Genome Project (2003).

PCR has been used to amplify DNA from 14,000-year-old fossil bones of saber-toothed cats preserved in asphalt. Such studies help scientists compare these extinct animals to various living cat species in order to better understand cat evolution.

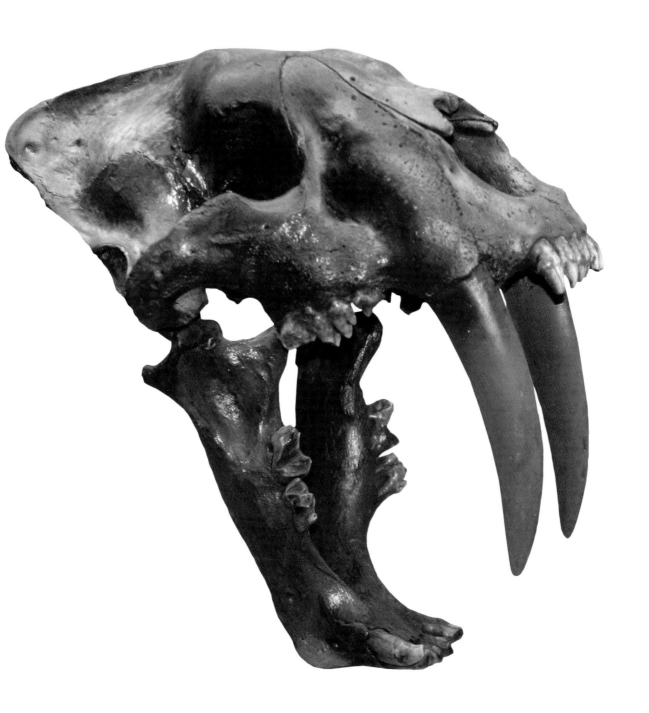

Peptic Ulcers and Bacteria

Marcellus Donatus of Mantua (1538–1602), **John Lykoudis** (1910–1980), **John Robin Warren** (b. 1937), **Barry James Marshall** (b. 1951)

In 1586, Italian physician Marcellus Donatus of Mantua was among the first to document open sores in the lining of the stomach after performing an **autopsy**. Until recently, peptic ulcers of the stomach and neighboring duodenum were believed to be caused by stress and diet. Today, we know that a majority of such ulcers are caused by *Helicobacter pylori*, a spiral-shaped bacterium that thrives in the acidic environment of the stomach. Medical acceptance of the bacterial cause resulted from the pioneering efforts of Australian researchers Robin Warren and Barry Marshall. In 1984, to help convince his skeptical colleagues, Marshall actually drank the contents of a petri dish containing *H. pylori*, and five days later he developed gastritis (inflammation of the stomach lining).

Ulcers may cause abdominal pain and vomiting of blood. Perforation of the stomach or duodenum can be life-threatening. When *H. pylori* colonizes the stomach, it can cause chronic inflammation and increase or decrease gastrin secretion, which controls the amount of acid in the stomach. *H. pylori* can be detected by stomach or duodenum cultures, blood tests (for antibodies), stool tests (for antigens), and a urea breath test, in which the patient ingests radioactive urea. If radioactive carbon dioxide is detected in the breath, it is likely that *H. pylori* has digested the carbon-containing urea. *H. pylori* is thought to be transmitted though food, water, and human saliva. However, only a minority of people with *H. pylori* actually develop ulcers, for reasons that may involve genetic predisposition and the varying virulence of *H. pylori* strains.

Treatment of *H. pylori* includes the combination of antibiotics, bismuth compounds, and proton-pump inhibitors that reduce stomach acidity. Interestingly, in 1958, Greek physician John Lykoudis developed his own antibiotic treatment for ulcers, but his work was largely shunned by other physicians.

Peptic ulcers can also be caused by **aspirin**, ibuprofen, and other NSAIDs (nonsteroidal anti-inflammatory drugs). NSAIDs can decrease the production of prostaglandins (hormonelike molecules), which normally stimulate the production of protective mucus in the stomach.

SEE ALSO Brunner's Glands (1679), Autopsy (1761), Observations of St. Martin's Stomach (1833), Penicillin (1928), and Medical Self-Experimentation (1929).

Artistic rendition of H. pylori *with its four to six flagella (whiplike tails), which allow the bacterium to move through the mucus lining to reach the stomach epithelium.*

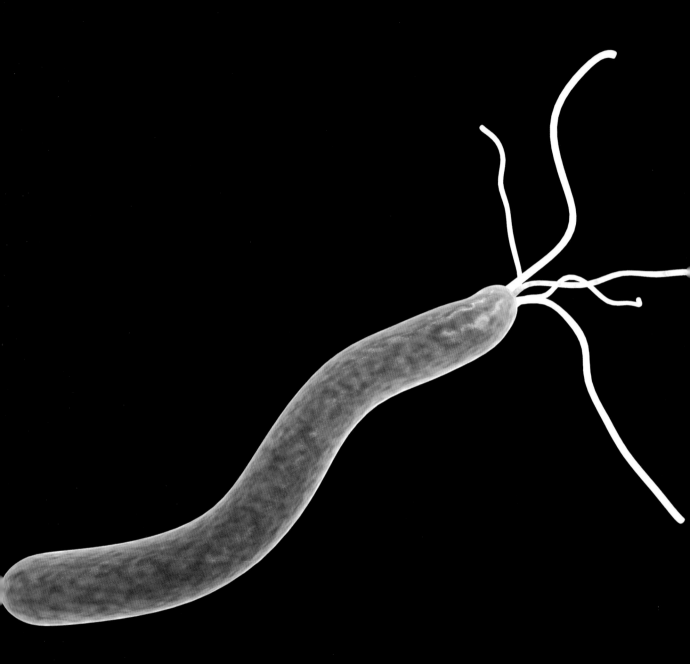

Telomerase

Elizabeth Helen Blackburn (b. 1948), Carolyn Widney "Carol" Greider (b. 1961)

The chromosomes in our cells are each made of a long coiled **DNA** molecule wrapped around a protein scaffold. The ends of each chromosome have a special protective cap called a telomere that contains a sequence of bases represented as TTAGGG. Although the enzyme that copies DNA for cell division cannot quite copy to the very end of each chromosome, the telomere compensates for this potential flaw because the endpieces are simply TTAGGG, potentially repeated more than 1,000 times. However, with each cell division, a portion of the telomere is lost through this erosion process, and when the telomere becomes too short, the chromosome can no longer be replicated in these "old" cells. Many body cells enter a state of senescence (inability to divide) after about 50 cell divisions in a culture dish.

In 1984, while studying the microscopic protozoan *Tetrahymena*, biologists Carol Greider and Elizabeth Blackburn discovered telomerase, an enzyme with an RNA component that can counteract the chromosome erosion and elongate the telomeres by returning TTAGGG to the chromosome ends. Telomerase activity is very low in most somatic (nonreproductive) cells, but it is active in fetal cells, adult germ cells (which produce **sperm** and egg), immune system cells, and tumor cells—all of which may divide regularly. These discoveries suggest a connection between telomerase activity and both aging and **cancer**. Thus, various experiments are underway to test the idea of triggering telomerase activation or inactivation in order to either increase lifespan (by making cells immortal) or inhibit cancers (by changing immortal, continuously dividing cells to mortal ones). Several premature-aging diseases in humans are associated with short telomeres, and telomerase activation has been discovered in a majority of human tumors. Note that because the single-celled, freshwater *Tetrahymena* organism has active telomerase, it can divide indefinitely—and is, essentially, immortal.

Greider and Blackburn write, "In the early 1980s, scientists would not have set out to identify potential anticancer therapies by studying chromosome maintenance in *Tetrahymena*. . . . In studies of nature, one can never predict when and where fundamental processes will be uncovered."

SEE ALSO Causes of Cancer (1761), Chromosomal Theory of Inheritance (1902), Cancer Chemotherapy (1946), HeLa Cells (1951), and DNA Structure (1953).

Mice that are engineered to lack telomerase become prematurely old but return to health when the enzyme is replaced. Researchers can use certain stains to study development and degeneration of bone and cartilage in mice.

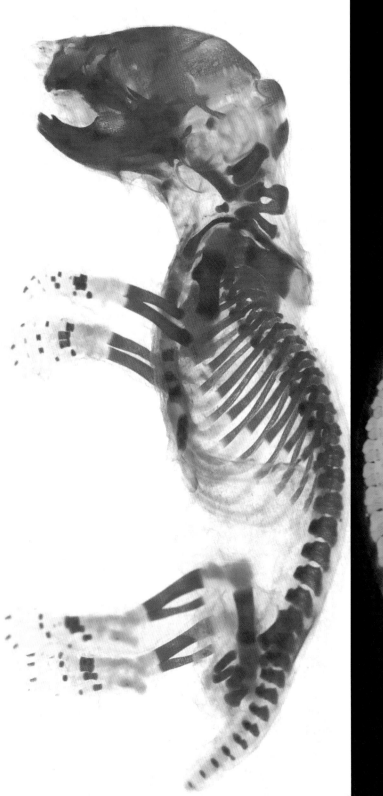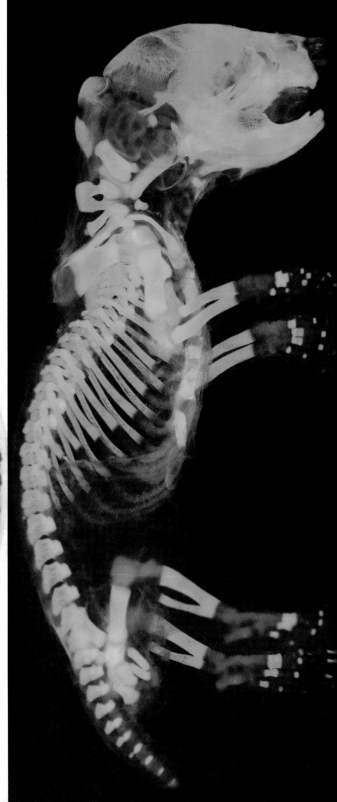

Small Bowel Transplant

The small intestine, or small bowel (SB), is a long, snaking tube that extends from the stomach to the large intestine. Roughly 20 feet (6 meters) in length, most of the digestion and absorption of food takes place in this organ. Cells in the inner wall of the SB secrete various enzymes, but most of the digestive enzymes are secreted by the pancreas and enter the SB via the pancreatic duct. Cells in intestinal villi (fingerlike projections in the inner wall) transport nutrients from inside the SB into capillaries, and blood vessels then circulate the nutrients to the organs of the body.

Although SB transplants have been attempted since the 1960s, results were often so discouraging due to donor rejection of the foreign tissue that this entry is dated at 1987, when Japanese researchers published a paper on Tacrolimus (also called FK-506), a novel immunosuppressant discovered in soil containing the bacteria *Streptomyces tsukubaensis* in 1984. The introduction of Tacrolimus led to a rise in the number of successful transplants. Further increases in patient survival came later, with additional improvements in drug therapies to reduce transplant rejection.

The SB is one of the most difficult organs to transplant because of its heavy colonization with microorganisms, strong expression of antigens, and large numbers of white blood cells. Before transplants are attempted due to intestinal failure, physicians first try total parenteral nutrition (TPN), in which liquid nutrition is directly provided through a catheter inserted into a vein. Unfortunately, long-term TPN can lead to complications, including liver failure, bone disorders, infections, and vein damage related to the catheter insertion.

Reasons for SB failure include Crohn's disease (an inflammation of the SB), necrotizing enterocolitis (tissue death in infants), and Hirschsprung's disease (paralyzed bowel). Donor intestines usually come from individuals who have died, although some intestinal segments from living-donor relatives have been transplanted. Additionally, SB transplants are sometimes performed together with transplants of other organs, such as the liver.

SEE ALSO Tissue Grafting (1597), Brunner's Glands (1679), Corneal Transplant (1905), Kidney Transplant (1954), Bone Marrow Transplant (1956), Liver Transplant (1963), Lung Transplant (1963), Hand Transplant (1964), Pancreas Transplant (1966), Heart Transplant (1967), Cyclosporine (1972), Face Transplant (2005), and Growing New Organs (2006).

Roughly 20 feet (6 meters) in length, the small intestine is the long, snaking tube (toward the front of this picture) that extends from the stomach to the large intestine.

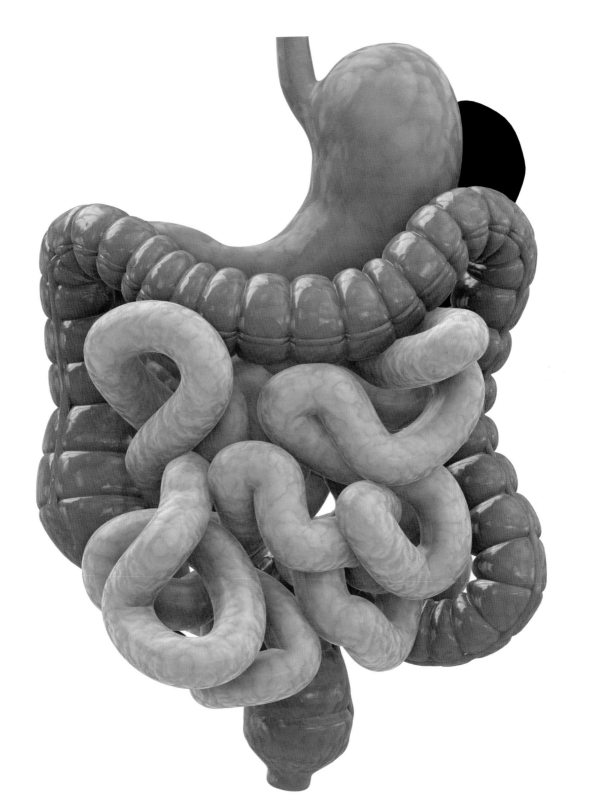

Gene Therapy

William French Anderson (b. 1936)

Many diseases result from defects in our genes, which are our units of heredity that control traits ranging from eye color to our susceptibility to **cancer** and asthma. For example, **sickle-cell anemia**, which produces abnormal red blood cells, arises from a single deleterious change in the **DNA** sequence of a gene.

Gene therapy is a young discipline that involves the insertion, alteration, or removal of genes in human cells to treat disease. One form of gene therapy involves the use of a virus that is engineered to contain a useful human gene. The virus inserts this gene into a defective human cell (usually at a random location in the host's DNA), and this new gene manufactures a properly functioning protein. If a **sperm** or egg were modified, the change would be passed to offspring, with profound ethical implications for the human race.

The first approved gene therapy procedure in the United States occurred in 1990, to treat a four-year-old girl who was suffering from a rare immune disorder known as adenosine deaminase (ADA) deficiency that made her vulnerable to infections. American researcher W. French Anderson and colleagues treated white blood cells withdrawn from her body with the gene she lacked, returned the cells to her body, and hoped the cells would produce the enzyme she needed. Although the cells safely produced the enzyme, the cells failed to give rise to healthy new cells. Gene therapy was later used to successfully treat ADA deficiency, other forms of severe immune deficiency (e.g., "bubble boy" disease), AIDS (by genetically altering T cells to resist HIV viruses), and Parkinson's disease (by reducing symptoms). Nevertheless, the procedure carries risks in some cases. Several of the children in an immune deficiency study contracted leukemia, since viral insertion of genes into a host cell can sometimes disrupt normal gene function. Also, the viral carriers of the genes (or the cells that harbor the newly implanted gene) may be attacked by the host immune's system, rendering the treatment ineffective. At worst, a strong immune attack can kill a patient.

SEE ALSO Mendel's Genetics (1865), Inborn Errors of Metabolism (1902), Cause of Sickle-Cell Anemia (1949), DNA Structure (1953), Autoimmune Diseases (1956), Levodopa for Parkinson's Disease (1957), Nanomedicine (1959), Oncogenes (1976), and Epigenetics (1983).

Hemophilia is caused by a mutation in a single gene on the X chromosome. Hemophiliacs bleed profusely when cut. Show here is Queen Victoria of the United Kingdom (1819–1901), who passed this mutation to numerous royal descendants.

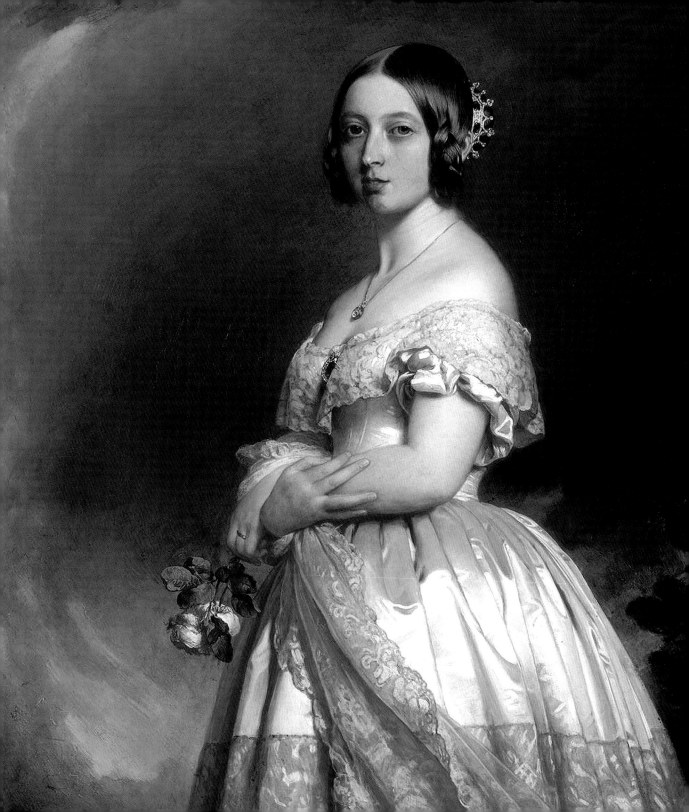

Do Not Resuscitate

Karen Ann Quinlan (1954–1985)

Civil rights leader Martin Luther King Jr. once said, "The quality, not the longevity, of one's life is what is important." Indeed, through the recent few decades, profound debates have ensued regarding when a physician should let a terminally ill or comatose patient die. Law Professor William A. Woodruff writes, "As medical technology progressed to the point where a patient's vital signs could be sustained almost indefinitely, society began to question the value of these advancements. If the patient was permanently comatose, unable to interact with his environment . . . and unable to function at even a basic cognitive level, what purpose was served in keeping him alive?"

This kind of question led to the establishment of modern do-not-resuscitate (DNR) orders in the United States and other countries. These legal documents allow patients (or other designees) to specify that resuscitation should not be attempted when a person suffers cardiac or respiratory arrest. One important step to DNRs in the United States was the 1975 legal case in which the New Jersey Supreme Court upheld the right of the father of comatose Karen Quinlan to have her removed from artificial ventilation. In 1991, the U.S. Patient Self-Determination Act forced **hospitals** to honor a patient's decision about his or her health care, and competent patients had the right to refuse treatment. Thus, if a DNR order is present, advanced cardiac life support will not be used, and **cardiopulmonary resuscitation** will not be attempted.

Of course, DNRs introduce a certain complexity into the health-care system. For example, with the advent of DNRs, if a patient is resuscitated in a hospital against the patient's wishes, a "wrongful life" lawsuit could be filed. In the case of *Payne v. Marion General Hospital* (1990), a court ruled against a physician who issued a DNR order at the request of a patient's relatives. The court found that the patient was competent a few minutes before his death and, thus, should have been consulted.

SEE ALSO Hospitals (1784), Nursing (1854), Informed Consent (1947), Cardiopulmonary Resuscitation (1956), Hospice (1967), and Near-Death Experiences (1975).

Syringe pumps in an intensive care unit (ICU) may be used to administer painkillers and antiemetics (medication to suppress vomiting) to reduce patient suffering. ICUs also include mechanical ventilators to assist breathing through an endotracheal tube or a tracheotomy.

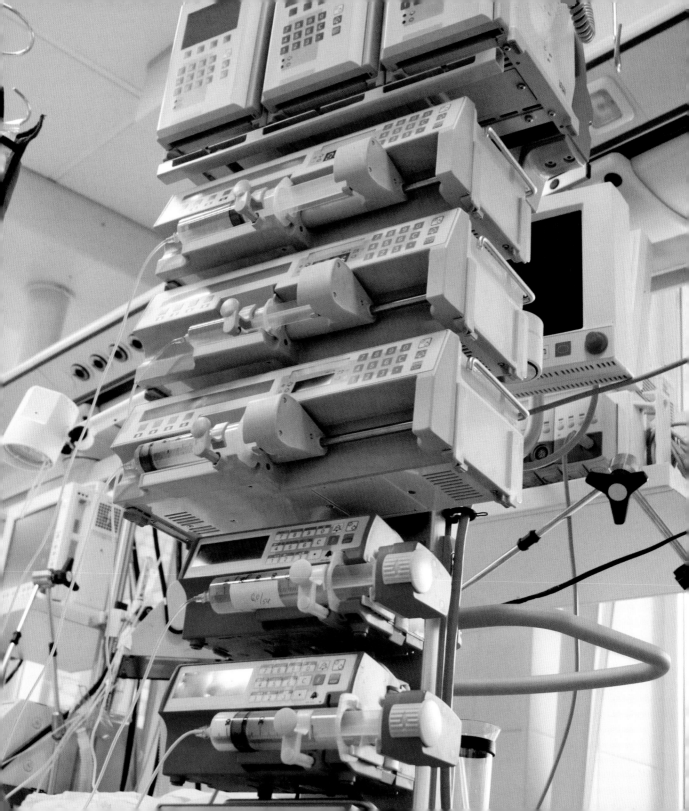

RNA Interference

Andrew Zachary Fire (b. 1959), **Craig Cameron Mello** (b. 1960)

"A small, transparent worm seems an unlikely character in one of the most exciting science stories of the late twentieth century," writes science journalist Kat Arney. "But without these tiny wrigglers—known to scientists as *Caenorhabditis elegans*—[American biologists] Andrew Fire and Craig Mello would not have earned the 2006 Nobel Prize in Physiology or Medicine."

As background, genes are specified by the **DNA** (deoxyribonucleic acid) in chromosomes in our cells. DNA information can be copied into mRNA (messenger ribonucleic acid), and proteins can subsequently be synthesized using the information in the mRNA. In 1998, Fire, Mello, and colleagues described a method in which they could selectively suppress specific **gene** activity after exposing worms to the appropriate RNA sequences in a process referred to as RNA interference (RNAi).

In organisms such as plants, fruit flies, and worms, RNAi can be initiated in the laboratory by using long double-stranded RNAs (dsRNAs) that correspond to a target gene to be inactivated. Once inside cells, dsRNAs get chopped into smaller interfering RNAs (siRNAs) by an enzyme called Dicer that exists in cells. The siRNAs assemble into RNA-induced silencing complexes (RISCs, a complex of proteins including the Argonaute protein). With the help of Argonaute, the RISCs then attack, cleave, and destroy mRNAs that correspond to the siRNA sequences, thus silencing the expression of a target gene. In mammals, scientists do not use the long dsRNAs because they are seen as foreign genetic material and trigger a powerful immune response. However, by bypassing Dicer and using the shorter appropriate siRNAs, scientists can experiment with RNAi in mammals.

Normal human cells probably use RNAi to defend against viruses—as demonstrated in plants and invertebrates—and to direct gene expression and development of cells. Note that microRNAs are the short RNA fragments naturally generated in cells. Researchers are hopeful that RNAi can be used in medical therapies, including the control of **cancer** (by silencing genes in tumor cells), treatment of neurodegenerative diseases, and antiviral therapies.

SEE ALSO Causes of Cancer (1761), Mendel's Genetics (1865), DNA Structure (1953), Reverse Transcriptase and AIDS (1970), Oncogenes (1976), Epigenetics (1983), and Polymerase Chain Reaction (1983).

Researchers first described the use of RNA interference to selectively suppress specific genes in the worm Caenorhabditis elegans, *shown here using fluorescence confocal microscopy methods to highlight the occurrence of two proteins in a living specimen.*

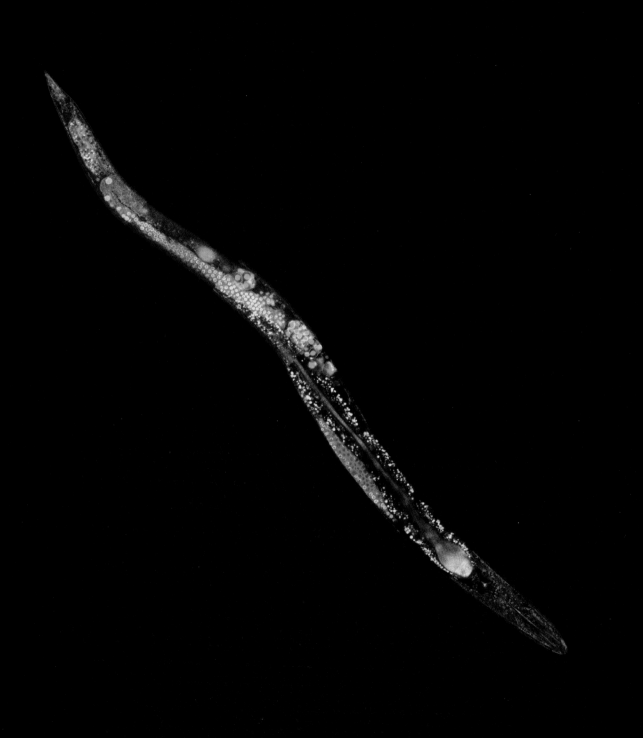

Robotic Surgery

Mani Menon (b. 1948)

Journalist David Von Drehle eloquently describes his observations of robotic surgery: "There's a major surgery in progress . . . but you can't see a patient [or] surgeon. There must be a scalpel wielder here somewhere, but all you can see is people sitting at machines in near darkness. The largest of the machines is a weird behemoth in the center of the room, spiderlike, shrouded in plastic sleeves."

One of the most popular forms of robotic surgery resembles **laparoscopic surgery**, also referred to as keyhole surgery or minimally invasive surgery, performed through small incisions. However, instead of the surgeon hovering above the patient and directly manipulating the tubelike devices inserted into a patient's abdomen, robotic surgery allows the surgeon to sit comfortably at a console and manipulate instruments attached to several robotic arms, while viewing three-dimensional images transmitted from within the patient's body. Robotic surgery can have advantages beyond laparoscopic surgery, which already minimizes blood loss and pain while accelerating patient recovery time. For example, robotic surgery can suppress the surgeon's hand tremors. Large hand movement can be scaled to provide more accuracy over tiny movements and manipulations. As mentioned in the entry "**Telesurgery**," robotic surgery also allows a surgeon to perform an operation on a patient in a separate location through the use of high-speed communication networks.

In 2000, American surgeon Mani Menon was the first surgeon in the United States to use a robot to remove a **cancerous** prostate gland, and he established the nation's first center for robotic prostatectomy that same year. Today, robot-assisted laparoscopy is used for hysterectomies, repair of heart mitral valves, hernia repairs, gallbladder removals, and much more. Von Drehle notes how easy it is to visualize the surgical area using these approaches: "The abdomen is a lovely place to be a robot because surgeons can inflate the region like a balloon using carbon dioxide and then light the space like a film studio."

SEE ALSO Sutures (3000 B.C.), Halstedian Surgery (1904), Endoscope (1954), Laparoscopic Surgery (1981), and Telesurgery (2001).

The da Vinci Surgical System employs robots to help perform complex operations using a minimally invasive approach. (©2012, Intuitive Surgical, Inc.)

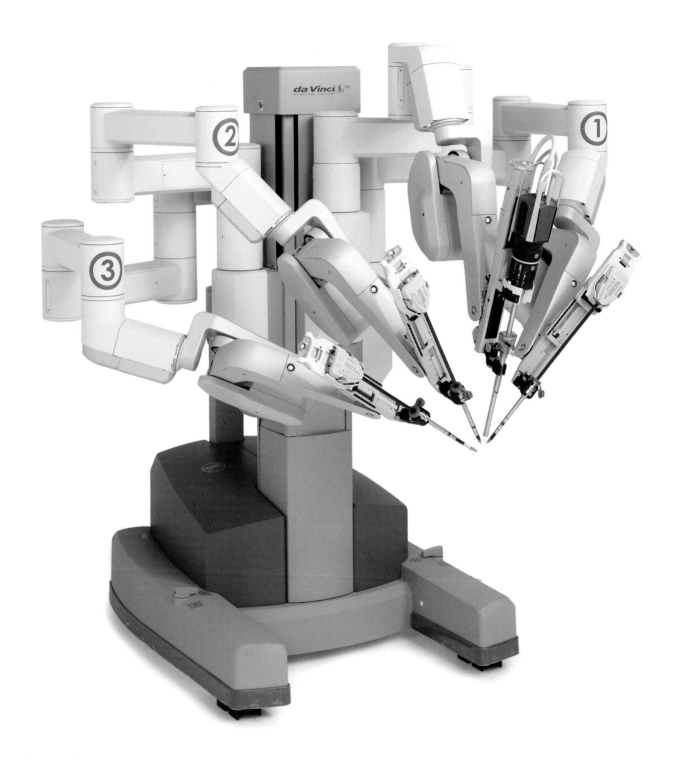

Telesurgery

Jacques Marescaux (b. 1948), **Mehran Anvari** (b. 1959)

Telesurgery allows a surgeon to perform an operation on a patient in a separate location through the use of high-speed communication networks and multiarmed robots. On September 7, 2001, the first transatlantic surgical procedure was performed between New York City and Strasbourg, France, with a separation of nearly 4,300 miles (7,000 km). French surgeon Jacques Marescaux led the **laparoscopic surgery** from New York as he operated on a 69-year-old woman in France who required gallbladder removal (see entry "**Endoscope**"). Fiber-optic communications between the two countries allowed Marescaux's hand movements to be conveyed to robotic surgical instruments equipped with an endoscopic camera, and images from the camera were transmitted back to Marescaux. The average delay was 150 milliseconds in each direction, which was sufficiently small to permit effective surgery.

In 2003, Iranian-born Mehran Anvari, a Canadian laparoscopic surgeon, helped perform the world's first telerobotics-assisted surgery between **hospitals** in Canada. Anvari's hand, wrist, and finger movements were translated from a console to control the endoscopic camera and surgical instruments in the abdomen of the patient about 250 miles (400 kilometers) away in order to perform a Nissen fundoplication (surgery to treat chronic acid reflux).

Latency—the time delay between the surgeon moving her hands and the remote robotic arms responding—can make telesurgery difficult in many scenarios. On the other hand, telesurgery may help provide specialized surgical expertise to a patient who does not have to travel beyond her local hospital. Telesurgery may also be useful on the battlefield and, someday, for missions in space. Robot-assisted surgery (see entry "**Robotic Surgery**") eliminates the normal hand tremors of the surgeon, who may remain seated during the operation in a comfortable position.

Today, robot surgeries have been performed numerous times for such operations as prostate removal and the repair of blockages between the kidney and the ureter. Robotic devices are being developed to supply increasingly sophisticated force feedback to the surgeon's hands, so that she can better "feel" the remote tissues.

SEE ALSO Sutures (3000 B.C.), Halstedian Surgery (1904), Endoscope (1954), Laparoscopic Surgery (1981), and Robotic Surgery (2000).

In 2007, researchers tested surgical robots that communicated with an unmanned aerial vehicle over a California desert. This overhead data link between robots and remote surgeons may be useful on battlefields or in rural or remote telesurgery.

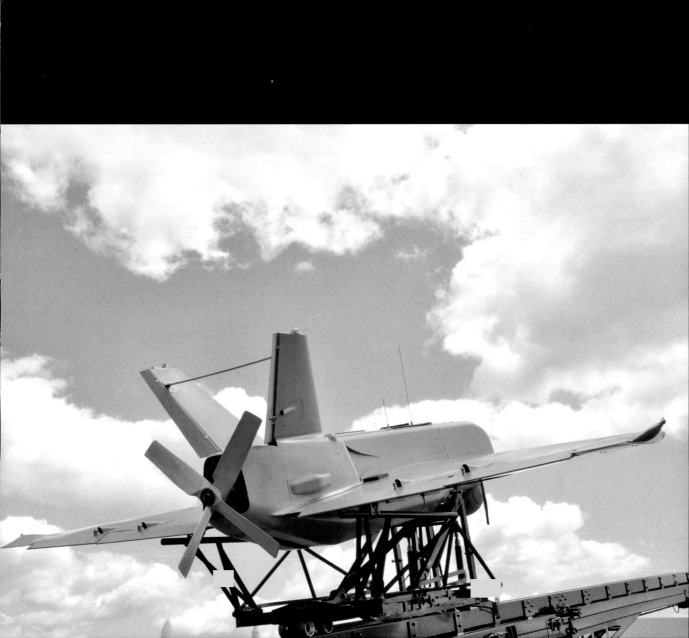

Human Genome Project

James Dewey Watson (b. 1928), **John Craig Venter** (b. 1946), **Francis Sellers Collins** (b. 1950)

The Human Genome Project (HGP) is an international effort to determine the genetic sequence of the approximately three billion chemical base pairs in our **DNA** and to gain insight into its roughly 20,000 genes. Genes are units of heredity and embodied as stretches of DNA that code for a protein or an RNA molecule that has a particular function. The HGP began in 1990 under the leadership of American molecular biologist James Watson and, later, under American physician-geneticist Francis Collins. A parallel effort was conducted by American biologist Craig Venter, founder of Celera Genomics. Not only does this DNA sequence help us understand human disease, it also helps elucidate the relationship between humans and other animals.

In 2001, Collins spoke regarding the publication of a majority of the human genome: "It's a history book: a narrative of the journey of our species through time. It's a shop manual: an incredibly detailed blueprint for building every human cell. And it's a transformative textbook of medicine: with insights that will give health-care providers immense new powers to treat, prevent, and cure disease." A more complete sequence, announced in 2003, is considered to be a watershed moment in the history of civilization.

To help generate the human genetic sequence, the genome was first broken into smaller fragments, and these pieces were inserted into bacteria in order to make many copies and create a stable resource, or library, of DNA clones. Assembling the larger sequences from fragments required sophisticated computer analyses.

Except for identical twins, individual human genomes differ, and future research will continue to involve the comparison of sequences of different individuals to help scientists better understand the role of genetics in disease and differences among humans. Only about 1 percent of the genome's sequence codes for proteins. The number of genes in humans falls between the number for grape plants (~30,400 genes) and for chickens (~16,700 genes). Interestingly, nearly half of the human genome is composed of transposable elements, or jumping DNA fragments that can move around, on, and between chromosomes.

SEE ALSO Chromosomal Theory of Inheritance (1902), DNA Structure (1953), Epigenetics (1983), and Polymerase Chain Reaction (1983).

Going beyond the HGP, results from the Neanderthal Genome Project allow researchers to compare human genomes to sequences from Neanderthals, our close evolutionary relatives who became extinct around 30,000 years ago.

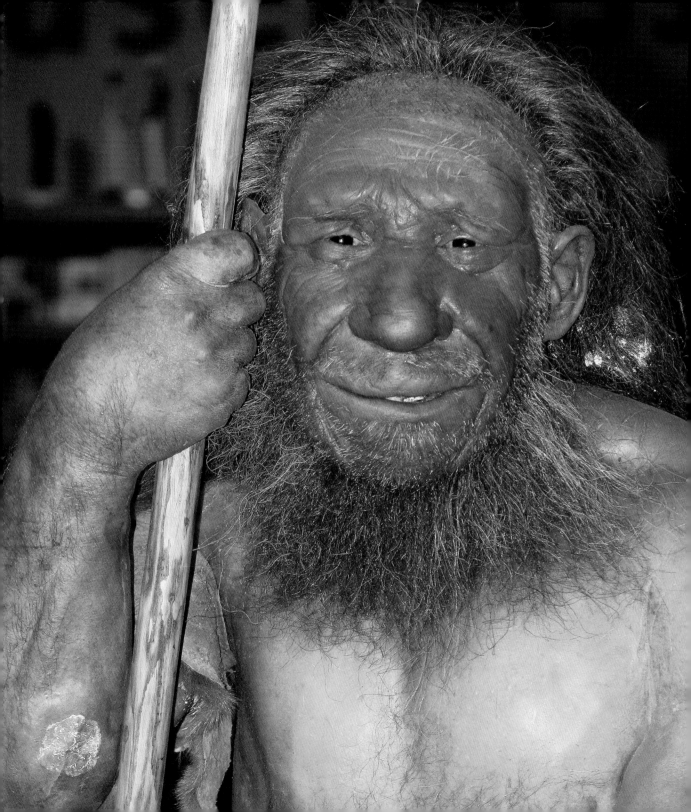

Face Transplant

Jean-Michel Dubernerd (b. 1941), **Bernard Devauchelle** (b. 1950)

Isabelle Dinoire's dog tore off her face in May 2005—after she had taken a sedative and fallen on the ground. "When I woke up, I tried to light a cigarette and I did not understand why it was not staying between my lips. It was then that I saw the pool of blood and the dog beside it! I went to see myself in the mirror, . . . It was too horrible."

In order to give Dinoire a new face, the world's first partial face transplant was carried out in 2005 by a team led by French surgeons Bernard Devauchelle and Jean-Michel Dubernerd. They successfully attached the nose, lips, and chin of another woman who had committed suicide hours before the surgery.

Not long ago, the idea of transplanting entire faces or hands between people who were genetically different would have seemed an impossible challenge. These composite tissue allotransplantations (CTAs), as they are formally called, require the use of modern immunosuppressants, so that the recipient tissues do not reject the donor tissue, along with the joining of numerous blood vessels and nerves. In contrast to solid-organ allografts, such as a **liver transplant**, a face transplant may involve many diverse tissues (such as muscles, tendons, nerves, bones, vessels, and skin) that may make tissue rejection an even greater challenge.

Since the time of Dinoire's face transplant, a variety of face transplants have been performed, some with even greater regions of the face, including tear ducts and eyelids. In the United States, a face transplant was performed on Connie Culp in 2008 that included most nasal sinuses, the upper jaw, and even teeth from a brain-dead donor. (Culp had been shot in the face by her husband.) People with face transplants must take antirejection drugs for life but can regain motion of facial muscles along with skin sensation. The implanted face does not resemble the donor's face because of underlying bone structure differences between the donor and recipient.

SEE ALSO Tissue Grafting (1597), Cranial Nerves Classified (1664), Corneal Transplant (1905), Prosopagnosia (1947), Kidney Transplant (1954), Bone Marrow Transplant (1956), Liver Transplant (1963), Lung Transplant (1963), Hand Transplant (1964), Pancreas Transplant (1966), Heart Transplant (1967), Cyclosporine (1972), Small Bowel Transplant (1987), and Human Cloning (2008).

Model of some of the key facial structures, including muscles, lips, and bone. Composite tissue allotransplantations, featuring such diverse tissues, may make tissue rejection an even greater challenge than for organ transplants involving less diverse tissues.

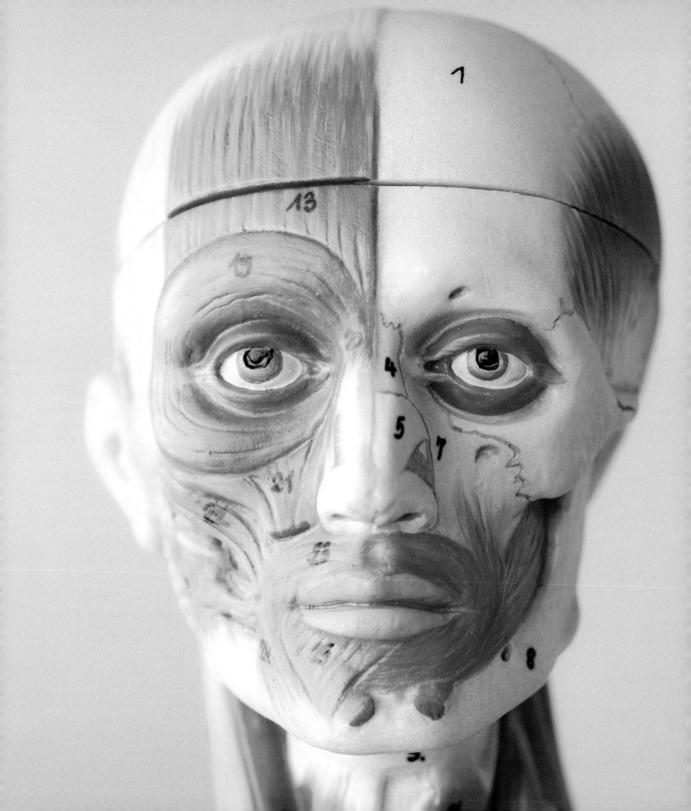

Growing New Organs

Anthony Atala (b. 1958)

"Imagine . . . creating an organ in the lab that can be transplanted into a patient without risk of rejection," writes CBS News correspondent Wyatt Andrews. "It sounds like science fiction, but . . . it's the burgeoning field of regenerative medicine, in which scientists are learning to harness the body's own power to regenerate itself, with astonishing results."

In 2006, a team of researchers led by physician Anthony Atala at the Wake Forest University School of Medicine in North Carolina created the world's first lab-grown organ—a urinary bladder—and successfully transplanted it into a child. A normal bladder has an outer layer of muscles, a middle layer of collagen (connective tissue), and an inner lining of urothelial cells that are impermeable to urine.

In the field of regenerative medicine, living functional tissues and organs are constructed for use in the human body. Atala engineered bladders for young people with defective bladders due to spina bifida, which also involves spinal cord defects. The children's tiny, rigid bladders often forced urine back toward the kidneys, leading to kidney damage. Traditionally, replacement bladders were constructed with portions of the child's bowel. However, because the bowel tissue is meant to *absorb* chemicals, these recipients face a higher risk of **cancer** and abnormally high calcium levels.

In order to carry out the engineered bladder transplant, Atala removed some muscle and urothelial cells from a child's bladder, allowed the cells to grow for several weeks outside the body in petri dishes, and then "painted" the muscle cells onto the outside of a bladder-shaped scaffolding made of collagen. He painted the inside of the scaffolding with urothelial cells. Next, this crude bladder was placed in a nutrient broth and incubated for ten days. The resultant bladder was then successfully attached to the child's original ureters at top and sphincters (circular muscles) at bottom. Scientists are currently exploring the creation of other artificial organs and tubes using similar kinds of methods. In 2011, a patient received a synthetic trachea (windpipe) that was created in a lab with the patient's own stem cells.

SEE ALSO Tissue Grafting (1597), Corneal Transplant (1905), Kidney Transplant (1954), Bone Marrow Transplant (1956), Nanomedicine (1959), Liver Transplant (1963), Lung Transplant (1963), Pancreas Transplant (1966), Heart Transplant (1967), Cyclosporine (1972), Small Bowel Transplant (1987), and Human Cloning (2008).

Schematic illustration of a male human bladder with a cancerous growth. The smaller organ beneath the bladder is the prostate gland, which surrounds the urethra.

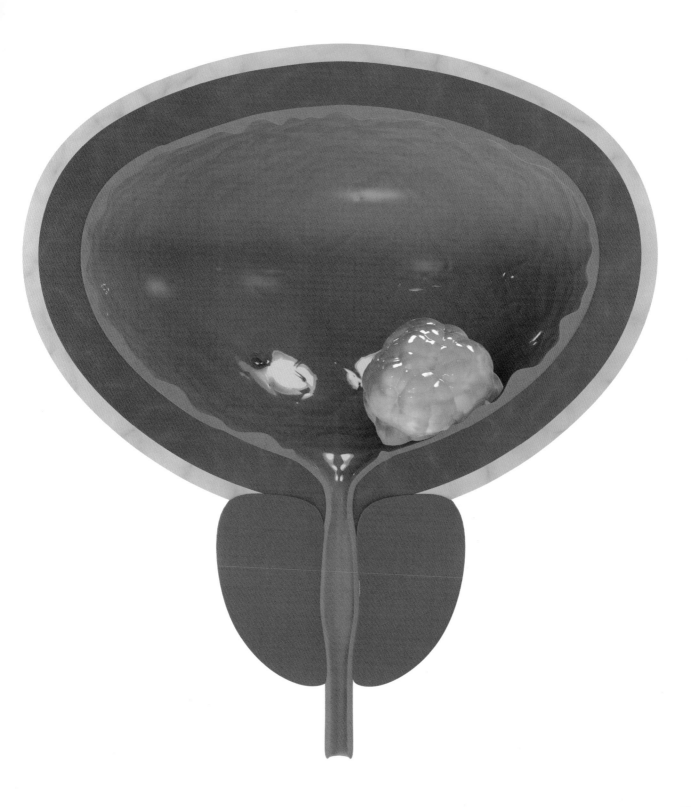

Human Cloning

Science educator Regina Bailey writes, "Imagine a world where cells can be created for therapeutic treatment of certain diseases or whole organs can be generated for transplants. . . . Humans could duplicate themselves or make exact copies of lost loved ones. . . . [Cloning and biotechnology] will define our time for future generations." In 2008, an ethical storm was already brewing when American scientist Samuel Wood became the first man to clone himself.

Reproductive human cloning refers to the production of a person who is essentially genetically identical to another. This may be accomplished by somatic cell nuclear transfer (SCNT), a process in which the nucleus of a donor adult cell is inserted into an egg cell whose nucleus has been removed, which may result in a developing embryo implanted in a womb. A new organism can also be cloned by splitting the early embryo, so that each portion becomes a separate organism (as happens with identical twins). With therapeutic human cloning, the clone is not implanted, but its cells serve a useful purpose, such as growing new tissues for transplantation. These patient-specific tissues do not trigger the immune response.

In 1996, Dolly, a sheep, became the first mammal to be successfully cloned from an adult cell. In 2008, Wood successfully created five embryos using **DNA** from his own skin cells, which might have been a source of embryonic stem cells used to repair injuries and cure diseases. Embryonic stem cells are capable of becoming any kind of cell in the human body. For legal and ethical reasons, the five embryos were destroyed. Following the news of human cloning, a Vatican representative condemned the act, stating, "This ranks among the most morally illicit acts." Other methods for collecting stem cells do not require cloning of embryos. For example, skin cells can be reprogrammed to create induced pluripotent stem cells (iPS), with no embryo needed, which might serve as possible sources for various replacement tissues destroyed by degenerative diseases.

SEE ALSO Abortion (70), Tissue Grafting (1597), Separation of Conjoined Twins (1689), Searches for the Soul (1907), DNA Structure (1953), Bone Marrow Transplant (1956), First Test-Tube Baby (1978), and Growing New Organs (2006).

Long discussed in science fiction, human cloning may become relatively easy to accomplish in the future. A Vatican representative condemned early experiments as ranking "among the most morally illicit acts."

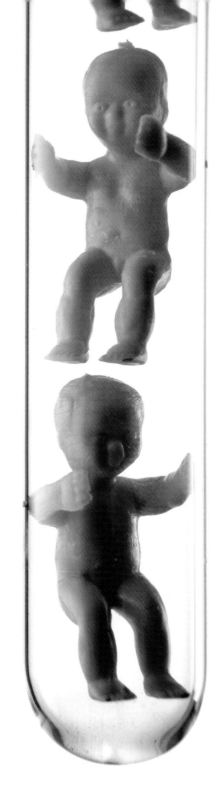

Notes and Further Reading

I've compiled the following list that identifies some of the material I used to research and write this book, along with sources for many quotations. As many readers are aware, Internet websites come and go. Sometimes they change addresses or completely disappear. The website addresses listed here provided valuable background information when this book was written.

If I have overlooked an interesting or pivotal moment in medicine that you feel has not been fully appreciated, please let me know about it. Just visit my website *pickover.com*, and send me an e-mail explaining the idea and how you feel it influenced medicine.

General Reading

Adler, R., *Medical Firsts*, Hoboken, NJ: Wiley, 2004.

Craft, N., *The Little Book of Medical Breakthroughs*, NY: Metro Books, 2010.

DeJauregui, R., *100 Medical Milestones that Shaped World History*, San Mateo, CA: Blue Wood Books, 1998.

Ellis, H., *Operations that Made History*, London: Greenwich Medical Media, 1996.

Loudon, I., *Western Medicine*, NY: Oxford University Press, 1997.

Porter, R., ed., *Cambridge Illustrated History of Medicine*, NY: Cambridge University Press, 2009.

Porter, R., *Timetables of Medicine*, NY: Black Dog & Leventhal, 2000.

Simmons, J., *Doctors & Discoveries*, Boston: Houghton Mifflin, 2002.

Straus, E., Straus, A., *Medical Marvels*, Amherst, NY: Prometheus, 2006.

Wikipedia Encyclopedia, *wikipedia.org*.

Introduction

Cunningham, A., *The Anatomist Anatomis'd*, Surrey, UK: Ashgate, 2010.

Kemp, M., Wallace, M., *Spectacular Bodies*, Berkeley, CA: University of California Press, 2000.

Lenzer, J., Brownlee, S., *tinyurl.com/5wbnlsw*.

Simmons, J., *Doctors & Discoveries*, Boston: Houghton Mifflin, 2002.

The Great Courses, *tinyurl.com/4f5asmc*.

Witch Doctor, 10,000 B.C.

Adler, R., *Medical Firsts*, Hoboken, NJ: Wiley, 2004.

Krippner, S., in *The Complete Idiot's*

Guide to Shamanism, Scott, G., NY: Alpha, 2002.

Porter, R., ed., *Cambridge Illustrated History of Medicine*, NY: Cambridge University Press, 2009.

Trepanation, 6500 B.C.

Finger, S., *Origins of Neuroscience*, NY: Oxford University Press, 1994.

Urinalysis, 4000 B.C.

Armstrong, J., *Kidney Intl.* **71**:384; 2007.

Sutures, 3000 B.C.

Kirkup, J. *The Evolution of Surgical Instruments*, Novato, CA: Norman, 2006.

Circumcision, 2400 B.C.

Bryk, F., *Circumcision in Man and Woman*, Honolulu, HI: University Press, 2001.

Gollaher, D., *Circumcision*, NY: Basic Books, 2001.

Ayurvedic Medicine, 2000 B.C.

Magner, L., *A History of Medicine*, NY: Marcel Dekker, 1992.

Bloodletting, 1500 B.C.

In the 1800s, strange "mechanical leeches" were sometimes used. These spring-loaded devices simulated a leech's bite.

Greville Chester Great Toe, 1000 B.C.

The history of prosthetics for limb amputation can be traced to ancient civilizations, including ancient Egypt, Greece, India, Rome, and Peru. Poland, H., *tinyurl.com/47g7avl*.

Eye Surgery, 600 B.C.

The Bower Manuscript (fourth century A.D.) is the earliest surviving written material that contains the works of Sushruta.

James, P., Thorpe, N., *Ancient Inventions*, NY: Ballantine, 1995.

Koelbing, M., *Klin. Monatsbl. Augenheilkd.* **168**:103; 1976.

Sewage Systems, 600 B.C.

IN.gov, *tinyurl.com/482p73f*.

Hippocratic Oath, 400 B.C.

Adler, R., *Medical Firsts*, Hoboken, NJ: Wiley, 2004.

Huangdi Neijing, 300 B.C.

Unschuld, P., *Huang Di Nei Jing Su Wen*, Berkeley, CA: University of California Press, 2003.

Mithridatium and Theriac, 100 B.C.

Griffin, J., *Br. J. Clin. Pharmacol.* **58**:317; 2004.

Abortion, 70

RU-486 prevents implantation of the egg in the uterus or causes an abortion during the first nine weeks of pregnancy. The first law in the United States outlawing abortions after quickening (when the mother feels fetal movement) was passed in Connecticut in 1821. Some studies have shown that abortions do not occur more often in countries where abortions are legal than where they are illegal. Guenin, L., *Science* **292**:1659; 2001.

Dioscorides's *De Materia Medica*, 70

Mann, J., *Murder, Magic, and Medicine*, NY: Oxford University Press, 2000.

Avicenna's *Canon of Medicine*, 1025

Conrad, L., in *Companion Encyclopedia of the History of Medicine*, vol. 1, Bynum, W., Porter, R., eds., NY: Routledge, 1997.

Persecution of Jewish Physicians, 1161

Lerner, B., *tinyurl.com/qq67hz*.

Prager, D., Telushkin, J., *Why the Jews?*, NY: Touchtone, 2003.

TIME, *tinyurl.com/y9ej6dw*.

Al-Nafis's Pulmonary Circulation, 1242

Researchers who later theorized about pulmonary circulation include M. Servetus and R. Columbus (also Colombo).

Eyeglasses, 1284

In 1268, R. Bacon used scientific principles to show that lenses could be used to correct vision.

Magner, L., *A History of the Life Sciences*, NY: Marcel Dekker, 1979.

Biological Weapons, 1346

World Medical Association, *tinyurl. com/4gvudq8*.

Leonardo's Anatomical Drawings, 1510

Lambert, K., *tinyurl.com/4rhujfg*.

Museum of Science, *tinyurl.com/4zyjzw4*.

Paracelsus Burns Medical Books, 1527

Paracelsus was famous for his cocky manner, as exemplified in his writing: "Let me tell you this: every little hair on my neck knows more than you and all your scribes, and my shoe buckles are more learned than your Galen and Avicenna." Paracelsus felt that disease could be caused by poisons from the stars. C. Jung described him as "an ocean, or, to put it less kindly, a chaos, an alchemical melting-pot into which the human beings, gods, and demons . . . poured their peculiar juices."

Ball, P., *The Devil's Doctor*, NY: Farrar, Straus and Giroux, 2006.

Crone, H., *Paracelsus*, Melbourne: Albarello, 2004.

De Humani Corporis Fabrica, 1543

Adler, R., *Medical Firsts*, Hoboken, NJ: Wiley, 2004.

Saunders, J., O'Malley, C., *The Illustrations from the Works of Andreas Vesalius of Brussels*, NY: Dover, 1973.

Paré's "Rational Surgery," 1545

Keynes, G., *The Apologie and Treatise of Ambroise Paré*, London: Falcon, 1951.

Eustachi's Rescued Masterpieces, 1552

Cunningham, A., *The Anatomist Anatomis'd*, Surrey, UK: Ashgate, 2010.

Enersen, O., *tinyurl.com/4l47wdf*.

De Praestigiis Daemonum, 1563

Adler, R., *Medical Firsts*, Hoboken, NJ: Wiley, 2004.

Mora, G., in *History of Psychiatry and Medical Psychology*, Wallace, E., Gach, J., eds., NY: Springer; 2008.

Obstetrical Forceps, 1580

Epstein, R., *Get Me Out*, Norton, 2010.

Vickers, R., *Medicine*, Chicago: Heinemann Raintree, 2010.

Tissue Grafting, 1597

Common tissues suitable for grafting include skin, bones, tendons, and corneas. In 1823, German surgeon C. Bünger performed a free-skin graft to repair a nose.

Drawings of Pietro da Cortona, 1618

Norman, J., in *The Anatomical Plates of Pietro da Cortona*, NY: Dover, 1986.

Circulatory System, 1628

The hearts of cold-blooded animals, such as eels, were useful to Harvey because their hearts beat more slowly than mammalian hearts and allowed more careful observation. Harvey also showed that the pulse was caused not directly by the motion of the arteries but rather by a passive response from pressures caused by heart contractions. Other researchers also theorized about blood circulation, including M. Servetus, R. Columbus (also Colombo), and A. Cesalpino.

Adler, R., *Medical Firsts*, Hoboken, NJ: Wiley, 2004.

Murder and Wirsung's Duct, 1642

Howard, J., Hess, W., *History of the Pancreas*, NY: Springer, 2002.

Lymphatic System, 1652

Unlike the blood's circulatory system, the lymphatic system has no pumping organ. Weissmann, D., *tinyurl.com/4s8a9x5*.

Micrographia, 1665

Westfall, R., *Dictionary of Scientific Biography*, Gillispie, C., ed., NY: Scribner, 1970.

Discovery of Sperm, 1678

Some religious people wondered why God would be so wasteful of the homunculi, with so many preformed humans dying.

Discovery of Sarcoptes Scabiei, 1687

Ramos-e-Silva, M., *Intl. J. Dermatology* **37**:625; 1998.

Separation of Conjoined Twins, 1689

Overall, C., in *Feminist Ethics and Social and Political Philosophy*, Tessman, L., ed., NY: Springer, 2009.

Pulse Watch, 1707

Clendening, L., *Source Book of Medical History*, NY: Dover, 1960.

Gibbs, D., *Med. Hist.* **15**:187; 1971.

Mary Toft's Rabbits, 1726

Pickover, C., *The Girl Who Gave Birth to Rabbits*, Amherst, NY: Prometheus, 2000.

Cheselden's Osteographia, 1733

Kemp, M., Wallace, M., *Spectacular Bodies*, Berkeley, CA: University of California Press, 2000.

Neher, A., *Med. Hist.* **54**:517; 2010.

Albinus's Tables of the Human Body, 1747

Cunningham, A., *The Anatomist Anatomis'd*, Surrey, UK: Ashgate, 2010.

Schiebinger, L., in *The Making of the Modern Body*, Gallagher, C., Laqueur, T., eds., Berkeley, CA: University of California Press, 1987.

A Treatise on Scurvy, 1753

Bown, S., *Scurvy*, NY: St. Martin's, 2005.

Autopsy, 1761

In the United States, a medical examiner is a physician, but a coroner need not have medical qualifications. Among other things, the coroner is responsible for identifying the body, notifying next of kin, and signing the death certificate.

Causes of Cancer, 1761
Bloom, J., *Texas Monthly* 6:175; 1978.

Morgagni's "Cries of Suffering Organs," 1761
Simmons, J., *Doctors & Discoveries*, Boston: Houghton Mifflin, 2002.

Exploring the Labyrinth, 1772
Bainbridge, D., *Beyond the Zonules of Zinn*, Cambridge, MA: Harvard University Press, 2010.

Hospitals, 1784
Selzer, R., *Taking the World in for Repairs*, East Lansing, MI: Michigan State University Press, 1994.

Lavoisier's Respiration, 1784
Minet, C., *Nature* 86:95; 1911.

Digitalis, 1785
Major, R., *Classic Descriptions of Disease*, Springfield, IL: Charles C. Thomas, 1978.
Panda, H., *Hand Book on Herbal Drugs and Its Plant Sources*, Delhi: National Institute of Industrial Research, 2004.

Ambulance, 1792
Bell, R., *The Ambulance*, Jefferson, NC: McFarland, 2008.

Alternative Medicine, 1796
Rosenfield, A., foreword to *Traditional, Complementary and Alternative Medicine*, Bodeker, G., Burford, G., eds., Hackensack, NJ: World Scientific, 2006.

Smallpox Vaccination, 1798
Despite his success, Jenner did not know of the cellular mechanism of immunity, which involves white blood cells. Initially, his work was attacked and ridiculed.
Mulcahy, R., *Diseases*, Minneapolis, MN: Oliver Press, 1996.
Riedel, S., *Proc. Bayl. Univ. Med. Cent.* 18:21; 2005.

Stethoscope, 1816
In the early 1850s, A. Leared and G. P. Camman invented the binaural stethoscope (with two earpieces). Note that the stiffer a membrane, the higher its natural frequency of oscillation and the more efficiently it operates at higher frequencies. The ability of a chest-piece to collect sound is roughly proportional to its diameter. Larger diameters are also more efficient at capturing lower frequencies.

Higher frequencies are diminished by tubing that is too long. Other physics principles of stethoscopes are discussed in Constant, J., *Bedside Cardiology*, NY: Lippincott Williams & Wilkins, 1999.
Porter, R., *The Greatest Benefit to Mankind*, NY: Norton, 1999.

Blood Transfusion, 1829
Hurt, R., *The History of Cardiothoracic Surgery*, Pearl River, NY: Parthenon, 1996.

Medical Specialization, 1830
Asimov, I., *I. Asimov*, NY: Bantam, 1995.
Weisz, G., *Divide and Conquer*, NY: Oxford University Press, 2006.

Anatomy Act of 1832, 1832
For his crimes, Burke was sentenced, hanged, and dissected.

Intravenous Saline Solutions, 1832
A "normal saline" solution has nine grams of sodium chloride dissolved in one liter of water, thus providing about the same osmolarity (solute concentration) as blood.

General Anesthesia, 1842
In 1842, a student, W. Clarke, used ether to assist in a tooth extraction. The precise molecular effect of anesthesia is still a subject of research, and it appears that anesthetics affect the spinal cord and brain.

The Sanitary Condition of the Labouring Population of Great Britain, 1842
Winslow, C., *Science* 51:23; 1920.

Panum's "Measles on the Faroe Islands," 1846
The epidemic in the Faroe Islands was triggered by a cabinetmaker with measles who had journeyed from Copenhagen.

Semmelweis's Hand Washing, 1847
The lethal *Streptococcus* bacteria of septicemia could invade the uterus, which was made vulnerable and exposed by childbirth. Semmelweis referred to the cause as cadaverous particles. American physician O. W. Holmes Sr. also argued that puerperal fever spread from patient to patient via physician contact, and he suggested that physicians clean their instruments.
Carter, K., Carter, B., *Childbed Fever*, New Brunswick, NJ: Transaction Publishers, 2005.

Appendectomy, 1848
Craft, N., *The Little Book of Medical Breakthroughs*, NY: Metro Books, 2010.

Ophthalmoscope, 1850
In 1847, English inventor C. Babbage created an ophthalmoscope similar to the one developed and promoted by von Helmholtz. Retinal changes may be associated with diabetes mellitus, syphilis, leukemia, and brain and kidney diseases.
McKendrick, J., *Hermann Ludwig Ferdinand Von Helmholtz*, NY: Longmans, 1899.

Hypodermic Syringe, 1853
Duce, A., Hernández, F., *Hernia* 3:103; 1999.

Broad Street Pump Handle, 1854
Guynup, S., *tinyurl.com/2fu6z*.

Nursing, 1854
Henderson, V., *ICN Basic Principles of Nursing Care*, Geneva, Switzerland: International Council of Nurses, 2004.

Cell Division, 1855
R. Remak also discovered that new cells are formed by the division of preexisting cells. F. Raspail coined the phrase *omnis cellula e cellula*.
Simmons, J., *The Scientific 100*, NY: Kensington, 1996.

Treatment of Epilepsy, 1857
A *magnetoencephalogram* (MEG) may also be used to evaluate epilepsy. J. Jackson

made early seminal contributions to the understanding of epilepsy.

Gray's Anatomy, 1858

Later editions included X-ray plates and electron micrographs, and were organized in terms of regions of the body rather than systems.

Cerebral Localization, 1861

In more than 95 percent of right-handed men, language and speech appear to be mediated by the brain's left hemisphere. D. Ferrier performed tests on brains from various animals to map sensory and motor areas. Other important names in the history of cerebral localization include F. du Petit, J. Jackson, and C. Wernicke.

Germ Theory of Disease, 1862

Pasteur's vaccinations were notable in that he created them from weakened organisms. This was not the case in E. Jenner's use of cowpox to provide cross-immunity to smallpox. Pasteur's work influenced J. Lister and his quest to reduce infections during surgeries through antiseptic methods.

Antiseptics, 1865

Listerine mouthwash is named after Lister. Around 1862, the physician G. Tichenor used alcohol as an antiseptic for wounds. Clark, F., *Med. Libr. & Hist. J.* 5:145; 1907.

Medical Thermometer, 1866

In 1654, F. II de' Medici made sealed tubes that could be used as thermometers that were not perturbed by changes in atmospheric pressure. Medical thermometers were not quickly adapted in the American Old West, because the designs were fragile and broke in the physician's saddlebags.

Cause of Leprosy, 1873

Mycobacterium lepromatosis also causes leprosy (Hansen's disease).

Modern Brain Surgery, 1879

Fox, M., *Lucky Man*, NY: Hyperion, 2002.

Cesarean Section, 1882

Sewell, J., *tinyurl.com/4plwedj.*

Koch's Tuberculosis Lecture, 1882

Skeletal evidence suggests that tuberculosis has plagued humanity since prehistoric times. In 2008, roughly 1.3 million people died from tuberculosis. *Nobelprize.org, tinyurl.com/4rv5vak.*

Salpingectomy, 1883

Ellis, H., in *Schein's Common Sense Emergency Abdominal Surgery*, Schein, M., Rogers, P., Assalia, A., eds., NY: Springer, 2010.

Cocaine as Local Anesthetic, 1884

Hardy, T., Hardy, F., *Thomas Hardy*, Hertfordshire, UK: Wordsworth, 2007 (originally published in 1928).

Antitoxins, 1890

Linton, D., *Emil von Behring*, Philadelphia: American Philosophical Society, 2005.

Neuron Doctrine, 1891

Shepherd, G., *Foundations of the Neuron Doctrine*, NY: Oxford University Press, 1991.

Discovery of Viruses, 1892

In 1901, W. Reed and colleagues recognized the first human virus, yellow fever virus.
Adler, R., *Medical Firsts*, Hoboken, NJ: Wiley, 2004.

Discovery of Adrenaline, 1893

J. Abel isolated a benzoyl derivative of adrenaline before Takamine's discoveries. Later, it was determined that Takamine's adrenaline was probably impure and a mixture of adrenaline and noradrenaline (norepinephrine). The sympathetic nervous system triggers the synthesis of adrenaline precursors. Around 1904, F. Stolz synthesized adrenaline without using any animal extracts, making adrenaline the first hormone to be synthesized artificially. Note that other hormones are produced in the thyroid gland, ovaries, and testes. Hormones may also, for example, regulate growth, metabolism, and hunger cravings. Carmichael, S., *tinyurl.com/64v45a4.*

Cause of Bubonic Plague, 1894

The first outbreaks of the plague in China occurred in the early 1330s. The plague was reported in Constantinople in 1347.
Cantor, N., *In the Wake of the Plague*, NY: Free Press, 2001.
Marriott, E., *Plague*, NY: Holt, 2003.
Moote, L., Moote, D., *The Great Plague*, Baltimore, MD: Johns Hopkins University Press, 2004.

D. D. Palmer and Chiropractic, 1895

Schneider, E., Hirschman, L., *What Your Doctor Hasn't Told You and the Health-Store Clerk Doesn't Know*, NY: Penguin, 2006.

X-rays, 1895

Prior to Röntgen's work, N. Tesla began his observations of X-rays (at that time still unknown and unnamed).
Haven, K., *100 Greatest Science Inventions of All Time*, Westport, CT: Libraries Unlimited, 2005.

Cause of Malaria, 1897

G. Grassi and colleagues demonstrated that only *Anopheles* mosquitoes transmitted the disease to humans. Malaria can cause red blood cells to become sticky and cause blockages. Chloroquine is also used in the treatment or prevention of malaria.
Poser, C., Bruyn, G., *An Illustrated History of Malaria*, Pearl River, NY: Parthenon, 1999.
Rosenberg, C., foreword to *The Making of a Tropical Disease*, Packard, R., Baltimore, MD: Johns Hopkins University Press, 2007.

Aspirin, 1899

Shorter, E., in *Cambridge Illustrated History of Medicine*, Porter, R., ed., NY: Cambridge University Press, 2009.

Defibrillator, 1899

In 1956, P. Zoll demonstrated that defibrillation could be successfully applied across the closed chest. M. Mirowski and colleagues developed the first ICDs. Other important researchers in the history of defibrillation include C. Kite, N. Gurvich, B. Lown, C. Wiggers, and W. Kouwenhoven.

Hearing Aids, 1899

Acoustic chairs were sometimes used in the 1700s, consisting of hollow armrests that would channel sounds to openings near the sitter's ears.

Psychoanalysis, 1899

C. Jung, A. Adler, and S. Freud are considered to be among the principal founding fathers of modern psychology. The philosopher K. Popper argued that psychoanalysis is pseudoscience, and some studies suggest that outcomes from psychotherapy are no different from placebo controls. The first occurrence of the word *psychoanalysis* appears in 1896. Freud developed his initial ideas in *Studies of Hysteria*, cowritten with J. Breuer.
Hart, M., *The 100*, NY: Kensington, 1992.
Reef, C., *Sigmund Freud*, NY: Clarion Books, 2001.
Storr, A., *Feet of Clay*, NY: The Free Press, 1996.

Chromosomal Theory of Inheritance, 1902

Today we know that the number of a creature's chromosomes is quite varied—humans have 46, chimpanzees 48, horses 64, and gypsy moths 62.

Cause of Sleeping Sickness, 1902

Petersen, M., *Our Daily Meds*, NY: Farrar, Straus and Giroux, 2008.

Vascular Suturing, 1902

Carrel lost respect from some peers when he witnessed a healing at the religious shrine at Lourdes and suggested that some medical cures may not be explainable by science. His views on eugenics were also controversial.

Electrocardiograph, 1903

Einthoven's thin needle was created by attaching quartz to an arrow on a bow. Heat was applied to the quartz, and the arrow flew across the room to pull the quartz into an amazingly thin string. A light shining on the needle recorded a trace on photographic paper.

Radiation Therapy, 1903

French photographer A. Saint Victor also discovered radioactivity. By increasing the presence of oxygen in a tumor, greater numbers of damaging free radicals are produced. Stereotactic radiosurgery uses very accurate methods for targeting beams of radiation. In general, multiple beams may be used to target a cancer from many angles. Proton beams can spare surrounding healthy tissues because protons deposit much of their energy at the end of their path. Gamma rays are sometimes used in radiotherapy and are produced by decay of cobalt 60 or other elements, or by linear accelerators.

Corneal Transplant, 1905

V. Filatov popularized the use of cadaver corneas for transplants.

"Analytic" Vitamin Discovery, 1906

Initially, Eijkman thought of the brown rice hulls as curing beriberi and not that beriberi was caused by the *absence* of a chemical. In 1912, C. Funk identified vitamin B1 as the missing substance. The ancient Chinese, Greeks, and Egyptians were aware that certain foods cured certain diseases. For example, livers were recommended by several ancient cultures to cure night blindness.
Combs, G., *The Vitamins*, Burlington, MA: Elsevier Academic Press, 2007.
Haven, K., *100 Greatest Science Discoveries of All Time*, Westport, CT: Libraries Unlimited, 2007.

Alzheimer's Disease, 1906

Around half of early-onset AD patients have inherited gene mutations. The gene for AB precursor protein is located on chromosome 21, and people with Down syndrome who have an extra copy of this gene almost always exhibit AD by 40 years of age. Studies suggest that those who drink large amounts of coffee have a reduced risk of dementia later in life. Medical marijuana may also delay AD. Some studies suggest that head injuries earlier in life increase the risk for AD later in life. Other early discoverers of AD include O. Fischer, F. Bonfiglio, G. Perusini, and S. Fuller.

Imprisonment of Typhoid Mary, 1907

Because the physicians mistakenly believed that removing her gallbladder could eliminate the disease, they asked Mallon if they could take out the organ. She refused, thinking that the doctors might be attempting to kill her.

Chlorination of Water, 1910

Darnall Army Medical Center, *tinyurl. com/48evjwo*.

Erhlich's Magic Bullets, 1910

Simmons, J., *The Scientific 100*, NY: Kensington, 1996.

Fluoridated Toothpaste, 1914

Colorado Brown Stain occurred when the very young (two or three years old) had consumed too much fluoride. Fluoride strengthens teeth while they are developing and protects the teeth after they have erupted into the mouth.

Neurotransmitters, 1914

A single neuron can release more than one kind of neurotransmitter. A single kind of neurotransmitter can inhibit or excite depending on the receptor present. When a neutron transmitter binds to a receptor, it may open channels to facilitate the flow of ions.

Human Growth Hormone, 1921

The pituitary releases HGH when it receives a signal from the hypothalamus in the form of HGH-releasing hormone. Release can also be triggered by stress and fasting. HGH also regulates other glands in the body. Tragically, some batches of corpse pituitary glands caused Creutzfeldt-Jakob

encephalopathy in recipients.
Angier, N., *tinyurl.com/4mafjag*.

Banishing Rickets, 1922
Studies suggest that too much or too
little vitamin D may cause premature
aging. Vitamin D acts throughout the
body to regulate cell growth and slow the
progression of some autoimmune diseases
and cancers.

Commercialization of Insulin, 1922
N. Paulescu was the first to isolate
insulin, but his impure form was
never used on patients. The story of
the discovery of insulin is associated
with some jealousy and ill will. When
Banting and J. J. R. Macleod won
the Noble Prize for work on insulin,
Banting gave a share of his winnings
to Best, whom he thought was unjustly
overlooked. J. Collip helped purify the
insulin extracts. Diabetes may cause
cardiovascular disease and damage to the
retina. Autoimmune attack is one of the
main causes of type 1 diabetes, which
is also called juvenile diabetes. Insulin
also controls the conversion of glucose
to glycogen in muscles and the liver. In
ancient days, diabetes was diagnosed by
tasting sugar in the urine.

Welbourn, R., in *Companion
Encyclopedia of the History of Medicine*,
vol. 1, Bynum, W., Porter, R., eds., NY:
Routledge, 1997.

Truth Serum, 1922
Rejali, D., *Torture and Democracy*,
Princeton, NJ: Princeton University
Press, 2007.

Human Electroencephalogram, 1924
Bear, M., Connors, B., Paradiso, M.,
Neuroscience, NY: Lippincott, 2006.

Modern Midwifery, 1925
Hanson, K., in *Images of Pastoral Care*,
Dykstra, R., ed., St. Louis, MO: Chalice
Press, 2005.
Sullivan, N., *tinyurl.com/4gf6qwt*.

Liver Therapy, 1926
PA is a possible cause when the patient's
blood contains large and immature
RBCs. Treatment includes B12
supplementation. When RBCs become
old and die, the spleen breaks down the
RBCs, and iron is returned to the blood,
where it is carried to the bone marrow for
use in newly formed RBCs. PA can also
cause nerve damage.

Iron Lung, 1928
DeJauregui, R., *100 Medical Milestones
that Shaped World History*, San Mateo,
CA: Blue Wood Books, 1998.
Eiben, R., in *Polio*, Daniel, T., Robbins,
F., Rochester, NY: University of
Rochester Press, 1999.

Penicillin, 1928
Although it was once believed that
antibiotics in a natural setting are a means
for bacteria or fungi to better compete with
bacteria in the soil, American biochemist
S. Waksman suggested that these
microbial products are a "purely fortuitous
phenomenon" and "accidental."

IUD, 1929
Some IUDs irritate the lining of the uterus,
making it difficult for an embryo to implant.
A string descends from the IUD into the
vagina, enabling the user or the physician to
ensure the IUD is in place, and facilitating
its removal by a physician. IUDs do not
prevent sexually transmitted diseases.

Medical Self-Experimentation, 1929
Freed, D., *Lancet* **330**:746; 1987.

Stanley's Crystal Invaders, 1935
Creager, A., *The Life of a Virus*, Chicago:
University of Chicago Press, 2001.

Sulfa Drugs, 1935
Although penicillin was discovered before
sulfa drugs, the medical applications were
not realized until after sulfa drugs were used
in treatments. Also note that P. Ehrlich
and colleagues had earlier discovered that
arsenic could be used to treat syphilis, but
this was not 100 percent effective.

Grundmann, E., *Gerhard Domagk*,
Münster: Lit Verlag, 2005.

Antihistamines, 1937
The H_2 receptors are used by drugs such as
cimetidine (Tagamet) that inhibit gastric acid
secretion. H_1 antihistamines can be used to
counter nausea and motion sickness.

Healy, D., *The Creation of
Psychopharmacology*, Cambridge, MA:
Harvard University Press, 2002.

Cause of Yellow Fever, 1937
Crosby, M., *The American Plague*, NY:
Berkley, 2007.

Electroconvulsive Therapy, 1938
Cody, B., *tinyurl.com/4hv3kh4*.
Hartmann, C., *Psychiatr. Serv.* **53**:
413; 2002.

Dialysis, 1943
In peritoneal dialysis, dialysate is
added to the body's natural peritoneal
(abdominal) cavity, and toxins diffuse
through the body's peritoneal membrane
into the dialysate, which is then removed
from the body.

Maher, J., *Replacement of Renal Function
by Dialysis*, Dordrecht, Netherlands:
Editor Kluwer, 1989.

Blalock-Taussig Shunt, 1944
Nuland, S., *Doctors*, NY: Black Dog &
Leventhal, 2008.

Transorbital Lobotomy, 1946
Freeman often used electroshock to
anesthetize lobotomy patients. Women
had lobotomies at twice the rate of men.

Enersen, O., *tinyurl.com/4gk77wa*.

Informed Consent, 1947
The Declaration of Helsinki originally
distinguished between therapeutic
research (which might be beneficial for
the patient) and nontherapeutic research
(to obtain medical knowledge not likely to
benefit the patient).

Randomized Controlled Trials, 1948
Comparative effectiveness research can
sometimes be useful when performed

using electronic medical records of large health networks.

Enkin, M., preface to *Randomized Controlled Trials*, Jadad, A., Enkin, M., Malden, MA: BMJ Books, 2007.

Cause of Sickle-Cell Anemia, 1949

SCT is highest in West Africa, where it has provided a selective advantage against malaria. Studies of mice with SCT suggest that levels of heme—a component of hemoglobin—in the blood plasma play a role in the parasite being able to cause disease. Also, the increased concentration of carbon monoxide in such mice stabilized hemoglobin, leading to reduced immune pathology.

Mammography, 1949

Chemotherapy damages the DNA in cancer cells but, unfortunately, also in fast-growing normal cells. Other important researchers in the history of mammography include S. Warren and J. Gershon-Cohen.

Antipsychotics, 1950

With antipsychotic drugs, the voices in patients' heads might still be present but recede from center stage and are less worrisome. The newer medicines are often referred to as atypical drugs. Clozapine can also lead to extreme weight gain. All antipsychotic drugs make seizures more likely. J. Hamon also conducted early research on chlorpromazine.

Graedon, J., Graedon, T., *tinyurl. com/4f3z6b7*.

Turner, T., *Brit. Med. J.* **334**:7; 2007.

HeLa Cells, 1951

Skloot, R., *The Immortal Life of Henrietta Lacks*, NY: Crown, 2010.

Skloot, R., *tinyurl.com/y8h5trq*.

Tobacco Smoking and Cancer, 1951

Other important early studies involving smoking and cancer include the research of Americans E. L. Wynder and E. A. Graham, as well as a 1939 German study.

Wolfson, M., *The Fight Against Big Tobacco*, Hawthorne, NY: Aldine Transaction, 2001.

Amniocentesis, 1952

As medicine progresses, these techniques may be increasingly used to correct diseases in the developing embryo and thus decrease the need for considering termination of any pregnancy. Fetal blood sampling is sometimes performed to study cells in the umbilical cord.

Magill, F., *Great Events from History*, Hackensack, NJ: Salem Press, 1991.

Artificial Heart Valves, 1952

Other key individuals in the history of artificial heart valves include A. Carpentier, N. Starr-Braunwald, and D. Harken.

DNA Structure, 1953

DNA may be used to assess hereditary risk for certain diseases. Gene therapy, in which healthy genes are inserted into human cells, continues to be researched for treatment of diseases. Understanding gene regulation, in which genes become active and inactive, is crucial to our understanding of DNA function.

Ridley, M., jacket flap for *DNA*, Krude, T., ed., NY: Cambridge University Press, 2004.

Heart-Lung Machine, 1953

Stanley, A., *Mothers and Daughters of Invention*, Piscataway, NJ: Rutgers University Press, 1995.

Endoscope, 1954

Fanu, J., *The Rise and Fall of Modern Medicine*, NY: Carroll & Graf, 2000.

Birth-Control Pill, 1955

The mini-pill was introduced in the early 1970s, and it contained only progestin. It prevented pregnancy solely through changes in the cervix and uterus. Other key scientists in the development of the pill are J. Rock and M. C. Chang.

Placebo Effect, 1955

Placebo treatments of gastric ulcers have often been as effective as acid-secretion inhibitor drugs, as confirmed by stomach endoscopy. Many recent clinical trials of antidepressant medications have shown that sugar pills can provide the same relief.

Shapiro, A., Shapiro, E., in *The Placebo Effect*, Harrington, A., ed., Cambridge, MA: Harvard University Press, 1999.

Polio Vaccine, 1955

H. Koprowski was also an important figure in the history of polio research. The various vaccines require more than one dose. In 1955, Cutter Laboratories produced some vaccines that were contaminated with live polio virus, causing around 260 cases of polio. One advantage of the OPV is that sterile needles are not necessary.

Offit, P., *The Cutter Incident*, New Haven, CT: Yale University Press, 2005.

Bone Marrow Transplant, 1956

Other diseases treated with bone marrow transplants (hematopoietic stem cell transplants) include sickle-cell anemia, lymphoma, and multiple myeloma. Stem cells have antigens on their surfaces and can be rejected just like any transplanted organ. Recipients of stem cells generally require immunosuppressive drugs to reduce graft-versus-host disease. Donor cells can come from bone marrow, the peripheral circulating blood, or umbilical cord blood. If bone marrow is extracted from the patient, it may be "purged" to remove any residual malignant cells before implantation. Bone marrow transplants were the first form of stem cell therapy.

Carrier, E., Ledingham, G., *100 Questions & Answers about Bone Marrow and Stem Cell Transplantation*, Sudbury, MA: Jones & Bartlett Learning, 2004.

Cardiopulmonary Resuscitation, 1956

Resuscitation with compressions only is less effective in children than adults.

Levodopa for Parkinson's Disease, 1957

Dopamine does not cross the blood-brain barrier. G. Cotzias developed effective levodopa therapies in 1967. PET scans can be useful for studying PD.

Medical Ultrasound, 1957

Higher frequencies can be used to provide greater image clarity, but do not penetrate as deeply into the body as lower-frequency ultrasound. Piezoelectric materials are used to produce the ultrasounds. The amount of reflected waves depends on the relative densities of the tissues at interfaces. Many other physicians and technologists contributed to the development of medical ultrasound.
Khurana, A., in *Donald's Practical Obstetric Problem*, Misra, R., ed., New Delhi: Edward Arnold Publishers, 2009.

Hip Replacement, 1958

In 1960, S. Baw pioneered the use of ivory hip parts.
Neary quoted in Elliott, J., *tinyurl. com/4d3nrqw*.

Pineal Body, 1958

Strassman, R., *DMT*, Rochester, VT: Park Street Press, 2000.

Structure of Antibodies, 1959

Monoclonal antibodies, derived from a single immune cell, have been found that recognize certain human cancers.

Laser, 1960

Hecht, J., *Understanding Lasers*, Piscataway, NJ: IEEE Press, 2008.

Thymus, 1961

Marks, G., *Encyclopedia of Jewish Food*, Hackensack, NJ: Wiley, 2010.

Cryonics, 1962

In the 1970s, researchers demonstrated some electrical activity in cat brains after several years of storage at –20 °C.
Alam, H., *tinyurl.com/4h3kku2*.

Thalidomide Disaster, 1962

TIME, tinyurl.com/yg5y8m7.

Cognitive Behavioral Therapy, 1963

Mathematician J. Nash is famous for claiming that he was able to overcome his schizophrenia to a large degree by a reasoning process in which he was able to persuade himself of the improbability of the conclusions he was making. By adjusting his thinking about his delusions and the voices he heard, he was able to diminish their hold over him.

Beta-Blockers, 1964

Propranolol was sold under the brand name Inderal.

Hand Transplant, 1964

Some hand recipients receive bone marrow cells from the donor to help "reeducate" the recipient's immune system to decrease tissue rejection.

Pancreas Transplant, 1966

The digestive enzymes produced by the donor pancreas may drain into the patient's intestine or bladder. The transplant can eliminate the need for insulin shots and decreases the secondary problems of diabetes.

CAT Scans, 1967

Mathematician J. Radon formulated fundamental algorithms used in reconstructing CT images.

Heart Transplant, 1967

Fitzpatrick, L., *tinyurl.com/ylrlnmp*.

Reverse Transcriptase and AIDS, 1970

Once the DNA copy of the retroviral RNA is inserted into the host DNA, this "provirus" becomes a permanent part of the infected cell's genome. Alas, the inhibitor drugs often become ineffective because retroviruses mutate rapidly, making the proteases and RTs difficult to attack. Antiviral drugs are taken in combination. The first extensively studied retrovirus was a tumor virus of birds, isolated in 1911 by P. Rous. In 1979, R. Gallo discovered the first human retrovirus, HTLV-1. Retroviruses have been implicated in some prostate cancers.

Cyclosporine, 1972

Microbiologist J. F. Borel also played an important role in the discovery of cyclosporine while at Sandoz. Although the world was excited by the first successful heart transplant, in 1967, this patient survived only 18 days, and other patients also became victims of their own immune system.
Hollingham, R., *Blood and Guts*, NY: Thomas Dunne Books, 2009.
Werth, B., *The Billion-Dollar Molecule*, NY: Simon & Schuster, 1995.

Statins, 1973

More cholesterol in the bloodstream comes from the liver's synthesis of cholesterol than from diet. Cholesterol is an important component of membranes and is also used for creating hormones. HDL carries cholesterol back to the liver. Endo reasoned that fungi probably produced inhibitors for cholesterol-producing enzymes as a way to defend themselves against bacteria, which had cholesterol in their cell walls. Interestingly, atherosclerotic plaques can still form even in individuals who do not have high blood cholesterol levels.
Landers, P., *tinyurl.com/4drujob*.

Oncogenes, 1976

Usually, cancer involves a multistep process in which cells acquire several mutations that together lead to increased proto-oncogene function and/or decreased TS gene function.

Cochlear Implants, 1977

CIs do not restore normal hearing, and after CI implantation, patients must undergo therapy to help them adapt to the new sounds. W. House also played a key role in the history of CIs. Today, CIs are often fitted to both ears.

Magnetic Resonance Imaging (MRI), 1977

NMR (nuclear magnetic resonance) was first described in 1937 by physicist I. Rabi. In 1945, physicists F. Bloch and E. Purcell refined the technique. In 1966, R. Ernst developed Fourier transform (FT) spectroscopy and showed how RF pulses could be used to create a spectrum of NMR signals as a function of frequency. P. Lauterbur and P. Mansfield received the Nobel Prize for their role in producing images from magnetic resonance scans. Patients with pacemakers and certain metal implants often should not be scanned because of the effect of the magnet.

First Test-Tube Baby, 1978
TIME, tinyurl.com/ye3zju7.

Fetal Surgery, 1981
Camosy, P., quoted in *The Making of the Unborn Patient*, Caspar, M., Piscataway, NJ: Rutgers University Press, 1998.

Laparoscopic Surgery, 1981
The term *thoracopy* is sometimes used to refer to keyhole surgery performed in the chest. C. Nezhat was also important in the development of video laparoscopy.
Spaner S., Warnock, G., *J. Laparoendosc. Adv. Surg. Tech. A*, 7:369; 1997.

Prions, 1982
Gajdusek was able to transmit kuru to primates and show that kuru had an incubation period of several years. In the 1980s, the "mad cows" had eaten pieces of sheep that had scrapie. Scrapie causes sheep to rub the wool off their bodies. Note that in some cases, the dangerous PrP-Sc seems to arise simply by a chance natural event in the body.

Telomerase, 1984
Telomerase is a reverse transcriptase that creates single-stranded DNA from single-stranded RNA as a template. J. Szostak was also involved in the discovery of telomerase. Shortened telomeres have been associated with Alzheimer's disease, cardiovascular disease, diabetes, cancer, childhood trauma, and prolonged depression.
Greider, C., Blackburn, E., *Scien. Amer.* 274:92; 1996.

Do Not Resuscitate, 1991
Woodruff, W., *The Army Lawyer*, 4: 6; 1989.

RNA Interference, 1998
RNAi also plays a role in protecting cells against transposons, jumping pieces of genetic material that can damage a cell's DNA. One challenge for therapeutic use of RNAi includes unwanted "off-target" effects in which siRNAs inhibit nontargeted mRNAs. RNAi may also involve the alteration of chromatin structure and promotion of DNA methylation. RNAi can be passed on for several generations in worms.
Arney, K., in *Defining Moments in Science*, Steer, M., Birch, H., Impney, A., eds., NY: Sterling, 2008.

Robotic Surgery, 2000
Other uses of robotic surgery involve the computer-directed milling of artificial parts (e.g., hip joints).
Drehle, D., *tinyurl.com/2ee7njs.*

Telesurgery, 2001
With telediagnosis, MRI scans in the United States may be sent electronically to a radiologist overseas and findings quickly returned. Augmented reality allows images to be superimposed atop a surgeon's view of an operating field, for example, to make inner structures "visible" on the surface of an organ.

Human Genome Project, 2003
Donovan, A., Green, R., *The Human Genome Project in College Curriculum*, Lebanon, NH: Dartmouth, 2008.

Face Transplant, 2005
Face transplants are not only cosmetic; they can allow a person to eat and drink through the mouth, which may not have been possible before the transplant. Antirejection drugs increase a recipient's chances of cancer.

Growing New Organs, 2006
Scaffolds may be constructed of more than one material, some of which may eventually biodegrade and dissolve away. Engineered urethras are successfully created by adding muscle cells to the inside of a tube-mesh and endothelial cells to the outside. The cells come from the patients' bladders.
Andrews, W., *tinyurl.com/37z4wf.*

Human Cloning, 2008
In reproductive cloning, the clone is not truly identical since the somatic (body) cell may contain mutations in the DNA, as well as specific methylation patterns. Also, the mitochondrial DNA comes from the donor egg. Note also that the environments in the uterus and in the egg play a role in the development of an embryo and shape some of its characteristics. In plants, clones can be made simply by cuttings of plants. Some variety of grapes used today for making wine are clones of grapes that first appeared 2,000 years ago. For research purposes, cloning can be used to create animals with the same genetic blueprint and thus eliminate many variables during experiments. Areas for possible use include the treatment of Alzheimer's, Parkinson's, and other degenerative diseases.

Researchers have made iPS cells from blood and skin and then induced these iPS cells into becoming heart muscles and brain and spinal-cord neurons. Such cells might be used to replace damaged heart tissue. Perhaps by cloning healthy heart cells and injecting them into damaged regions of the heart, certain kinds of heart disease can be ameliorated.

After SCNT, the nucleus-egg combination is stimulated with electricity to trigger cell division.
Bailey, R., foreword to Gralla, J., Gralla, P., *Complete Idiot's Guide to Understanding Cloning*, NY: Alpha, 2004.

Index

Photo Credits

Because several of the old and rare illustrations shown in this book were difficult to acquire in a clean and legible form, I have sometimes taken the liberty of applying image-processing techniques to remove dirt and scratches, enhance faded portions, and occasionally add a slight coloration to a black-and-white figure in order to highlight details or to make an image more compelling. I hope that historical purists will forgive these slight artistic touches and understand that my goal was to create an attractive book that is aesthetically interesting and alluring to a wide audience. My love for the incredible depth and diversity of topics in medicine and history should be evident through the photographs and drawings.